Pregnancy and Allergy

Editor

EDWARD S. SCHULMAN

IMMUNOLOGY AND ALLERGY
CLINICS OF NORTH AMERICA

https://www.immunology.theclinics.com/

February 2023 • Volume 43 • Number 1

ELSEVIER

1600 John F. Kennedy Boulevard • Suite 1800 • Philadelphia, Pennsylvania, 19103-2899

http://www.theclinics.com

IMMUNOLOGY AND ALLERGY CLINICS OF NORTH AMERICA Volume 43, Number 1

February 2023 ISSN 0889-8561, ISBN-13: 978-0-323-96171-4

Editor: Taylor Hayes
Developmental Editor: Jessica Cañaberal

Immunology and Allergy Clinics of North America (ISSN 0889–8561) is published quarterly by Elsevier Inc., 360 Park Avenue South, New York, NY 10010-1710. Months of issue are February, May, August, and November. Periodicals postage paid at New York, NY and additional mailing offices. Subscription prices are $365.00 per year for US individuals, $704.00 per year for US institutions, $100.00 per year for US students and residents, $445.00 per year for Canadian individuals, $100.00 per year for Canadian students, $895.00 per year for Canadian institutions, $470.00 per year for international individuals, $895.00 per year for international institutions, $220.00 per year for international students. To receive student/resident rate, orders must be accompanied by name of affiliated institution, date of term, and the *signature* of program/residency coordinator on institution letterhead. Orders will be billed at individual rate until proof of status is received. Foreign air speed delivery is included in all *Clinics* subscription prices. All prices are subject to change without notice. **POSTMASTER**: Send address changes to *Immunology and Allergy Clinics of North America,* Elsevier Health Sciences Division, Subscription Customer Service, 3251 Riverport Lane, Maryland Heights, MO 63043. **Customer Service: 1-800-654-2452 (U.S. and Canada); 314-447-8871 (outside U.S. and Canada). Fax: 314-447-8029.** E-mail: journalscustomerservice-usa@elsevier.com (for print support); journalsonlinesupport-usa@elsevier.com (for online support).

Reprints. For copies of 100 or more, of articles in this publication, please contact the Commercial Reprints Department, Elsevier Inc., 360 Park Avenue South, New York, New York 10010-1710. Tel. 212-633-3874, Fax: 212-633-3820, E-mail: reprints@elsevier.com.

Immunology and Allergy Clinics of North America is covered in MEDLINE/PubMed (Index Medicus), Current Contents/Life Sciences, Science Citation Index, ISI/BIOMED, Chemical Abstracts, and EMBASE/Excerpta Medica.

Contributors

EDITOR

EDWARD S. SCHULMAN, MD
Professor Emeritus of Medicine, Former Chair, Allergy, Pulmonary, Critical Care, and Sleep Medicine, Director, Allergy, Asthma and Airway Research Center, Drexel University College of Medicine, Philadelphia, Pennsylvania, USA

AUTHORS

CEM AKIN, MD, PhD
Clinical Professor of Medicine, Department of Internal Medicine, Division of Allergy and Immunology, Michigan Medicine, University of Michigan, Michigan, USA

NONIE ARORA, MD, MBA
Department of Internal Medicine, Michigan Medicine, University of Michigan, Ann Arbor, Michigan, USA

RACHAEL BAIRD, MD
Women's Health Institute, Cleveland Clinic Foundation, Cleveland, Ohio, USA

LISA A. BECK, MD
Department of Dermatology, University of Rochester Medical Center, Rochester, New York, USA

CHARLES B. CAIRNS, MD
Walter H. and Leonore Annenberg Dean, College of Medicine, Professor of Medicine and Emergency Medicine, Senior Vice President, Medical Affairs, Drexel University, Philadelphia, Pennsylvania, USA

MICHAEL Z. CHENG, MD
Resident, Department of Otolaryngology–Head and Neck Surgery, Johns Hopkins School of Medicine, Johns Hopkins Bayview Medical Center, Baltimore, Maryland, USA

CHARLOTTE CUNNINGHAM-RUNDLES, MD, PhD
Division of Allergy and Immunology, Icahn School of Medicine at Mount Sinai, New York, New York, USA

RUTH P. CUSACK, MBBch
Department of Medicine, McMaster University, Hamilton, Ontario, Canada

ALAN GANDLER, MD
Assistant Professor, Department of Medicine, Division of Pulmonary, Allergy, and Critical Care, Perelman School of Medicine, University of Pennsylvania, Philadelphia, Pennsylvania, USA

GAIL M. GAUVREAU, PhD
Department of Medicine, McMaster University, Hamilton, Ontario, Canada

IRAM J. HAQ, MBBS, MRes, PhD
Translational and Clinical Research Institute, Newcastle University, Faculty of Medical Sciences, Newcastle University Medical School, Department of Paediatric Respiratory Medicine, Great North Children's Hospital, Newcastle Hospitals NHS Foundation Trust, Newcastle Upon Tyne, United Kingdom

MAEVE HOPKINS, MD
Women's Health Institute, Cleveland Clinic Foundation, Cleveland, Ohio, USA

LAURA JARDINE, AB, MBBChir, PhD
Newcastle University Medical School, Biosciences Institute, Newcastle University, Faculty of Medical Sciences, Haematology Department, Freeman Hospital, Newcastle Hospitals NHS Foundation Trust, Newcastle Upon Tyne, United Kingdom

MEGAN E. JENSEN, BNutrDiet (Hons), PhD, AdvAPD
Priority Research Centre for Healthy Lungs, University of Newcastle, Newcastle, New South Wales, Australia; Hunter Medical Research Institute, Callaghan, New South Wales, Australia

JEAN KIM, MD, PhD
Associate Professor, Department of Otolaryngology–Head and Neck Surgery, Department of Medicine, Division of Allergy and Clinical Immunology, Johns Hopkins School of Medicine, Johns Hopkins Bayview Medical Center, Baltimore, Maryland, USA

ANNA KOVALSZKI, MD
Clinical Associate Professor of Medicine, Department of Internal Medicine, Division of Allergy and Immunology, Michigan Medicine, University of Michigan, Ann Arbor, Michigan, USA

MONICA KRAFT, MD
Murray M. Rosenberg Professor of Medicine and Systems Chair, Samuel Bronfman Department of Medicine, Icahn School of Medicine at Mount Sinai, Mount Sinai Health System, New York, New York, USA

MARGARET M. KUDER, MD, MPH
Department of Allergy and Clinical Immunology, Respiratory Institute, Cleveland Clinic Foundation, Cleveland, Ohio, USA

LEAH LAAGEIDE, MD
Department of Dermatology, University of Rochester Medical Center, Rochester, New York, USA

DAVID M. LANG, MD
Department of Allergy and Clinical Immunology, Respiratory Institute, Cleveland Clinic Foundation, Cleveland, Ohio, USA

JULIE MIRPURI, MD
Division of Neonatal-Perinatal Medicine, UT Southwestern Medical Center, Dallas, Texas, USA

VANESSA E. MURPHY, BMedChem (Hons), PhD
Priority Research Centre for Healthy Lungs, University of Newcastle, Newcastle, New South Wales, Australia; Hunter Medical Research Institute, Callaghan, New South Wales, Australia

ROBERT NACLERIO, MD
Department of Otolaryngology–Head and Neck Surgery, Johns Hopkins School of Medicine, Johns Hopkins Bayview Medical Center, Baltimore, Maryland, USA

JENNIFER A. NAMAZY, MD
Allergy and Immunologist, Division of Allergy, Asthma and Immunology, Scripps Clinic Medical Group, Department of Allergy and Immunology, Scripps Clinic, San Diego, California, USA

ELEANOR M. POPE, BA
Department of Dermatology, University of Rochester Medical Center, Rochester, New York, USA

COURTNEY L. RAMOS, DO
Allergy and Immunology Fellow, Division of Allergy, Asthma and Immunology, Scripps Clinic Medical Group, San Diego, California, USA

MARC A. RIEDL, MD, MS
Professor of Medicine, Division of Rheumatology, Allergy and Immunology, Department of Medicine, University of California, San Diego, La Jolla, California, USA

MICHAEL SCHATZ, MD
Department of Allergy and Immunology, Kaiser Permanente, San Diego, California, USA

INA SCHIM VAN DER LOEFF, MBBS, PhD
Newcastle University Medical School, Translational and Clinical Research Institute, Newcastle University, Faculty of Medical Sciences, Newcastle Upon Tyne, United Kingdom; Community Paediatrics, North Tyneside General Hospital, Northumbria Healthcare NHS Foundation Trust, North Shields, United Kingdom

EDWARD S. SCHULMAN, MD
Professor Emeritus of Medicine, Former Chair, Allergy, Pulmonary, Critical Care, and Sleep Medicine, Director, Allergy, Asthma and Airway Research Center, Drexel University College of Medicine, Philadelphia, Pennsylvania

THOMAS D.R. SPROAT, MBChB, MD
Department of Paediatric Respiratory Medicine, Great North Children's Hospital, Newcastle Hospitals NHS Foundation Trust, Neonatal Unit, Royal Victoria Infirmary, Newcastle Hospitals NHS Foundation Trust, Newcastle Upon Tyne, United Kingdom

KATHERINE STUMPF, MD
Department of Pediatrics, Division of Neonatal-Perinatal Medicine, UT Southwestern Medical Center, Dallas, Texas, USA

CHRISTIANE E. WHETSTONE, BSc
Department of Medicine, McMaster University, Hamilton, Ontario, Canada

ROSALIND J. WRIGHT, MD, MPH
Professor of Pediatrics, Department of Environmental Medicine and Public Health, Institute for Exposomic Research, New York, New York, USA

ERIKA J. YOO, MD, FCCP
Associate Professor, Department of Medicine, Division of Pulmonary, Allergy, and Critical Care Medicine, Jane and Leonard Korman Respiratory Institute, National Jewish Health, Sidney Kimmel Medical College, Thomas Jefferson University, Philadelphia, Pennsylvania, USA

SHOULING ZHANG, MD
Division of Allergy and Immunology, Icahn School of Medicine at Mount Sinai, New York, New York, USA

Contents

Building an immune system is a monumental task critical to the survival of the fetus and newborn. A functional fetal immune system must complement the maternal immune system in handling in utero infection; abstain from damaging non–self-reactions that would compromise the materno-fetal interface; mobilize in response to infection and equip mucosal tissues for pathogen exposure at birth. There is growing appreciation that immune cells also have noncanonical roles in development and specifically may contribute to tissue morphogenesis. In this review we detail how hemato-poietic and lymphoid organs jointly establish cellular constituents of the immune system; how these constituents are organized in 2 mucosal sites-gut and lung-where early life immune function has long-term conse-quences for health; and how exemplar diseases of prematurity and inborn errors of immunity reveal dominant pathways in prenatal immunity.

Physiologic changes during pregnancy have implications for both upper and lower airway function. Upper airway resistance increases, and total lung capacity decreases. Upper airway symptoms increase; some women develop pregnancy-induced rhinitis and there is an increased prevalence of sleep-disordered breathing compared to prepregnancy. Longitudinal studies examining changes in upper and lower airway function parameters are limited, particularly in women with asthma. Some studies have observed reduced lung function with advancing gestation; however, changes are small and unlikely to be of major clinical significance. Spirom-etry is therefore a useful tool for clinical assessment of women with asthma during pregnancy.

This review article explores the available literature on the association of maternal nutrient intake with development of allergies in offspring. It exam-ines the mechanisms for maternal diet–mediated effects on offspring im-munity and dissects recent human and animal studies that evaluate the role of both maternal macro- and micronutrient intake on offspring suscep-tibility to asthma, eczema, food allergy, and atopy.

Disease programming reflects interactions between genes and the environment. Unlike the genome, environmental exposures and our response to exposures change over time. Starting in utero, the respiratory system and related processes develop sequentially in a carefully timed cascade, thus effects depend on both exposure dose and timing. A multitude of environmental and microbial exposures influence respiratory disease programming. Effects result from toxin-induced shifts in a host of molecular, cellular, and physiologic states and their interacting systems. Moreover, pregnant women and the developing child are not exposed to a single toxin, but to complex mixtures.

Pregnancy can induce significant upper airway distress in women by the induction of rhinitis of pregnancy (ROP). Pregnancy can also exacerbate underlying rhinopathies. Little is known regarding the pathophysiology of the ROP. Diagnosis of other coexistent rhinopathies is key. Treatment regimens closely mirror standard treatments for other rhinopathies that are independent of pregnancy and are generally accepted as safe. Early recognition of the progression of rhinitis in the pregnant patient into complications of rhinosinusitis is important to prevent harm to both mother and fetus.

Asthma is one of the most common potentially serious medical problems to complicate pregnancy. Optimal management of asthma during pregnancy is thus important for both mother and baby. Treating asthmatic women requires understanding the effects of pregnancy on the course of asthma, and, conversely, the effects of asthma on pregnancy outcomes. Successful management also requires an understanding the barriers to asthma control in this population of patients. Evidence has shown that it is essential that the allergist-immunologist, obstetrician, and patient work as a team during pregnancy to achieve optimal maternal and neonatal outcomes.

One-third of women with asthma have deterioration of their asthma during pregnancy, and one-fourth of pregnant women with asthma will experience severe exacerbations necessitating emergency department (ED) visits or hospitalizations. Early recognition of acute severe asthma, including life-threatening status asthmaticus, and aggressive medical interventions with β2-agonists, anticholinergic agents, and systemic corticosteroids are necessary to treat maternal airway bronchoconstriction, support maternal and fetal oxygenation, and avoid adverse fetal outcomes. This review describes management of acute severe asthma in pregnancy, including status asthmaticus, in the ED and intensive care unit.

Margaret M. Kuder, Rachael Baird, Maeve Hopkins, and David M. Lang

Anaphylaxis in pregnancy is a rare event, but has important implications for the pregnant patient and fetus. The epidemiology, pathophysiology, diagnosis, and treatment all carry important considerations unique to the pregnant patient. Common culprits of anaphylaxis are primarily medications, particularly antibiotics and anesthetic agents. Diagnosis can be difficult given the relative lack of cutaneous symptoms, and normal physiologic changes in pregnancy such as low blood pressure and tachycardia. Apart from patient positioning, treatment is similar to that of the general population, with a focus on prompt epinephrine administration.

Eleanor M. Pope, Leah Laageide, and Lisa A. Beck

The safe management of allergic skin disorders during pregnancy is essential to maternal and fetal health. Poorly controlled allergic skin disease affects the health of mother and child. This article reviews the disease course and treatment of atopic dermatitis, chronic urticaria, and allergic contact dermatitis in pregnancy. It focuses on topical and systemic therapies in the context of pregnancy and breastfeeding. Because disease activity may vary in pregnancy, prescription stewardship is imperative; a balance among disease control, minimum effective dosing, and medication safety profiles should be maintained. Secondary complications and risks to maternal or infant health should also be avoided.

Shouling Zhang and Charlotte Cunningham-Rundles

An overview of primary antibody immunodeficiency in pregnancy is presented. Indications for immunoglobulin replacement therapy (IGRT), dosing, and safety considerations are highlighted. Uses of immunizations and antimicrobial therapy are also discussed. In general, IGRT, both intravenous and subcutaneous, is considered safe in pregnancy.

Marc A. Riedl

In recent years, hereditary angioedema (HAE) management has substantially advanced but also become more complex with additional therapeutic options. Pregnancy significantly influences the clinical symptoms of HAE in many women because of estrogen effects or other physiologic factors, and also introduces important safety concerns related to HAE medications. Management of HAE during pregnancy requires clinicians to be familiar with the potential clinical course, triggers, and recommended treatment strategies to provide guidance and optimal medical management to women and families affected by the condition. This review provides an overview of data, considerations, and recommendations related to HAE and pregnancy.

Mastocytosis is a rare neoplastic disorder of the mast cell lineage resulting in unregulated proliferation and activation of mast cells. Symptoms worsen in about one-third of pregnant patients. Treatment focuses on management of symptoms with antimediator therapy (H1 & H2 antihistamines, glucocorticoids, and epinephrine, if required). Medication selection requires care during labor and delivery. Although it is generally considered safe to use a medication patient tolerated before, some common medications may need to be avoided or used with caution (eg, codeine, morphine, nonsteroidal antiinflammatory drugs, vancomycin) if the patient does not have any history of exposure to them.

Poorly controlled asthma can affect neonatal outcomes including congenital anomalies, which can be reduced with appropriate asthma care during pregnancy. Although there is a concern regarding the safety of asthma medication use during pregnancy and congenital anomalies, the risk of uncontrolled asthma outweighs any potential risks of controller and reliever medication use. Patient education before and during pregnancy is critical to ensure good compliance to therapy and reduce the risk of poor asthma control.

Asthma, allergic rhinitis, chronic urticaria, and atopic dermatitis are common diseases that affect hundreds of thousands of pregnant women each year. The authors discuss the use of biologics in women who are pregnant or lactating, indications, available safety information, and knowledge gaps. There are pregnant patients for which standard treatment is either inadequate or contraindicated; in those cases, monoclonal antibodies (biologics) should be considered despite the unknown risk to the fetus. In severe asthma, omalizumab is the best studied with reassuring available safety data. Insufficient safety data exist on mepolizumab, reslizumab, benralizumab, dupilumab, and tezepelumab use during pregnancy and lactation.

It is known that poor asthma control is common in pregnancy, and asthma in general disproportionally affects underserved communities. However, there is a paucity of data examining strategies to improve asthma control specifically among pregnant women from vulnerable populations. Identified barriers to optimal asthma care in other underserved groups include health literacy, financial constraints, cultural differences, and poor environmental controls. These deficiencies may also be targets for multimodal interventions geared toward improving asthma outcomes for underserved women during pregnancy.

IMMUNOLOGY AND ALLERGY CLINICS OF NORTH AMERICA

SERIES OF RELATED INTEREST

Medical Clinics
https://www.medical.theclinics.com/

THE CLINICS ARE AVAILABLE ONLINE!
Access your subscription at:
www.theclinics.com

Preface

"Doctor...I'm Pregnant"!

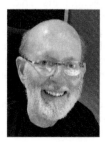

Edward S. Schulman, MD
Editor

Suddenly she turned, smiled, and said, "Dr Schulman, I'm eight weeks pregnant." "Mazel tov." I scurried to review her problem list, medication list, and my last note. I panicked slightly. Sound familiar? Was my patient taking potentially toxic meds during this first trimester? Is my knowledge up-to-date? Can I confidently counsel her, answering her many questions?

When I accepted Elsevier's offer to edit this issue of *Immunology and Allergy Clinics of North America* on pregnancy, I envisioned a one-stop-shopping, state-of-the-art guide. I listed key topics and then sought to enlist trusted A-list authors to produce a definitive sourcebook. Distinguished colleagues in the realms of basic immunology, otolaryngology, dermatology, epidemiology, pharmacology, allergy, nutrition, immune disorders, and pulmonary emergency medicine shared that vision. I am very grateful to them.

The issue starts with the immune system's gestational development and goes on to a review of adaptations that the maternal upper and lower airways make during pregnancy. The following articles cover nutrition and the influence of maternal exposures, known as the exposome, on the child's immune outcomes.

Next is the management of upper-airway disorders, chronic asthma, and *status asthmaticus gravidus*. Then comes anaphylaxis in pregnancy followed by the pregnancy considerations of common allergic skin disorders, primary antibody deficiency, hereditary angioedema, and mastocytosis. The final articles deal with the risks associated with drugs, especially biologics. The culminating article discusses the potential for improving pregnancy outcomes in underserved communities.

Editing this issue proved to be a valuable learning opportunity. Each article yielded vital takeaways that stuck with me. The emergence of the immune system during gestation is a monumental and beautiful task. Understanding it has undergone quantum leaps. Spirometry remains a useful clinical tool because, despite anatomical changes, there are no important differences in the maternal forced expiratory volume

Immunol Allergy Clin N Am 43 (2023) xiii–xiv
https://doi.org/10.1016/j.iac.2022.09.002
0889-8561/23/© 2022 Published by Elsevier Inc.

immunology.theclinics.com

in 1 second or forced vital capacity during pregnancy. However, sleep-disordered breathing is underdiagnosed. Moreover, maternal nutrient intake may influence the offspring's microbiome and especially its susceptibility to allergy. Since its effects are both internal and external, the quality of the exposome is vital to the development of fetal immunity.

The origins of rhinitis in pregnancy are complex, not hormonal alone. If the clinician stresses the importance of NOT STOPPING asthma medications and if the patient heeds the point, then asthma remains highly controllable during pregnancy. Proper medication management will not harm the baby while controlling asthma. In the case of severe asthma, it is critical to monitor oxygenation in both the patient and the fetus. Pregnancy-induced changes in the patient's anatomy make intubation complicated and mechanical ventilation challenging.

In anaphylaxis, we must "think outside the box" during pregnancy because there are many factors in addition to drugs that may cause it. Allergic skin disorders require a balance among the elements of medication safety profiles, minimum effective dosing, and disease control.

Even though primary immune defects of antibody production do not preclude a normal pregnancy, immunoglobulin replacement therapy must account for placental transfer of a variety of factors, including immunoglobulin G. Hereditary angioedema symptoms are highly unpredictable. Therefore, HAE and obstetric specialists must collaborate closely. While mastocytosis does not contraindicate pregnancy, careful medication management is essential, especially in anesthesia usage at the time of delivery.

This issue ends with a detailed discussion on the safety of medications, especially biologics. It is vitally important to optimize care strategies in low-resourced areas. High health care costs, morbidity, and mortality must be minimized.

In closing, I want to thank the very helpful people at Elsevier and our roster of outstanding authors who prepared this issue of the *Immunology and Allergy Clinics of North America*.

Edward S. Schulman, MD
200 West Washington Square, #2707
Philadelphia, PA 19106, USA

E-mail address:
es29@drexel.edu

Gestational Development of the Human Immune System

Laura Jardine, AB, MBBChir, PhD[a,b,*], Ina Schim van der Loeff, MBBS, PhD[c],
Iram J. Haq, MBBS, PhD[c,d], Thomas D.R. Sproat, MBChB, MD[e]

KEYWORDS

• Development • Prenatal • Immunity • Human

KEY POINTS

• Fetal immune cells are generated by multiple hematopoietic organs in 3 phases
• Phase 1 generates innate immune cells with noncanonical roles supporting tissue morphogenesis; phase 2 diversifies innate immune effectors and phase 3 generates adaptive immunity
• Immune development is compartmentalizedin specific tissues, for example, memory T cells are concentrated in the gut
• Innate immune activation has negative consequences on development
• From the second trimester, regulatory T cells are required to balance adaptive immune development

INTRODUCTION

Immune cells are generated through hematopoiesis (**Fig. 1**). The initial "primitive" wave of hematopoiesis occurs in the yolk sac (YS) at around 2 to 3 postconception weeks (PCW), and provides mostly megakaryocyte, erythroid and a limited array of myeloid cells (macrophages) from short-lived YS precursors.[1-3]

Definitive hematopoietic stem cells (HSCs) arise in the dorsal aorta of the embryo at 3 to 4PCW, and subsequently seed the fetal liver.[4] Fetal liver hematopoiesis, by 7PCW, produces megakaryocyte and erythroid cells, along with a diverse array of

[a] Biosciences Institute, Newcastle University, Faculty of Medical Sciences, Newcastle Upon Tyne NE2 4HH, United Kingdom; [b] Haematology Department, Freeman Hospital, Newcastle Hospitals NHS Foundation Trust, Newcastle Upon Tyne, United Kingdom; [c] Translational and Clinical Research Institute, Newcastle University, Faculty of Medical Sciences, Newcastle Upon Tyne NE2 4HH, United Kingdom; [d] Department of Paediatric Respiratory Medicine, Great North Children's Hospital, Newcastle Hospitals NHS Foundation Trust, Newcastle Upon Tyne, United Kingdom; [e] Neonatal Unit, Royal Victoria Infirmary, Newcastle Hospitals NHS Foundation Trust, Richardson Road, Newcastle Upon Tyne NE1 4LP, United Kingdom
* Corresponding author. Newcastle University Medical School, 3rd floor William Leech Building, Framlington Place, Newcastle Upon Tyne NE2 4HH, United Kingdom.
E-mail address: Laura.Jardine@ncl.ac.uk

Immunol Allergy Clin N Am 43 (2023) 1–15
https://doi.org/10.1016/j.iac.2022.05.009
0889-8561/23/© 2022 Elsevier Inc. All rights reserved.
immunology.theclinics.com

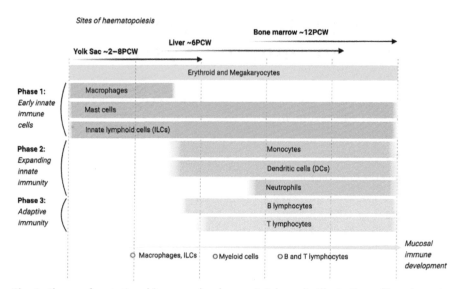

Fig. 1. Phases of gestational immune development. Schematic illustration of how hematopoietic organs produce immune cells in three phases, and how these phases are recapitulated in building mucosal immune systems for example, gut and lung. (Created with BioRender.com.)

innate immune cells: monocyte, mast cell, dendritic cell (DC), early granulocytes, natural killer (NK) and innate lymphoid cells (ILC).[1]

Both T and B cell progenitors are present in small numbers at 7PCW.[1] Initial B cell maturation occurs in the liver, while T cell maturation requires the thymus. The first naïve B cells emerge in the liver around 12 to 13PCW[5] and the first single positive T cells in the thymus around 11 to 12PCW.[6]

The long bones, which will become lifelong sites of hematopoiesis, are predominantly cartilage in the first trimester.[7] At 10 to 11PCW, definitive (HSCs) seed the bone marrow (BM) and hematopoiesis is rapidly established.[5] By 12PCW, the BM produces all the immune cell types seen in the liver, but allows for expansion of B lymphopoiesis, and greater diversification of the myeloid lineage, with neutrophil maturation and a full array of DC subsets produced.[8]

YS, fetal liver, and BM are not the only sites of immune cell production. The spleen, a tissue that retains hematopoietic potential during postnatal life,[9] supports erythroid, megakaryocyte, myeloid, and B lymphoid production.[10,11] Sites without appreciated hematopoietic potential, such as skin, kidney, lung, are thought to support *in situ* maturation because lineage-committed progenitors and complete spectra of differentiating cell states simultaneously exist.[10,11] Maturing B cells, for example, have been confirmed to exist outside blood vessels in the submucosa of gut[10] and the dura mater of the meninges.[12]

The use of single-cell multiomics technologies has provided unprecedented resolution to insights from studying human prenatal tissues (reviewed in[13]). As the access to healthy fetal tissues after 20PCW is extremely rare, limited detail of the second half of human gestation has been generated via this approach. Fetal blood sampling has provided some information on steady-state immune development.[14,15] While preterm samples may provide insights, they are confounded by the transformative influence of birth on the immune system.[16] From the information available, gestation immune development can be divided into three phases: first, a phase of early innate immune cells (macrophages, mast cells, ILC progenitors) before 8PCW; second, a phase of expanding innate immunity (monocytes, neutrophils, NK cells, and DCs) before 14PCW; and third, a phase of adaptive immunity (T and B lymphocytes) from 14PCW (see **Fig. 1**).

BUILDING AN IMMUNE REPERTOIRE
Phase 1: Early Innate Immune Cells

Macrophages are widely appreciated as tissue-resident mononuclear phagocytes that engulf and present antigens. Macrophages also perform a wide range of homeostatic functions, with diverse and highly adapted macrophage subpopulations found in tissues. Of relevance to development, macrophage subtypes prune synapses,[17] support vascular development[18] and facilitate erythropoiesis.[18–20] Macrophages in some tissue niches, such as microglia in the brain, derive from YS precursors and self-renew *in situ* during postnatal life.[21] In other tissues, such as gut, macrophages, derive from a combination of YS precursors and circulating monocytes.[21] Changes in macrophage heterogeneity occur across gestation, with early macrophages (8–10PCW) expressing proinflammatory genes (*NKFB1, FOS, JUN*) and later macrophages (12–16PCW) expressing genes associated with scavenger function and immune defense, such as complement components and antigen-presenting molecules.[10] The early inflammatory state could represent a maturation stage, as transient activation (with *NFKB1, FOS* and *JUN* expression) occurs during the generation of induced pluripotent stem cell-derived macrophages *in vitro* and coincides with a shift away from a naive chromatin landscape.[22] Later macrophages more reflect the functional specialization that occurs after maturation under the influence of tissue-specific cues.

Mast cells are characterized by metachromatic granules, which mediate rapid allergic inflammation when cross-linked IgE triggers their release.[23] The earliest mast cells in mice and humans have neither granules[1,24] nor complete IgE receptors.[1] As with macrophages, YS-derived mast cells can persist long-term in some tissues but be replaced by later hematopoiesis in others.[24,25] Mast cells express genes associated with endothelial cell recruitment (*CXCL3, CXCL2,* and *CXCL8*)[10] and are reported to support angiogenesis in postnatal life,[23] but their role in prenatal vascular development is not yet known.

The term ILCs covers a spectrum of innate immune cells that mirror T lymphocytes in terms of function and cytokine expression; with NK cells the equivalent of cytotoxic T cells and ILC1,2 and 3 the equivalent of helper Th1, Th2, and Th3 subsets.[26] ILCs are integral lymphoid and nonlymphoid tissue components, which provide immunity via rapid cytokine secretion, and shape the tissue microenvironment by cross-talk with immune and stromal cells.[26] In both mice and humans, the earliest committed ILC state is the ILC precursor, found in fetal liver and BM but also in mucosal tissues such as gut.[1,8,27,28] The ILC precursor emerges around the same time in embryonic gut and liver.[27,28] Maturation from ILC precursor to differentiated ILC subset has been demonstrated.[27–29] Murine parabiosis studies support relatively low-levels of ILC turnover, in comparison to rapid turnover of NK cells,[30] but definitive studies on ILC-subset maintenance in tissues in steady-state and inflammation across development are lacking. The early dedication to ILC production most likely reflects their importance in lymphoid tissue and Peyer's patch morphogenesis (specifically via a group 3 ILC termed lymphoid tissue inducer (LTi) cells[31]). In postnatal life, ILCs are important in maintaining epithelial barrier production, for example, IL-22 production by ILC3 maintains intestinal stem cells during mucosal damage.[32] They also partici-pate in epithelial remodeling during infection.[33,34] Further work is required to establish whether ILC influence on the epithelium begins during development.

The common themes between these 3 rather different immune cell groups are that they are tissue-resident, long-lived, and provide crosstalk between tissue structural cells and the immune system. By producing these cells during Phase 1 of immune development, they become embedded within the fabric of tissues from early in organogenesis.

Phase 2: Expanding Innate Immunity

Monocytes are circulating innate immune cells that can phagocytose, produce proin-flammatory cytokines and differentiate into macrophages and DCs, facilitating roles in inflammation resolution and wound-healing.[35] Monocytes remain around 3% of blood leukocytes throughout pregnancy,[14] but the monocyte count increases linearly with gestational age.[15] Monocytes are first detected in embryonic liver,[1,8] but subsequently emerge in fetal BM.[8] Prenatal and postnatal monocytes differ in distribution, heteroge-neity, and function. Monocytes are frequent in fetal tissues such as skin, but not in adult counterparts.[10,36] In postnatal life, human monocytes are conventionally divided into CD14^{++}CD16$^-$ classical monocytes, CD14^{++}CD16$^+$ intermediate and CD14$^+$CD16^{++} nonclassical monocytes,[37] whereas only classical monocytes are seen in fetal liver and BM.[1,8] Fetal monocytes are capable of phagocytosis, reactive oxygen species production and inflammatory cytokine response on stimulation, however, with direct *in vitro* comparisons against adult monocytes, the magnitude of these responses differs.[38]

Neutrophils are scarce in second trimester fetal blood, accumulating to postnatal levels during the third trimester;[14] however, neutrophil maturation can be detected in the BM from 12PCW, suggesting that limited release may occur.[8] Lower expression of CD18 and CD62L on fetal neutrophils[38] potentially supports BM retention and reduced migration into peripheral tissues, respectively.[39,40] Functionally, fetal neutro-phils are capable of slightly reduced phagocytosis but equivalent reactive oxygen species production compared with adult neutrophils,[38] perhaps indicating that neutro-phils could damage fetal tissues unless compartmentalized.

While NKs fall under the umbrella of ILCs and are observed in "Phase 1" of immune cell production, arising in YS and fetal liver,[1] they do not express genes relating to cytolytic function until the second trimester BM hematopoiesis.[8,10] *In vitro* functional assays confirm the poor cytolytic function of fetal liver NK cells but demonstrate that they do degranulate and produce TNFα and IFNγ on stimulation.[41] Functional differences between fetal liver and fetal BM NK cells still require confirmation.

DCs are innate immune cells that trigger adaptive immune responses by migrating to draining lymph nodes and presenting antigens to naive T cells. They are principally divided into plasmacytoid DCs, that are poised for IFNα production, and 2 subsets of myeloid DCs (DC1 and DC2), that have subspecialized roles in postnatal immune response.[42] Prenatal functional differences between human DC subsets are largely unexplored. DC1, DC2, and pre-pDCs emerge in fetal liver,[1] but a more adult-like spectrum of DC types occurs in fetal BM.[8] DCs are proportionally more abundant in second-trimester spleen, skin, and lung than in equivalent adult tissues.[43] They can be found in afferent lymphatics and draining lymph nodes after 16PCW.[43] Fetal DCs respond to toll-like receptor (TLR) agonists and stimulate naive T cell proliferation like their adult counterparts.[43] They differ in their cytokine-production and their influence on T cell polarization, with IL-4 production and regulatory T cells generation (Treg) more common after exposure to fetal DCs.[43] In part, fetal DCs regulate T cell responses through Arginase-2 production, which depletes the L-Arginine required for TNFα synthesis.[43]

During this second phase of immune system development, the first innate immune effectors emerge. These effectors are capable of inflammatory, cytolytic, and phagocytic responses, although with differences from adult counterparts. Given the potential for tissue damage, a range of protective strategies exist, including compartmentalization, delayed acquisition of cytolytic function, and altering the immune response via metabolite depletion.

Phase 3: Adaptive Immunity

B and T lymphocytes in fetal blood increase progressively during the second trimester.[44] Immunoglobulin heavy chain (IgH) and TCR repertoires are initially skewed, but diversity increases with age, approaching the levels seen in healthy infants by the end of the beginning of the third trimester.[44] Specific B and T cell responses to prenatal infection and immunization can be effectively generated *in vivo*,[45–47] and robust secretion of cytokines and cytolytic molecules can be demonstrated on *ex vivo* stimulation of T cells.[48,49] Tregs serve an important role in restraining T cell responses in utero, particularly those against maternal alloantigens, and are more abundant in fetal than adult lymphoid tissue.[49,50]

Fetal mature T cells include CD4, CD8, Treg and unconventional subsets.[10,51] All develop in the thymus and are absent in the case of congenital athymia.[52] The earliest thymic outputs, at 7-9PCW, are dominated by unconventional T cells.[6,10] Unconventional and conventional T cells use the same progenitors but diverge due to differences in signaling resulting from spatial location within the thymic medulla and the cell types they encounter.[10,51] While *EOMES* and *TBX21*-expressing type 1, and *RORC* and *CCR6*-expressing type 3 innate T cells are only found prenatally, *PDCD1*-expressing CD8αα cells rebound after birth and peak in childhood.[10] Unconventional T cells can elicit the full spectrum of effector T cell responses, including cytokine and chemokine production and cytotoxicity.[10,53] The key differences from conventional T cells are the types of triggering antigen, the rapidity and the localization of the response.[10,53] Unconventional T cells recognize a broad spectrum of both self and microbial antigens. They constitutively express activation markers (CD44, CD69), and many subsets are clonally expanded before antigen exposure, allowing abundant production of cytokines minutes after stimulation.[53,54] Many unconventional T cells are tissue-resident.[10,53] Their presence may afford some mucosal tissue readiness for pathogen exposure at birth. As a role in wound-healing has been described,[55] unconventional T cells could participate in tissue remodeling during tissue morphogenesis.

Fetal nonprogenitor B cells include immature B cells, mature B cells, plasma cells, and B1 cells.[10] B1 cells, only recently identified in humans, are specified in early development.[10,56] Their characteristic function is to spontaneously secrete IgM antibody, serving as a reservoir of immediate defense against infection. The B cell receptor (BCR) repertoire of B1 cells is selected to enrich for BCRs against common pathogen motifs and against self-antigens, such as Annexin V and phosphatidylcholine, present in the membrane of apoptotic cells.[56,57] This self-reactivity allows B1 IgM to participate in clearance of cell debris, and IL-10 production to inhibit inflammatory responses.[56] Fetal plasma cells are rare and predominantly IgM-specific,[10] in keeping with reports of low-level IgM predominant circulating plasma cells in neonates.[58] While in postnatal life, T-cell dependent B cell activation in germinal centers promotes affinity maturation and class-switch recombination, alternative pathways of B-cell help must be exploited in fetal life because germinal centers have not yet developed.[59]

While the mechanisms remain elusive, a functional difference exists between neonatal and later B cells, with long-term protective responses particular to later-developing cells.[58]

This third phase of immune development sees a diverse adaptive immune repertoire established, with unconventional T and B1 lymphocytes poised for immediate response to pathogen and polyclonal naive T and B cells prepared for pathogen-specific response.

BUILDING A MUCOSAL IMMUNE SYSTEM

Innate and adaptive immune development in gut and its dysregulation in necrotizing enterocolitis (NEC)

The developing gut progresses from a simple tube at 3-4PCW, to a structure with distinct regions and with local variation between crypts and villi at 12PCW.[60] At around the same time, the fetus begins to swallow amniotic fluid and the developing mucosa receives its first environmental exposures.[61] The basic immune landscape of the gut is established early in the second trimester and is stable in composition until infancy.[62,63] Adaptive immune cells are the most abundant type, with antigen-presenting cells collectively the next largest fraction and NK cells and ILC together comprising 1/3 of cells.[62–64] Of T cells, naïve, memory and regulatory cells are present.[62–64] CD4 T cells in gut express the expected tissue residency markers CD69 and CD103.[62,63] The naïve T cells express CD31, indicative of recent thymic egress,[62,64] and have high clonal diversity by the early second trimester (14–20PCW). Intriguingly, around half of gut CD4 T cells are CCR7-CD45RA-memory cells, compared with fewer than 5% in liver or spleen.[64] Several studies have confirmed that memory cells are both clonally expanded and prepared for effector function.[62–64] The presence of clonally expanded memory cells implies that the presentation of immunogenic antigen occurs *in utero*. Clones with overlapping specificities can be found, even within the relatively small number of fetal samples studied, suggesting that a common antigen exposure is responsible, potentially maternal diet-derived or possibly microbial.[63] Whether or not there is a fetal microbiota has been hotly debated. Using a combination of sensitive sequencing methods, fetal tissue culture, and imaging, the presence of bacteria in the developing fetal gut has been demonstrated. While mesenteric lymph node T cells could be activated on reexposure to bacterial antigens, it is not yet known whether gut memory T cells are pathogen-specific.[65] Memory CD4 T cells express Th1 cytokine genes,[62,63] releasing IFNγ, IL2, and TNFα when stimulated ex vivo.[64] TNFα has been reported to support epithelial development.[63]

NEC almost exclusively affects preterm infants and offers an insight into the immunologic deficiencies of fetal gut mucosa. NEC is characterized by an inflamed, necrotic bowel which can rapidly progress to severe illness and death.[66] Bacterial invasion of the bowel wall occurs, likely due to a combination of weak inter-epithelial cell tight junctions and an underdeveloped mucus layer.[67,68] Innate immune activation, due to an augmented mucosal response to gram-negative bacteria and a tolerogenic T cell response, leads to widespread intestinal cell inflammation and death.[68] NEC incidence is inversely related to gestation, associated with microbial dysbiosis and the absence of breast milk.[69,70] These 3 elements are interlinked with both the immune landscape and response. For example, the preterm gut has an increased response to lipopolysaccharide (LPS), found in gram-negative bacteria.[71] An increased abundance of gram-negative bacteria preceding NEC is thought to trigger this response.[72] Composed largely of innate immune cells, the second trimester gut is well-equipped with TLR-4-expressing macrophages and DCs that respond to LPS. Human milk offers protection against NEC, not only by reducing the TLR-4 response, but by providing bacteria and immune-modulating proteins.[73] Human milk feeding promotes the growth of *Bifidobacterium* in the neonatal gut,[74] and an increased abundance of *Bifidobacterium* within protects against NEC.[70] Certain carbohydrates (human milk oligosaccharides (HMOs)) are present in human milk purely to improve the growth of *Bifidobacterium*, with the presence of a specific HMOs in maternal breast milk implicated in reduced risk of NEC development.[67,75] Provision of a probiotic containing *Bifidobacterium* species alters the infants T helper response by reducing the Th2 and Th17 responses in favor of Th1 responses.[76] While postnatal environmental influences have been shown to affect gut mucosal immune development, it is less clear about antenatal influences. However, in a mice model whereby maternal mice were supplemented with an aryl hydrocarbon receptor (AHR) ligand, it has been demonstrated that offspring had attenuated AHR signaling in the intestine, affording protection from NEC.[77] This offers compelling evidence that maternal diet in mammals may have a direct effect on gut mucosal immune development; however, further work is required to explore this concept in humans.

Lung immune development and its impact on morphogenesis, infection susceptibility, and allergic disease

There are 4 key stages of mammalian lung development: pseudoglandular, canalicular, saccular, and alveolar, whereby the first 3 are completed during fetal development and alveolarization continues after birth.[78] The lung buds form around 5PCW and undergo branching to first specify bronchial epithelium (5–16PCW) and later alveolar epithelium (>16PCW).[79] Immune cells accompany this process from the earliest stages, with macrophages and ILC progenitors present at 5-6PCW and myeloid cells accumulating rapidly from 9 to 11PCW.[11] B, T, and NK lymphoid cells reach prominence around 15PCW and constitute greater than 20% of cells by 16PCW.[11] In contrast, lymphoid cells remain less than 2% until birth in mice.[80]

Studies in human development have not yet revealed tissue-specific properties of lung immune cells that allow for a functioning mucosal immune system at birth or explored the crosstalk between immune and nonimmune cells in lung development. Single-cell and *in situ* multiomics of the adult lung have identified specific niches for lung immune cells, such as the submucosal glands as a site for T, B, and plasma cell localization, and have characterized stromal cell types that regulate immune cell infiltration, such as bronchial "immune recruiting" fibroblasts.[81] The challenge will now be to explore how much of this organization is initiated prenatally.

Studies in mice have demonstrated the heterogeneity of myeloid cells and their roles in lung development. Embryonic macrophages are highly proliferative and localized to developing blood vessels, suggesting a role in supporting pulmonary vascular growth.[80] Discrete populations emerge in later gestation, with distinct roles in immune regulation and surveillance, innate defense, tissue remodeling and structural airway development.[80,82] Activation of fetal lung macrophages can inhibit the expression of genes required for lung development, leading to preterm birth and perinatal death.[83] Liver-derived monocytes migrate to the lung and remain relatively immature in the healthy murine fetus, maturing to alveolar macrophages on GM-CSF exposure at birth.[84] Immune activation, for example, due to chorioamnionitis, can accelerate this maturation.[85] While this response may be to prepare the fetus for premature birth, arrested maturation of lung morphogenesis in the form of Bronchopulmonary dysplasia (BPD) can occur.[86] BPD is a complication of extreme prematurity, whereby inflammation, mechanical ventilation and prolonged oxygen requirements are associated with the cessation of lung development during the canalicular and saccular stages, resulting in a reduction in alveoli available for gas exchange.[87]

At birth, the physiologic environment within the lung changes dramatically. What was once fluid-filled and hypoxic rapidly transforms into an air-filled normoxic environment. Postnatal physiologic changes, such as increase in pulmonary vascular blood flow and changes in oxygen tension, together with microbial colonization, are associated with immune maturation and function (reviewed in[88]). An example is increased IL-33 production by lung epithelium, which recruits ILC2s to the lung.[82,89,90] Together with basophils, IL13-producing ILC2s promote type-2 immune responses in alveolar macrophages and DCs.[82,89,90] This type-2 bias results in delayed neonatal response to bacterial infections.[89] Respiratory syncytial virus (RSV) morbidity, to which neonates are particularly susceptible, is associated with heightened IL-13-production and impaired CD8 T cell response compared with older children.[88,91] RSV-induced Th2 cytokine production by Tregs can increase susceptibility to experimental allergic disease.[92]

INFERRING DOMINANT PATHWAYS FROM INBORN ERRORS OF IMMUNITY (IEI)

Monogenic disorders of the immune system can shed light on important molecular and cellular pathways of the developing immune system. These IEI tend to present in infancy, although some are also associated with fetal loss and prematurity.

Damaging Effects of Unrestrained Type I Interferon

Type I interferons are essential for human antiviral immunity. The absence of interferon-α/β receptor (IFNAR) or signal transducer and activator of transcription 2 (STAT2), key mediators of type I interferon signaling, causes fatal susceptibility to viral disease in childhood.[93,94] Interferons also regulate cell activation, proliferation, and death. Interferon signaling as part of the normal immune response to *in utero* TORCH infections may contribute to the pregnancy complications caused by such infections.[95] TORCH is an acronym for a group of infectious agents that cause *in utero* infections: Toxoplasma, Other (HIV, Syphilis, Zika virus), Rubella, Cytomegalovirus, and Herpes Simplex virus. There is a significant overlap between TORCH infections and Mendelian disorders of interferon overactivity, such as disorders of the IFNAR signaling pathway[96–99] and Aicardi-Goutières syndrome.[100] These pseudo-TORCH syndromes typically present with encephalopathy, cerebrospinal fluid lymphocytosis, and basal ganglia calcification.

Fetal immune cells capable of IFNα production, such as NK cells, emerge during the first trimester. A fetal source of IFNa is implicated in prenatal pathology as *Ifnar1* $\pm$ mice born to *Ifnar1-/-* mothers suffer impaired placental development during Zika virus infection and have shorter survival than their *Ifnar1-/-* littermates.[101] Regulatory mechanisms to protect fetal and reproductive tissues from material interferon exposure, include overexpression of G-protein-coupled estrogen receptor 1 (GPER1).[102] Infection of fetal tissues with TORCH or overactivity of interferon signaling pathways must overwhelm such protective mechanisms.

Immunodysregulation polyendocrinopathy enteropathy X-linked (IPEX) syndrome and Omenn syndrome: the need for a balanced T cell compartment.

IPEX syndrome is caused by mutations in FOXP3,[103] an essential transcription factor for the development and function of thymic Tregs.[104–106] FOXP3-deficient Tregs are unable to inhibit T cell proliferation and cytokine production.[105] IPEX is clinically heterogeneous, but most patients present soon after birth with type 1 diabetes, enteropathy and eczema.[107] IPEX families are frequently affected by male pregnancy loss,[108–114] typically due to fetal hydrops. Although the pathophysiology is not completely understood, some reports attribute hemolytic anemia, and others have described increased extramedullary hematopoiesis.[114] A study of 2 newborns with IPEX who died soon after birth showed extensive T cell enrichment as well as chronic inflammation of the pancreas with oligoclonal T cell enrichment, suggestive of antigen-driven autoimmunity before birth.[115]

Omenn syndrome is a disorder of T cell development that typically presents in infancy with life-threatening infection, erythroderma, lymphadenopathy, hepatosplenomegaly, diarrhea, and eosinophilia. Patients lack B cells and have oligoclonal, activated, autologous T cells.[116] The syndrome is usually caused by hypomorphic mutations in recombination-activation (RAG) genes, although severe combined immunodeficiencies (SCID) with defects in ADA, IL7Ra, IL2Rg, ARTEMIS, and DNA ligase also exist.[117] Omenn-associated RAG mutations reduce, but do not completely abolish their function as mediators of V(D)J recombination, the process by which T cell repertoire diversity is generated.[118,119] While complete absence of RAG activity presents as T^-B^- SCID,[120] partial RAG activity permits some T cells to develop and leave the thymus.[119] Environmental factors, including infection, may contribute to the evolution of some immune dysregulatory features, such as erythroderma, by triggering the expansion of clonotypic autoreactive T cells.[121] Impaired barrier immunity contributes to susceptibility to severe infection.

These syndromes demonstrate the importance of a regulated T cell compartment to prenatal immune homeostasis. In Omenn syndrome, patients experience both infection susceptibility from impaired conventional T cell function and graft-versus-host-disease-like pathology from impaired Treg function. The prenatal consequences of IPEX, whereby the defect is specific to Tregs, underscore the importance of Treg function during early development.

SUMMARY

Despite the difficulties of observing human gestational immune development, insights from high-resolution studies of fetal tissues have provided a detailed picture of how immune cells are generated at different time points and in different locations. There is a phased production of immune cells, with the specific innate immune cells required in early development most likely contributing to tissue morphogenesis. The details of these noncanonical functions and how they vary between tissues require further investigation. Diverse innate immune effectors are then acquired before adaptive immune cell production escalates. Contrary to assumptions that the fetal immune system is "immature," the fetus is capable of generating specific immune responses to pathogens and vaccines and can activate with detrimental consequences on stimulation, or when homeostatic mechanisms are disturbed by IEI. A greater understanding of how the immune cell repertoire coordinates to maintain homeostasis and how this is disturbed by in utero infection, maternal immune activation and preterm birth will yield greater insights into the vulnerabilities of the fetal immune system and how it can be supported through the challenge.

ACKNOWLEDGMENTS

L. Jardine is an NIHR Academic Clinical Lecturer. I. Schim van der Loeff is an NIHR Academic Clinical Fellow. I.J. Haq is supported by funding provided by the Academy of Medical Sciences (SGL024 \ 1027).

DISCLOSURE

The authors disclose no conflicts of interest.

REFERENCES

1. Popescu DM, Botting RA, Stephenson E, et al. Decoding human fetal liver hematopoiesis. Nature 2019;574:365–71.
2. Copley MR, Eaves CJ. Developmental changes in hematopoietic stem cell properties. Exp Mol Med 2013;45:e55.
3. Ivanovs A, Rybtsov S, Ng ES, et al. Human hematopoietic stem cell development: from the embryo to the dish. Development 2017;144:2323–37.
4. Dzierzak E, Medvinsky A. The discovery of a source of adult hematopoietic cells in the embryo. Development 2008;135 2343–2346.
5. O'Byrne S, Elliott N, Rice S, et al. Discovery of a CD10-negative B-progenitor in human fetal life identifies unique ontogeny-related developmental programs. Blood 2019;134:1059–71.
6. Park JE, Botting RA, Domínguez Conde C, et al. A cell atlas of human thymic development defines T cell repertoire formation. Science 2020;367.
7. Charbord P, Tavian M, Humeau L, et al. Early ontogeny of the human marrow from long bones: an immunohistochemical study of hematopoiesis and its microenvironment. Blood 1996;87:4109–19.
8. Jardine L, Webb S, Goh I, et al. Blood and immune development in human fetal bone marrow and Down syndrome. Nature 2021;598:327–31.
9. Mende N, Bastos HP, Santoro A, et al. Unique molecular and functional features of extramedullary hematopoietic stem and progenitor cell reservoirs in humans. Blood 2022. https://doi.org/10.1182/blood.2021013450.
10. Suo C, Dann E, Goh I, et al. Mapping the developing human immune system across organs. Science 2022;376(6597). https://doi.org/10.1126/science.abo0510.
11. He P, Lim K, Sun D, et al. A human fetal lung cell atlas uncovers proximal-distal gradients of differentiation and key regulators of epithelial fates. bioRxiv 2022;474933. https://doi.org/10.1101/2022.01.11.474933.
12. Schafflick D, Wolbert J, Heming M, et al. Single-cell profiling of CNS border compartment leukocytes reveals that B cells and their progenitors reside in non-diseased meninges. Nat Neurosci 2021;24 1225–1234.
13. Park J-E, Jardine L, Gottgens B, et al. Prenatal development of human immunity. Science 2020;368:600–3.
14. Forestier F, Daffos F, Catherine N, et al. Developmental hematopoiesis in normal human fetal blood. Blood 1991;77:2360–3.
15. Christensen RD, Jensen J, Maheshwari A, et al. Reference ranges for blood concentrations of eosinophils and monocytes during the neonatal period defined from over 63 000 records in a multihospital health-care system. J Perinatology 2010;30:540–5.
16. Olin A, Henckel E, Chen Y, et al. Stereotypic Immune System Development in Newborn Children. Cell 2018;174:1277–92.e14.
17. Paolicelli RC, Bolasco G, Pagani F, et al. Synaptic pruning by microglia is necessary for normal brain development. Science 2011;333:1456–8.
18. Fantin A, Vieira JM, Gestri G, et al. Tissue macrophages act as cellular chaperones for vascular anastomosis downstream of VEGF-mediated endothelial tip cell induction. Blood 2010;116:829–40.
19. Li W, Guo R, Song Y, et al. Erythroblastic Island Macrophages Shape Normal Erythropoiesis and Drive Associated Disorders in Erythroid Hematopoietic Diseases. Front Cell Dev Biol 2021;0.

20. Theret M, Mounier R, Rossi F. The origins and non-canonical functions of macrophages in development and regeneration. Development 2019;146.
21. Ginhoux F, Guilliams M. Tissue-Resident Macrophage Ontogeny and Homeostasis. Immunity 2016;44:439–49.
22. Alsinet C, Nascimento Primo M, Lorenzi V, et al. Robust temporal map of human in vitro myelopoiesis using single-cell genomics. Nature Communications 2022; 13. https://doi.org/10.1038/s41467-022-30557-4.
23. Krystel-Whittemore M, Dileepan KN, Wood JG. Mast Cell: A Multi-Functional Master Cell. Front Immunol 2015;6:620.
24. Li Z, Liu S, Xu J, et al. Adult Connective Tissue-Resident Mast Cells Originate from Late Erythro-Myeloid Progenitors. Immunity 2018;49:640–53.e5.
25. Gentek R, Ghigo C, Hoeffel G, et al. Hemogenic Endothelial Fate Mapping Reveals Dual Developmental Origin of Mast Cells. Immunity 2018;48:1160–71.e5.
26. Vivier E, Artis D, Colonna M, et al. Innate Lymphoid Cells: 10 Years On. Cell 2018;174:1054–66.
27. Bando JK, Liang H-E, Locksley RM. Identification and distribution of developing innate lymphoid cells in the fetal mouse intestine. Nat Immunol 2015;16:153–60.
28. Elmentaite R, Kumasaka N, King HW, et al. Cells of the human intestinal tract mapped across space and time. Nature 2021;597:250–5.
29. Lim AI, Li Y, Lopez-Lastra S, et al. Systemic Human ILC Precursors Provide a Substrate for Tissue ILC Differentiation. Cell 2017;168:1086–100.e10.
30. Gasteiger G, Fan X, Dikiy S, et al. Tissue residency of innate lymphoid cells in lymphoid and nonlymphoid organs. Science 2015;350:981–5.
31. Mebius RE, Rennert P, Weissman IL. Developing Lymph Nodes Collect CD4 CD3 − LTβ Cells That Can Differentiate to APC, NK Cells, and Follicular Cells but Not T or B Cells. Immunity 1997;7 493–504.
32. Aparicio-Domingo P, Romera-Hernandez M, Karrich JJ, et al. Type 3 innate lymphoid cells maintain intestinal epithelial stem cells after tissue damage. J Exp Med 2015;212:1783–91.
33. von Moltke J, Ji M, Liang H-E, et al. Tuft-cell-derived IL-25 regulates an intestinal ILC2-epithelial response circuit. Nature 2016;529:221–5.
34. Monticelli LA, Sonnenberg GF, Abt MC, et al. Innate lymphoid cells promote lung-tissue homeostasis after infection with influenza virus. Nat Immunol 2011; 12:1045–54.
35. Patel AA, Yona S. Inherited and Environmental Factors Influence Human Monocyte Heterogeneity. Front Immunol 2019;10:2581.
36. Reynolds G, Vegh P, Fletcher J, et al. Developmental cell programs are co-opted in inflammatory skin disease. Science 2021;371.
37. Ziegler-Heitbrock L. Monocyte subsets in man and other species. Cell Immunol 2014;289:135–9.
38. Strunk T, Temming P, Gembruch U, et al. Differential maturation of the innate immune response in human fetuses. Pediatr Res 2004;56:219–26.
39. Gomez JC, Doerschuk CM. The role of CD18 in the production and release of neutrophils from the bone marrow. Lab Invest 2010;90:599–610.
40. Tedder TF, Steeber DA, Chen A, et al. The selecting: vascular adhesion molecules. The FASEB J 1995;9:866–73.
41. Angelo LS, Bimler LH, Nikzad R, et al. CXCR6+ NK Cells in Human Fetal Liver and Spleen Possess Unique Phenotypic and Functional Capabilities. Front Immunol 2019;0.
42. Reynolds G, Haniffa M. Human and Mouse Mononuclear Phagocyte Networks: A Tale of Two Species? Front Immunol 2015;6:330.

43. McGovern N, Shin A, Low G, et al. Human fetal dendritic cells promote prenatal T-cell immune suppression through arginase-2. Nature 2017;546:662–6.
44. Rechavi E, Lev A, Lee YN, et al. Timely and spatially regulated maturation of B and T cell repertoire during human fetal development. Sci Transl Med 2015;7: 276ra25.
45. Rastogi D, Wang C, Mao X, et al. Antigen-specific immune responses to influenza vaccine in utero. J Clin Invest 2007;117:1637–46.
46. King CL, Malhotra I, Mungai P, et al. B cell sensitization to helminthic infection develops in utero in humans. J Immunol 1998;160:3578–84.
47. Marchant A, Appay V, Van Der Sande M, et al. Mature CD8(+) T lymphocyte response to viral infection during fetal life. J Clin Invest 2003;111:1747–55.
48. Rayfield LS, Brent L, Rodeck CH. Development of cell-mediated lympholysis in human foetal blood lymphocytes. Clin Exp Immunol 1980;42:561–70.
49. Michaëlsson J, Mold JE, McCune JM, et al. Regulation of T Cell Responses in the Developing Human Fetus. The J Immunol 2006;176:5741–8.
50. Mold JE, Michaëlsson J, Burt TD, et al. Maternal alloantigens promote the development of tolerogenic fetal regulatory T cells in utero. Science 2008;322:1562–5.
51. Lee YJ, Jeon YK, Kang BH, et al. Generation of PLZF+ CD4+ T cells via MHC class II-dependent thymocyte-thymocyte interaction is a physiological process in humans. J Exp Med 2010;207:237–46.
52. Collins C, Sharpe E, Silber A, et al. Congenital Athymia: Genetic Etiologies, Clinical Manifestations, Diagnosis, and Treatment. J Clin Immunol 2021;41:881–95.
53. Mayassi T, Barreiro LB, Rossjohn J, et al. A multilayered immune system through the lens of unconventional T cells. Nature 2021;595:501–10.
54. Alonzo ES, Sant'Angelo DB. Development of PLZF-expressing innate T cells. Curr Opin Immunol 2011;23:220–7.
55. Toulon A, Breton L, Taylor KR, et al. A role for human skin-resident T cells in wound healing. J Exp Med 2009;206:743–50.
56. Baumgarth N. The double life of a B-1 cell: self-reactivity selects for protective effector functions. Nat Rev Immunol 2011;11:34–46.
57. Hayakawa K, Asano M, Shinton SA, et al. Positive selection of natural autoreactive B cells. Science 1999;285:113–6.
58. Blanco E, Pérez-Andrés M, Arriba-Méndez S, et al. Age-associated distribution of normal B-cell and plasma cell subsets in peripheral blood. J Allergy Clin Immunol 2018;141:2208–19.e16.
59. Barzanji AJ, Emery JL. Germinal centers in the spleens of neonates and stillbirths. Early Hum Dev 1978;1:363–9.
60. Elmentaite R, Ross ADB, Roberts K, et al. Single-Cell Sequencing of Developing Human Gut Reveals Transcriptional Links to Childhood Crohn's Disease. Dev Cell 2020;55:771–83.e5.
61. Grassi R, Farina R, Floriani I, et al. Assessment of fetal swallowing with grayscale and color Doppler sonography. AJR Am J Roentgenol 2005;185:1322–7.
62. Stras SF, Werner L, Toothaker JM, et al. Maturation of the Human Intestinal Immune System Occurs Early in Fetal Development. Dev Cell 2019;51:357–73.e5.
63. Schreurs RRCE, Baumdick ME, Sagebiel AF, et al. Human Fetal TNF-α-Cytokine-Producing CD4 Effector Memory T Cells Promote Intestinal Development and Mediate Inflammation Early in Life. Immunity 2019;50:462–76.e8.
64. Li N, van Unen V, Abdelaal T, et al. Memory CD4 T cells are generated in the human fetal intestine. Nat Immunol 2019;20:301–12.
65. Mishra A, Lai GC, Yao LJ, et al. Microbial exposure during early human development primes fetal immune cells. Cell 2021;184:3394–409.e20.

66. Battersby C, Santhalingam T, Costeloe K, et al. Incidence of neonatal necrotising enterocolitis in high-income countries: a systematic review. Arch Dis Child Fetal Neonatal Ed 2018;103:F182–9.
67. Bode L. Human Milk Oligosaccharides in the Prevention of Necrotizing Enterocolitis: A Journey From and Models to Mother-Infant Cohort Studies. Front Pediatr 2018;6:385.
68. Egozi A, Olaloye O, Werner L, et al. Single cell atlas of the neonatal small intestine with necrotizing enterocolitis. bioRxiv 2022. https://doi.org/10.1101/2022.03.01.482508.
69. Corpeleijn WE, de Waard M, Christmann V, et al. Effect of Donor Milk on Severe Infections and Mortality in Very Low-Birth-Weight Infants: The Early Nutrition Study Randomized Clinical Trial. JAMA Pediatr 2016;170:654–61.
70. Stewart CJ, Embleton ND, Marrs ECL, et al. Temporal bacterial and metabolic development of the preterm gut reveals specific signatures in health and disease. Microbiome 2016;4:67.
71. Hackam DJ, Sodhi CP. Toll-Like Receptor-Mediated Intestinal Inflammatory Imbalance in the Pathogenesis of Necrotizing Enterocolitis. Cell Mol Gastroenterol Hepatol 2018;6:229–38.e1.
72. Warner BB, Deych E, Zhou Y, et al. Gut bacteria dysbiosis and necrotising enterocolitis in very low birthweight infants: a prospective case-control study. Lancet 2016;387:1928–36.
73. Cacho NT, Lawrence RM. Innate Immunity and Breast Milk. Front Immunol 2017;8.
74. Stewart CJ, Ajami NJ, O'Brien JL, et al. Temporal development of the gut microbiome in early childhood from the TEDDY study. Nature 2018;562:583–8.
75. Masi AC, Embleton ND, Lamb CA, et al. Human milk oligosaccharide DSLNT and gut microbiome in preterm infants predicts necrotising enterocolitis. Gut 2021;70:2273–82.
76. Henrick BM, Rodriguez L, Lakshmikanth T, et al. Bifidobacteria-mediated immune system imprinting early in life. bioRxiv 2020. https://doi.org/10.1101/2020.10.24.353250.
77. Lu P, Yamaguchi Y, Fulton WB, et al. Maternal aryl hydrocarbon receptor activation protects newborns against necrotizing enterocolitis. Nat Commun 2021;12:1042.
78. Warburton D, El-Hashash A, Carraro G, et al. Lung organogenesis. Curr Top Dev Biol 2010;90:73–158.
79. Nikolić MZ, Sun D, Rawlins EL. Human lung development: recent progress and new challenges. Development 2018;145.
80. Domingo-Gonzalez R, Zanini F, Che X, et al. Diverse homeostatic and immunomodulatory roles of immune cells in the developing mouse lung at single cell resolution. Elife 2020;9.
81. Madissoon E, Oliver AJ, Kleshchevnikov V, et al. A spatial multi-omics atlas of the human lung reveals a novel immune cell survival niche. bioRxiv 2021;470108. https://doi.org/10.1101/2021.11.26.470108.
82. Cohen M, Giladi A, Gorki A-D, et al. Lung Single-Cell Signaling Interaction Map Reveals Basophil Role in Macrophage Imprinting. Cell 2018;175:1031–44.e18.
83. Blackwell TS, Hipps AN, Yamamoto Y, et al. NF-κB signaling in fetal lung macrophages disrupts airway morphogenesis. J Immunol 2011;187:2740–7.
84. Guilliams M, et al. Alveolar macrophages develop from fetal monocytes that differentiate into long-lived cells in the first week of life via GM-CSF. J Exp Med 2013;210:1977–92.

85. Kramer BW, Joshi SN, Moss TJM, et al. Endotoxin-induced maturation of mono-cytes in preterm fetal sheep lung. Am J Physiol Lung Cell Mol Physiol 2007;293: L345–53.
86. Jackson CM, Mukherjee S, Wilburn AN, et al. Pulmonary Consequences of Pre-natal Inflammatory Exposures: Clinical Perspective and Review of Basic Immu-nological Mechanisms. Front Immunol 2020;11:1285.
87. Davidson LM, Berkelhamer SK. Bronchopulmonary Dysplasia: Chronic Lung Disease of Infancy and Long-Term Pulmonary Outcomes. J Clin Med Res 2017;6.
88. Torow N, Marsland BJ, Hornef MW, et al. Neonatal mucosal immunology. Mucosal Immunol 2017;10:5–17.
89. Saluzzo S, Gorki A-D, Rana BMJ, et al. First-Breath-Induced Type 2 Pathways Shape the Lung Immune Environment. Cell Rep 2017;18:1893–905.
90. de Kleer IM, Kool M, de Bruijn MJW, et al. Perinatal Activation of the Interleukin-33 Pathway Promotes Type 2 Immunity in the Developing Lung. Immunity 2016; 45:1285–98.
91. Tregoning JS, Yamaguchi Y, Harker J, et al. The role of T cells in the enhance-ment of respiratory syncytial virus infection severity during adult reinfection of neonatally sensitized mice. J Virol 2008;82:4115–24.
92. Krishnamoorthy N, Khare A, Oriss TB, et al. Early infection with respiratory syn-cytial virus impairs regulatory T cell function and increases susceptibility to allergic asthma. Nat Med 2012;18:1525–30.
93. Duncan CJA, Mohamad SMB, Young DF, et al. Human IFNAR2 deficiency: Les-sons for antiviral immunity. Sci Transl Med 2015;7:307ra154.
94. Hambleton S, Goodbourn S, Young DF, et al. STAT2 deficiency and susceptibil-ity to viral illness in humans. Proc Natl Acad Sci U S A 2013;110:3053–8.
95. Yockey LJ, Iwasaki A. Interferons and Proinflammatory Cytokines in Pregnancy and Fetal Development. Immunity 2018;49:397–412.
96. Crow YJ, Stetson DB. The type I interferonopathies: 10 years on. Nat Rev Immu-nol 2021. https://doi.org/10.1038/s41577-021-00633-9.
97. Meuwissen MEC, Schot R, Buta S, et al. Human USP18 deficiency underlies type 1 interferonopathy leading to severe pseudo-TORCH syndrome. J Exp Med 2016;213:1163–74.
98. Gruber C, Martin-Fernandez M, Ailal F, et al. Homozygous STAT2 gain-of-func-tion mutation by loss of USP18 activity in a patient with type I interferonopathy. J Exp Med 2020;217.
99. Duncan CJA, Thompson BJ, Chen R, et al. Severe type I interferonopathy and unrestrained interferon signaling due to a homozygous germline mutation in. Sci Immunol 2019;4.
100. Aicardi J, Goutières F. A progressive familial encephalopathy in infancy with cal-cifications of the basal ganglia and chronic cerebrospinal fluid lymphocytosis. Ann Neurol 1984;15:49–54.
101. Yockey LJ, Jurado KA, Arora N, et al. Type I interferons instigate fetal demise after Zika virus infection. Sci Immunol 2018;3.
102. Harding AT, Goff MA, Froggatt HM, et al. GPER1 is required to protect fetal health from maternal inflammation. Science 2021;371:271–6.
103. Bennett CL, Christie J, Ramsdell F, et al. The immune dysregulation, polyendoc-rinopathy, enteropathy, X-linked syndrome (IPEX) is caused by mutations of FOXP3. Nat Genet 2001;27 20–21.
104. Khattri R, Cox T, Yasayko S-A, et al. An essential role for Scurfin in CD4 CD25 T regulatory cells. Nat Immunol 2003;4 337–342.

105. Hori S, Nomura T, Sakaguchi S. Control of Regulatory T Cell Development by the Transcription Factor Foxp3. Science 2003;299 1057–1061.
106. Fontenot JD, Gavin MA, Rudensky AY. Foxp3 programs the development and function of CD4+CD25+ regulatory T cells. Nat Immunol 2003;4:330–6.
107. Barzaghi F, Amaya Hernandez LC, Neven B, et al. Long-term follow-up of IPEX syndrome patients after different therapeutic strategies: An international multi-center retrospective study. J Allergy Clin Immunol 2018;141:1036–49.e5.
108. Xavier-da-Silva MM, Moreira-Filho CC, Suzuki E, et al. Fetal-onset IPEX: report of two families and review of literature. Clin Immunol 2015;156:131–40.
109. Louie RJ, Tan Q K-G, Gilner JB, et al. Novel pathogenic variants in FOXP3 in fetuses with echogenic bowel and skin desquamation identified by ultrasound. Am J Med Genet A 2017;173:1219–25.
110. Rae W, Gao Y, Bunyan D, et al. A novel FOXP3 mutation causing fetal akinesia and recurrent male miscarriages. Clin Immunol 2015;161:284–5.
111. Reichert SL, McKay EM, Moldenhauer JS. Identification of a novel nonsense mutation in theFOXP3gene in a fetus with hydrops-Expanding the phenotype of IPEX syndrome. Am J Med Genet A 2016;170 226–232.
112. Vasiljevic A, Poreau B, Bouvier R, et al. Immune dysregulation, polyendocrinopathy, enteropathy, X-linked syndrome and recurrent intrauterine fetal death. Lancet 2015;385:2120.
113. Shehab O, Tester DJ, Ackerman NC, et al. Whole genome sequencing identifies etiology of recurrent male intrauterine fetal death. Prenat Diagn 2017;37:1040–5.
114. Carneiro-Sampaio M, Moreira-Filho CA, Bando SY, et al. Front Pediatr 2020;0.
115. Allenspach EJ, Finn LS, Rendi MH, et al. Absence of functional fetal regulatory T cells in humans causes in utero organ-specific autoimmunity. J Allergy Clin Immunol 2017;140:616–9.e7.
116. de Saint-Basile G, Le Deist F, de Villartay JP, et al. Restricted heterogeneity of T lymphocytes in combined immunodeficiency with hypereosinophilia (Omenn's syndrome). J Clin Invest 1991;87:1352–9.
117. Villa A, Notarangelo LD, Roifman CM. Omenn syndrome: inflammation in leaky severe combined immunodeficiency. J Allergy Clin Immunol 2008;122:1082–6.
118. Fugmann SD, Lee AI, Shockett PE, et al. The RAG proteins and V(D)J recombination: complexes, ends, and transposition. Annu Rev Immunol 2000;18: 495–527.
119. Villa A, Santagata S, Bozzi F, et al. Partial V(D)J recombination activity leads to Omenn syndrome. Cell 1998;93:885–96.
120. Schwarz K, Gauss GH, Ludwig L, et al. RAG mutations in human B cell-negative SCID. Science 1996;274:97–9.
121. Villa A, Notarangelo LD. RAG gene defects at the verge of immunodeficiency and immune dysregulation. Immunol Rev 2019;287:73–90.

Longitudinal Changes in Upper and Lower Airway Function in Pregnancy

Vanessa E. Murphy, PhD[a,b,*], Megan E. Jensen, PhD, AdvAPD[a,b]

KEYWORDS

- Asthma • Rhinitis • Sleep-disordered breathing • Spirometry • Lung function
- Pulmonary function tests

KEY POINTS

- Blood volume increases and hormonal changes during pregnancy alter nasal mucosal secretions causing an increase in upper airway congestion and symptoms.
- Rhinitis symptoms affect at least 30% of women.
- The prevalence of snoring and sleep-disordered breathing increases in pregnancy.
- Lower airway function is reduced in pregnancy, but the magnitude of the changes is small.
- There are no clinically important changes in FEV_1 or FVC across pregnancy making spirometry a useful clinical tool to assess lung function.

INTRODUCTION

Pregnancy causes significant hormonal, mechanical, and circulatory changes, essential for meeting the increased metabolic demands of mother and fetus.[1] These include increases in cardiac output, pulmonary blood flow, circulating blood volume, oxygen consumption, carbon dioxide production, and basal metabolic rate. These pregnancy-related changes can impact the upper and lower airways (**Fig. 1**).

In the upper airway, there are significant changes to the nasopharynx and oropharynx, with mucosal changes including hyperemia, edema, plasma leakage, and glandular hypersecretion.[1] High levels of progesterone and estrogen in pregnancy are thought to cause fluid retention contributing to swelling around the neck, mucous membranes, and nasal passages, leading to narrowing of the oropharyngeal diameter and increases in upper airway resistance.[2]

[a] Priority Research Centre for Healthy Lungs, University of Newcastle, Newcastle, New South Wales, Australia; [b] Hunter Medical Research Institute, Level 2 West, c/- University of Newcastle, University Drive, Callaghan, New South Wales 2308, Australia
* Corresponding author. Hunter Medical Research Institute, Level 2 West, c/- University of Newcastle, University Drive, Callaghan, New South Wales 2308, Australia.
E-mail address: Vanessa.murphy@newcastle.edu.au

Immunol Allergy Clin N Am 43 (2023) 17–26
https://doi.org/10.1016/j.iac.2022.07.005
0889-8561/23/© 2022 Elsevier Inc. All rights reserved.

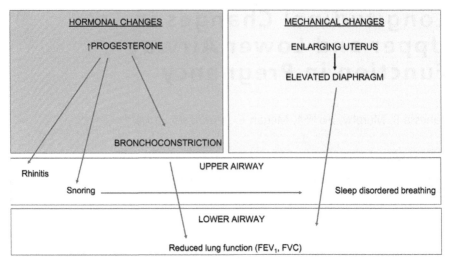

Fig. 1. Potential hormonal and mechanical effects of pregnancy on upper and lower airway function.

In the lower airways, pregnancy leads to changes in lung volumes including decreases in total lung capacity and functional residual capacity (FRC), reduced chest wall compliance, and increased tidal volume and minute ventilation. In addition, the chest wall undergoes significant structural changes in pregnancy. To accommodate the enlarging uterus, the diaphragm elevates ~4 cm, and the circumference of the lower rib cage increases by ~5 cm; these changes can alter respiration.

DISCUSSION
Pregnancy-Related Changes in Upper Airway Function

- Upper airway congestion and symptoms increase during pregnancy
- Likely due to pregnancy-induced increased blood volume leading to vascular engorgement of the nasal passages, and hormonal changes altering nasal mucosal secretions[3]

A 2004 study comprehensively examined nasal airway changes in 18 women using[4] anterior rhinoscopy, peak inspiratory nasal flow rate, acoustic rhinometry, and anterior rhinomanometry measurements, taken at 10 to 12, 20, and 32 to 36 weeks' gestation and 6 weeks postpartum. Significantly increased nasal congestion was observed from trimester 1 to 3, decreasing postpartum. The corresponding trend in decreased nasal volume was not significant. There was no longitudinal change in nasal flow rate. The authors hypothesized that the rise in serum progesterone and estrogen levels across pregnancy may be responsible for these changes.[4]

Using acoustic reflection, a 2003 study measured upper airway caliber (oropharyngeal junction area, mean pharyngeal area, and mean pharyngeal volume) in the seated, supine, and left lateral recumbent positions in 50 women in trimester 3 and 50 nonpregnant women.[5] Differences in upper airway dimensions in pregnant, versus nonpregnant, women included wider upper airways when seated, yet greater narrowing of the upper airways when moving from seated to supine.[5] This upper airway narrowing was likely due to decreased FRC and tracheal shortening in pregnancy.[5]

Narrower pharynxes at the oropharyngeal junction and smaller mean pharyngeal area and volume were observed in 37 pregnant women with, versus without, preeclampsia, when seated or supine.[5] These observations were consistent with previous studies demonstrating increased airflow limitation during sleep in women with pre-eclampsia.[6] Women who snored also had narrower oropharyngeal junction areas and mean pharyngeal areas when supine, compared to nonsnorers.[5] Upper airway narrowing during sleep can contribute to blood pressure surges; continuous positive airway pressure (CPAP) may improve sleep and blood pressure control in women with pre-eclampsia.[6]

A study by the same group among 100 pregnant women (50 of whom were followed postpartum) and 100 nonpregnant women found pregnant women had a smaller mean pharyngeal area when seated, supine, or lateral,[7] compared to nonpregnant and postpartum women. Narrower upper airways are potentially due to gestational weight gain, decreased FRC (due to diaphragmatic changes), or edema-induced swelling in the pharynx.[7]

Implications for Rhinitis

Allergic rhinitis is common and up to 30% of women have worse symptoms during pregnancy (**Box 1**).[8] In one study, 34% of women reported a worsening of nasal symptoms in pregnancy, whereas 15% had an improvement and 45% had no change.[9] Treatment is similar to the nonpregnant population—avoiding triggers and using nasal corticosteroids and antihistamines.[10] Considered first-line therapy, intranasal corticosteroids have a safety profile comparable to inhaled corticosteroids.[11,12] A 2016 systematic review found no high-quality studies available on rhinitis treatment during pregnancy, therefore providing expert panel recommendations such as the use of nasal corticosteroids for chronic rhinosinusitis maintenance therapy.[13]

Box 1
Upper airway disorders in pregnancy

Rhinitis symptoms affect ≥30% of women and may be due to:
- Pre-existing rhinitis
- Pregnancy rhinitis
- Eosinophilic nonallergic rhinitis
- Nasal polyposis
- Viral or bacterial infection
- Rhinitis medicamentosa.

Pregnancy-induced rhinitis is a nonallergic rhinitis that first appears in pregnancy and generally resolves within 2 weeks of birth.

There is an increased frequency of sleep disordered breathing during pregnancy, especially in women with risk factors including:
- Obesity
- Hypertension
- Advanced maternal age

Obstructive sleep apnea (OSA) screening is recommended between 12 and 18 weeks' gestation.[65]

OSA is associated with poor perinatal outcomes, including:
- Low birth weight
- Pre-eclampsia
- Gestational hypertension
- Premature birth
- Cesarean section
- Gestational diabetes

A recent study of 681 women found that 32% experienced pregnancy-induced rhinitis.[14] Although unknown, the mechanisms may be via changes in nasal hyperre-activity or hormones. Treatment for pregnancy rhinitis includes elevating the head while sleeping and nasal saline washes.

Implications for Sleep-Disordered Breathing

Sleep-disordered breathing (SDB) refers to episodes of increased upper airway resistance during sleep, defined by $\geq$ 5 episodes of apnea or hypopnea/hour of sleep (ie, an apnea-hypopnea index of $\geq$5) (see **Box 1**).[15] Improvements in apnea-hypopnea index and arterial oxyhemoglobin saturation were observed postnatally compared to late pregnancy, in 10 women with suspected SDB, suggesting an improvement in severity postpartum.[16] Snoring indicates further upper airway resistance and is more common in pregnancy (23%) than prepregnancy (4%). Snoring is associated with poorer perinatal outcomes including hypertension, pre-eclampsia, and fetal growth restriction,[17] likely due to increased systemic inflammation and oxidative stress from intermittent hypoxia.

A recent study of more than 2000 women found a prevalence of SDB of 4% in early pregnancy, and 6% in midpregnancy.[18] Women with SDB were more likely to be obese.[18] However, no associations independent of body mass index (BMI) were found for large-for-gestational age, or small-for-gestational age birth weights.[18] Other studies found increased risks of hypertensive disorders and gestational diabetes with increasing apnea-hypopnea index during pregnancy.[19]

Obstructive sleep apnea (OSA), a more serious form of SDB characterized by total or partial interruptions of airflow during sleep, results from upper airway obstructions generating a systemic inflammatory condition. OSA is likely underdiagnosed in pregnancy because of the complexity of conducting overnight polysomnography and the lack of validated questionnaires.[2] The prevalence of OSA increases in pregnancy, from 10% in trimester 1 up to 27% in trimester 3,[20] with obese women more likely to have OSA. A recent prospective study found that 43% of women with a BMI >35 kg/m^2 had OSA, of whom 14% had severe OSA.[21] Nasal CPAP is a well-tolerated and effective treatment during pregnancy, similar to the nonpregnant population. It may also be important to monitor weight during pregnancy, as this has implications for upper and lower airway changes.

Pregnancy-Related Changes in Lower Airway Function

- Spirometry is a common tool to measure lower airway function (**Box 2**). Whether spirometry values follow the same pattern during pregnancy in women with and without asthma is poorly understood because of limited large-scale studies **Box 2**.
- Hormonal variation and the enlarging uterus are the primary mechanisms implicated in maternal lung function changes during pregnancy.[22–24]

Changes in Lung Function in Pregnancy in Women Without Respiratory Disease

- Most studies report either no change or a small reduction in lung function with advancing gestation, and compared to nonpregnant women
- Studies are limited by poor quality, including a lack of longitudinal follow-up and small sample sizes

Many studies report that FEV_1 is reduced in pregnant, versus nonpregnant, women,[25–31] whereas other studies found no significant difference between these groups.[32–42] A Brazilian study examined pulmonary function in trimesters 1 and 3, among 120 pregnant women with normal lung function.[43] They found a significant

---

Box 2
Measurements of lower airway function

Spirometry is commonly used in assessment and monitoring of lung function.

Values are compared to a reference population to aid interpretation.[14]

Forced expiratory volume in one second (FEV_1)
- Maximum volume of air exhaled in the first second of a forced expiration from a position of full inspiration, expressed in liters, measured by spirometry

Forced vital capacity (FVC)
- Maximum volume of air exhaled with maximally forced effort from a maximal inspiration, expressed in liters, measured by spirometry

Peak Expiratory Flow (PEF)
- Maximum expiratory flow achieved from a maximum forced expiration, starting without hesitation from the point of maximal lung inflation, expressed in L/s or L/min

---

decrease in FEV_1 and FVC (% predicted and absolute values), but not FEV_1:FVC ratio, over gestation. FEV_1:FVC was lower in multiparous, versus nulliparous, women in early pregnancy.[43]

Conversely, a UK study found no significant difference in FEV_1, FVC, or peak expiratory flow rate (PEFR) in 203 pregnant, versus 22 nonpregnant, women,[42] and no differences between twin and singleton pregnancies.

A Norwegian study found that FVC increased progressively with gestational age in 80 pregnant women; however, the magnitude of the change was minor (2.1% over 21 weeks).[37] A study of 50 healthy women between 29 and 34 weeks, 50 healthy women more than 34 weeks' gestation, and 50 nonpregnant women matched for age and height found FVC was statistically lower in the late pregnancy group versus nonpregnant women, with no difference in FEV_1:FVC.[44] PEFR was lower in later versus earlier pregnancy, and statistically higher in nonpregnant, versus pregnant, women.[44]

FEV_1:FVC has been investigated in many pregnancy studies.[27,28,30,31,39] Neeraj and colleagues[27] did not find a significant group difference in FEV_1:FVC between 100 pregnant women in trimester 3, compared with 100 nonpregnant women. A later study by the same authors validated these findings[28] and found no difference between women less than 34, versus greater than 34, weeks' gestation. A recent study found a nonsignificant decrease in FEV_1:FVC in pregnant versus nonpregnant women.[39] Another Indian study reported similar results,[31] and observed no difference between singleton and twin pregnancies.

Puranik and colleagues found that PEF decreased significantly, at an average of 6.7 L/min/mo and 5.5 L/min/kg of weight gain, during pregnancy in 60 women,[34] with PEF lowest in month 9, versus nonpregnant women. A large-scale study of 1000 Nigerian women found PEF was reduced in pregnant, versus nonpregnant women, with this difference increasing with gestational age,[45] as have other studies.[25–29,31,35,41,46–50]

Other studies found no significant change in PEF during pregnancy.[38–40,42,51,52] The largest study by Purohit and Harsoda[51] found a nonsignificant progressive reduction with advancing gestation in 279 women, whereas 2 studies found PEF increased significantly with advancing gestation.[36,37] These conflicting results may reflect the limitations of using PEF to assess lung function changes over time and between groups. Although a commonly measured parameter, PEF has greater intrasubject variability compared to other parameters, such as FEV_1,[53,54] making it less reliable for group comparisons, and tends to underestimate pulmonary impairment.

An Australian study focused on the effect of asthma during pregnancy on lung function, also followed a cohort of women without respiratory disease, conducting spirometry at several time points during pregnancy.[55] Among 259 women, FVC% predicted decreased by 0.07% per week, whereas FEV_1% predicted decreased by 0.14% per week, a clinically insignificant change.[55]

Changes in Lung Function in Pregnancy in Women with Asthma

- Asthma symptoms and exacerbation risk can change in pregnancy
- There are few longitudinal studies of lung function in women with asthma during pregnancy
- A recent study showed no clinically important change in FEV_1 or FVC across gestation[55]

Asthma occurs in 8% to 12% of pregnant women,[56,57] and pregnancy has a variable effect on asthma disease severity; at least 20% of women have exacerbations requiring medical intervention.[58,59] Lung function assessment offers a useful tool to monitor maternal health, especially given the unpredictability of asthma during pregnancy. Lung function may also affect perinatal outcomes, with FEV_1 in women with asthma negatively associated with preterm birth, pregnancy-induced hypertension, and fetal growth. It is unknown if these relationships would be observed in women without asthma. Monitoring lung function during pregnancy, particularly in women with asthma, who are at increased risk of adverse perinatal outcomes and in whom the course of asthma is unpredictable during pregnancy, is therefore clinically relevant.[13,15–17]

Early studies were limited by small sample sizes and lack of repeat measures[60] and did not find changes in FEV_1 or FVC with advancing gestation.[61] Other studies have concluded that pulmonary function alters with advancing gestation. Beckmann found a significant progressive increase in PEF in 43 pregnant women with asthma, from 358.8 L/min in trimester 1, to 424.8 L/min in trimester 3.[62] A Portuguese study assessed lung function twice in pregnancy in 42 participants and a third time in 22 participants, with both asthma and allergic rhinitis.[63] At baseline, 28.6% of women had mild, moderate, or small airway obstruction; this classification was unaltered over the course of pregnancy. No correlation was observed between upper or lower airway symptom scores and FEV_1% predicted.[63]

An Australian study measured FEV_1, FEV_6, and FVC in 20 women with and 20 women without asthma, at several gestational time points.[22] Statistically significant decreases in absolute FEV_1, FEV_1% predicted, and FEV_1/FVC% at 21 to 28 weeks were detected compared to baseline (8–20 weeks), in both groups. However, lung function approached, or exceeded, baseline values by 29 to 40 weeks. These changes were exaggerated in women with asthma; FEV_1% was 4.6% lower at the first follow-up and 1.7% greater at the second. This study did not control for smoking history, which likely confounded the results.

The most comprehensive study to date examined the effect of advancing pregnancy, and its interaction with asthma, on FEV_1, FVC, and FEV_1:FVC in 1029 women during pregnancy.[55] Women with (n = 770) and without (n = 259) asthma had serial spirometry measurements during pregnancy. Multilevel mixed-effect regression modeling was used to analyze changes in lung function with gestational age, controlling for smoking, maternal weight status, and age. Baseline lung function was lower in women with asthma; however, the pattern of lung function over the remainder of pregnancy was only impacted marginally by either asthma or pregnancy itself. FVC% predicted decreased by 2.8% during pregnancy in both groups. Conversely, FEV_1% was relatively stable in women with asthma, but significantly decreased in women without asthma by 5.6% over pregnancy. FEV_1:FVC was unaffected, increasing marginally in women with asthma over the course of pregnancy, possibly as a consequence of active asthma management provided in the study. These results provide evidence to support the use of spirometry to assess lung function in pregnancy, because the impacts of pregnancy on spirometry indices were small and of limited clinical importance. However, the results cannot necessarily be applied to women with more severe asthma, or poorly controlled asthma.[55] Sensitivity analyses conducted in this study suggest maternal weight status is an important factor to consider in future studies, with baseline maternal obesity associated with reduced FEV_1, and the inclusion of maternal weight at each assessment of lung function marginally changing the estimates (although not the direction) of the effects of pregnancy on women with and without asthma.[55]

Another recent study among 275 pregnant women with active asthma found that those treated with inhaled corticosteroids and long-acting β-agonist, plus short-acting β-agonists had an 11% improvement in FEV_1 in trimester 3, compared to the trajectory of women using no asthma medication.[64] Spirometry was measured at less than 15 weeks, 20 to 22 weeks, and 30 to 32 weeks' gestation.[64] These findings suggest that appropriate use of medication improves lung function in pregnancy, consistent with the aforementioned study by Jensen *and colleagues*[55]

SUMMARY

Available evidence suggests upper airway changes may lead to an increase in rhinitis and SDB during pregnancy, with minimal reductions in lung function observed with advancing gestation. In particular, mild asthma has a limited impact on spirometry, making this a useful tool for clinical assessment and education during pregnancy.

CLINICS CARE POINTS

- Women with pre-eclampsia have increased airflow limitation during sleep, which may improve with CPAP
- One in 3 women with allergic rhinitis have an elevation in symptoms during pregnancy
- Intranasal corticosteroids are first-line therapy for allergic rhinitis during pregnancy, whereas nasal saline washes are useful for pregnancy-induced rhinitis
- Snoring is more common in pregnancy than pre-pregnancy and associated with maternal hypertension and fetal growth restriction
- Spirometry can be used to assess lung function in pregnant women with asthma, as any changes due to pregnancy are minimal and unlikely to be of clinical significance
- Measures of FEV_1 and FVC are more reliable than PEF

ACKNOWLEDGMENTS

The authors acknowledge the contribution of Jordan Ladwig to parts of the literature review on pulmonary function during pregnancy.

DISCLOSURE

Both authors have no conflicts of interest to declare. Dr V.E. Murphy is funded by a fellowship from the Medical Research Future Fund (Investigator Grant Application

ID 1196252). Dr M.E. Jensen is funded by the Peggy Lang Early Career Fellowship from the Hunter Children's Research Foundation.

REFERENCES

1. Hegewald MJ, Crapo RO. Respiratory physiology in pregnancy. Clin Chest Med 2011;32:1–13.
2. Joseph N, Shreeshaina, Loliem S B, et al. An assessment of risks associated with obstructive sleep apnea and its relationship with adverse health outcomes among pregnant women. A multi-hospital based study. Adv Respir Med 2020; 88:327–34.
3. Incaudo GA. Diagnosis and treatment of allergic rhinitis and sinusitis during pregnancy and lactation. Clin Rev Allergy Immunol 2004;27:159–77.
4. Philpott CM, Conboy P, Al-Azzawi F, et al. Nasal physiological changes during pregnancy. Clin Otolaryngol 2004;29(4):343–51.
5. Izci B, Riha RL, Martin SE, et al. The upper airway in pregnancy and pre-eclampsia. Am J Respir Crit Care Med 2003;167(2):137–40.
6. Edwards N, Blyton DM, Kirjavainen T, et al. Nasal continuous positive airway pressure reduces sleep-induced blood pressure increments in pre-eclampsia. Am J Resp Crit Care Med 2000;162:252–7.
7. Izci B, Vennelle M, Liston WA, et al. Sleep-disordered breathing and upper airway size in pregnancy and post-partum. Eur Respir J 2006;27:321–7.
8. Blaiss MS. Management of rhinitis and asthma in pregnancy. Ann Allergy Asthma Immunol 2003;90(6 Suppl 3):16–22.
9. Kircher S, Schatz M, Long L. Variables affecting asthma course during pregnancy. Ann Allergy Asthma Immunol 2002;89(5):463–6.
10. Pfaller B, Bendien S, Ditisheim A, et al. Management of allergic diseases in pregnancy. Allergy 2021;77(3):798–811.
11. Gilbert C, Mozzotta P, Loebstein R, et al. Fetal safety of drugs used in the treatment of allergic rhinitis: a critical review. Drug Saf 2005;28(8):707–19.
12. Gluck JC, Gluck PA. Asthma controller therapy during pregnancy. Am J Obstet Gynecol 2005;192(2):369–80.
13. Lal D, Jategaonkar AA, Borish L, et al. Management of rhinosinusitis during pregnancy: systematic review and expert panel recommendations. Rhinology 2016; 54:99–104.
14. Baudoin T, Simunjak T, Bacan N, et al. Redefining pregnancy-induced rhinitis. Am J Rhinol Allergy 2021;35:315–22.
15. Johns EC, Denison FC, Reynolds RM. Sleep disordered breathing in pregnancy: a review of the pathophysiology of adverse pregnancy outcomes. Acta Physiol (Oxf) 2020;229:e13458.
16. Edwards N, Blyton DM, Hennessy A, et al. Severity of sleep-disordered breathing improves following parturition. Sleep 2005;28:737–41.
17. Franklin KA, Holmgren PA, Jonsson F, et al. Snoring, pregnancy-induced hypertension and growth retardation of the fetus. Chest 2000;117:137–41.
18. Hawkins M, Parker CB, Redline S, et al. Objectively-assessed sleep-disordered breathing during pregnancy and infant birthweight. Sleep Med 2021;81:312–8.
19. Facco FL, Parker CB, Reddy UM, et al. Association between sleep-disordered breathing and hypertensive disorders of pregnancy and gestational diabetes mellitus. Obstet Gynecol 2017;129:31–41.
20. Pien GW, Pack AI, Jackson N, et al. Risk factors for sleep-disordered breathing in pregnancy. Thorax 2014;69:371–7.

21. Ghesquiere L, Deruelle P, Ramdane Y, et al. Obstructive sleep apnea in obese pregnant women: a prospective study. PLoS One 2020;15:e0238733.
22. Zairina E, Abramson MJ, McDonald CF, et al. A prospective cohort study of pulmonary function during pregnancy in women with and without asthma. J Asthma 2016;53(2):155–63.
23. LoMauro A, Aliverti A. Respiratory physiology of pregnancy. Breathe 2015;11:297–301.
24. Carlin A, Alfirevic Z. Physiological changes of pregnancy and monitoring. Best Pract Res Clin Obstet Gynaecol 2008;22:801–23.
25. Norregaard O, Schultz P, Ostergaard A, et al. Lung function and postural changes during pregnancy. Respir Med 1989;83(6):467–70.
26. Gupta L, Dixit R. A linear study of pulmonary function tests in normal pregnant and non-pregnant women. J Indian Med Assoc 2013;111(10):666–9.
27. Neeraj Sodhi C, Pramod J, Singh J, et al. Effect of advanced uncomplicated pregnancy on pulmonary function parameters of North Indian subjects. Indian J Physiol Pharmacol 2010;54(1):69–72.
28. Neeraj PJ, Singh J. Effect of advanced gestation on cellular activity in respiratory system in females: a study of alveolar ventilation parameters in pregnant women of North India. Int J Pharm Bio Sci 2012;3:31–7.
29. Panchal V, Dodiya D. Comparative study of dynamic lung function tests between third trimester pregnancy and non-pregnant women. Int J Res Med 2014;3:158–60.
30. Patil HJ, Deokar NA. Effect of advanced normal pregnancy on pulmonary function tests. IJAPB 2015;2:12–5.
31. Sidiqqui AH, Tauheed N, Ahmad A, et al. Pulmonary function in advanced uncomplicated singleton and twin pregnancy. J Bras Pneumol 2013;40:244–9.
32. Gazioglu K, Kaltreider NL, Rosen M, et al. Pulmonary function during pregnancy in normal women and in patients with cardiopulmonary disease. Thorax 1970;25:445–50.
33. Puranik BM, Kaore SB, Kurhade GA, et al. A longitudinal study of pulmonary function tests during pregnancy. Indian J Physiol Pharmacol 1994;38(2):129–32.
34. Puranik BM, Kurhade GA, Kaore SB, et al. PEFR in pregnancy: a longitudinal study. Indian J Physiol Pharmacol 1995;39(2):135–9.
35. Phatak MS, Kurhade GA. A longitudinal study of antenatal changes in lung function tests and importance of postpartum exercises in their recovery. Indian J Physiol Pharmacol 2003;47(3):352–6.
36. Kolarzyk E, Szot WM, Lyszczarz J. Lung function and breathing regulation parameters during pregnancy. Arch Gynecol Obstet 2005;272(1):53–8.
37. Grindheim G, Toska K, Estensen ME, et al. Changes in pulmonary function during pregnancy: a longitudinal cohort study. BJOG 2012;119(1):94–101.
38. Monga U, Kumari K. Pulmonary functions in Punjabi pregnant women. Indian J Physiol Pharmacol 2000;44:115–6.
39. Fadia A, Dhadse M. Dynamic pulmonary function tests in Indian pregnant and nonpregnant women. Int J Med Sci Public Health 2016;5:2114–7.
40. Dudhamal VB, Parate S. Study of pulmonary function test in different trimester of pregnancy. Int J Med Res Rev 2015;3:1239–45.
41. Yerneni S, Sajja S. Study of FEV1, VC and PEFR in different trimesters of pregnancy. Int J Res Health Sci 2014;2:41–6.
42. McAuliffe F, Kametas N, Costello J, et al. Respiratory function in singleton and twin pregnancy. Bjog 2002;109(7):765–9.
43. Pastro LDM, Lemos M, Fernandes FLA, et al. Longitudinal study of lung function in pregnant women: influence of parity and smoking. Clinics (Sao Paulo) 2017;72(10):595–9.

44. Gupta N, Verma SK, Dutta S. A comparative study to evaluate effect of advanced uncomplicated pregnancy on forced vital capacity and peak expiratory flow rate on healthy North Indian women. Natl J Physiol Pharm Pharmacol 2018;8:1451–6.

45. Chinko BC, Green KI. Peak expiratory flow rate of pregnant women in Port Harcourt. Int Res J Med Sci 2014;2:1–5.

46. Bansal M, Goyal M, Dhillon JK, et al. Longitudinal study of peak expiratory flow rate in pregnant women. NJIRM 2012;3:34–8.

47. Sunyal DK, Amin MR, Ahmed A, et al. Peak expiratory flow rate in pregnant women. J Bangladesh Soc Physiol 2007;2:20–3.

48. Memon MA, Memon SA, Bhura MS, et al. Change in peak expiratory flow rate in different trimesters of pregnancy. Rawal Med J 2012;37:243–6.

49. Teli A, Bagali S, Aithala M. A study of FVC, PEFR and MEP in different trimesters of pregnancy. IJBAR 2012;3:648–52.

50. Desphande H, Madkar C, Dahiya P. A study of pulmonary function tests in different stages of pregnancy. Int J Biol Med Res 2013;4:2713–6.

51. Purohit G, Harsoda JM. Peak expiratory flow rate with spirometry during pregnancy: rural Indian perspective. IJBAP 2014;3:195–9.

52. Brancazio LR, Laifer SA, Schwartz T. Peak expiratory flow rate in normal pregnancy. Obstet Gynecol 1997;89(3):383–6.

53. Vaughan MTR, Weber CRW, Tipton WR, et al. Comparison of PEFR and FEV1 in patients with varying degrees of airway obstruction. Effect of modest altitude. Chest 1989;95:558–62.

54. Choi IS, Koh YI, Lim H. Peak expiratory flow rate underestimates severity of airflow obstruction in acute asthma. Korean J Intern Med 2002;17:174–9.

55. Jensen ME, Robijn AL, Gibson PG, et al. Longitudinal analysis of lung function in pregnant women with and without asthma. J Allergy Clin Immunol Pract 2021;9:1578–85.

56. Rejno G, Lundholm C, Gong T, et al. Asthma during pregnancy in a population-based study - pregnancy complications and adverse perinatal outcomes. PLoS One 2014;9(8):e104755.

57. Sawicki E, Stewart K, Wong S, et al. Medication use for chronic health conditions by pregnant women attending an Australian maternity hospital. Aust N Z J Obstet Gynaecol 2011;51(4):333–8.

58. Murphy VE, Jensen ME, Powell H, et al. Influence of maternal BMI and macrophage activation on asthma exacerbations in pregnancy. J Allergy Clin Immunol Pract 2017;5(4):981–7.

59. Schatz M, Dombrowski MP, Wise R, et al. Asthma morbidity during pregnancy can be predicted by severity classification. J Allergy Clin Immunol 2003;112(2):283–8.

60. Stenius-Aarniala B, Piirila P, Teramo K. Asthma and pregnancy: a prospective study of 198 pregnancies. Thorax 1988;43(1):12–8.

61. Sims CD, Chamberlain GV, de Swiet M. Lung function tests in bronchial asthma during and after pregnancy. Br J Obstet Gynaecol 1976;83(6):434–7.

62. Beckmann CA. Peak flow values by gestation in women with asthma. Clin Nurs Res 2008;17(3):174–81.

63. Amaral L, Martins C, Coimbra A. Use of the Control of Allergic Rhinitis and Asthma Test and pulmonary function tests to assess asthma control in pregnancy. Aust N Z J Obstet Gynaecol 2018;58:86–90.

64. Rohn MCH, Stevens DR, Kanner J, et al. Asthma medication regimens in pregnancy: longitudinal changes in asthma status. Am J Perinatol 2021. https://doi.org/10.1055/s-0041-1727233.

65. Dominguez J, Krystal A, Habib A. Obstructive sleep apnea in pregnant women. Anesth Analg 2018;127:1167–77.

Maternal Macro- and Micronutrient Intake During Pregnancy

Does It Affect Allergic Predisposition in Offspring?

Katherine Stumpf, MD*, Julie Mirpuri, MD*

KEYWORDS

• Maternal diet • Allergy • Offspring • Vitamins • Eczema • Nutrients

KEY POINTS

• Maternal diet can influence offspring immune and microbiome development.
• Maternal diet may play a role in the allergic march in offspring.
• Maternal macronutrient intake, including fat, fiber, and carbohydrate, has recently been examined for association with susceptibility to offspring allergy.
• Maternal micronutrient supplementation with various vitamins and iron have been studied in several large trials for association with offspring allergy development.

INTRODUCTION

The in utero environment is not immune to the influence of maternal environmental exposures. One of the most dynamic maternal environmental exposures for the fetus results from variation in the maternal diet. The macro- and micronutrients in the maternal diet can vary based on choice, cultural background, food security, health-based dietary restrictions (eg, diabetic diet or cholestatic diet), and provider guidance (eg, supplementation of prenatal vitamins, folic acid, probiotics). The prevalence of challenge-proven food allergy[1] and atopic dermatitis[2] has increased in children, and environmental factors have been thought to play an important role in early programming.[3,4] Among these, maternal diet has been explored, and there is growing evidence that diet during pregnancy affects the allergic march in offspring. In this review, the authors briefly explore potential immune mechanisms of maternal diet–mediated effects on

Department of Pediatrics, Division of Neonatal-Perinatal Medicine, UT Southwestern Medical Center, 5323 Harry Hines Boulevard- Suite F3.302, Dallas, TX 75390-9063, USA
* Corresponding authors.
E-mail addresses: katherine.stumpf@utsouthwestern.edu (K.S.); Julie.mirpuri@utsouthwestern.edu (J.M.)

Immunol Allergy Clin N Am 43 (2023) 27–42
https://doi.org/10.1016/j.iac.2022.07.006
0889-8561/23/© 2022 Elsevier Inc. All rights reserved.

immunology.theclinics.com

offspring, then dissect the evidence for the modulation by specific macro- and micro-nutrients during pregnancy on susceptibility to allergy development in offspring, and finally conclude with a discussion of the implications for the health care provider in providing nutritional guidance to women before and during pregnancy.

Potential Mediators of Maternal Diet Effects on Offspring Immunity

Maternal diet can alter the neonatal and maternal microbiome

Diet is a significant modifier of the intestinal microbiome. Changes in diet can shift the intestinal microbiome, although whether dietary modifications transiently or permanently alter the microbiome is still being investigated.[5–7] Observational studies suggest that changes in the maternal diet modify both the maternal and offspring microbiome. Several prospective observational studies sampling the oral, vaginal, and intestinal microbiome of mothers with gestational diabetes (GDM) demonstrate that they are unique at the phylum and genus level from those of control mothers without GDM.[8–10] In addition, GDM offspring have a unique gut microbiome, with a specific decrease in Bacteroides, Corynebacterium, and Brevundimonas.[9] Whether these changes in the maternal microbiome are due to diet modification as a result of GDM diagnosis or hyperglycemia and metabolic derangements during pregnancy is still unclear, however. The microbiome is a potent modifier of the innate and adaptive immune response,[11–13] and early colonization changes as a result of maternal diet could influence the immune march in offspring[14] and susceptibility to allergies.

Maternal diet can modify in utero and postnatal metabolite exposure

Metabolites produced by bacterial breakdown of diet or directly introduced in the diet, such as indole, short-chain fatty acids, and retinoids, are known to modify immune development. There is also some evidence that the fetus is exposed to these metabolites in utero,[15–17] either via the placenta to the fetal blood or in the amniotic fluid. Postnatally, microbiota-derived and dietary metabolites are also present in breast milk,[18–20] are modified by maternal diet, and can influence offspring immune development.

Maternal diet can modify epigenetic signatures in utero

Several studies have demonstrated that maternal diet can modify epigenetic signatures in offspring, including changes in DNA methylation, histone modifications, and noncoding RNA.[21] These epigenetic changes can influence long-term immune development in offspring and potentially modify susceptibility to allergy.[22,23]

Macronutrients, Pregnancy, and Offspring Susceptibility to Allergy Development

Macronutrient intake during pregnancy and offspring allergy susceptibility: the evidence

Validated food questionnaires provided to women during pregnancy have been used to determine if dietary intake during pregnancy influences development of allergy in offspring. In a prospective cohort more than 1200 women were given a validated food propensity questionnaire during pregnancy to determine if dietary intake correlated with development of allergies in offspring up to the age of 4 years.[24] Offspring were categorized as having no allergy or having atopic dermatitis, asthma, wheezing, allergic rhinitis, and/or food allergy. The investigators found that consumption of vegetables and yogurt was associated with prevention of allergy in offspring, whereas consumption of fried potatoes, cold cereals, rice, and red meats were associated with increased propensity to develop allergy. Another similar study using food questionnaires showed that the Mediterranean diet during pregnancy was protective for persistent wheeze, atopic wheeze, and atopy in children who were followed-up up to 6 years old.[25] Although most of the human studies demonstrate association with the use of these validated questionnaires, animal studies complement these studies and demonstrate how specific macronutrients during pregnancy can affect immunity and development of allergies in offspring (**Table 1**).

High-fat diet during pregnancy and allergy development in offspring

In a German prospective birth cohort study (LISA), maternal diet during the last 4 weeks of pregnancy was collected using a food-frequency questionnaire, and association with development of eczema and allergic sensitization in offspring up to 2 years old was determined.[26] The investigators found that high intake of margarine and vegetable oils was positively associated with development of eczema in offspring, and high intake of deep-frying vegetable fat was positively related to sensitization against inhalant allergens. In contrast, high intake of fish was inversely associated with development of eczema in offspring. Lumia and colleagues similarly showed that the type of maternal fat intake during pregnancy was associated with risk for development of asthma in offspring. They showed that low maternal intake of linolenic acid and polyunsaturated fatty acids was associated with an increased risk of asthma in offspring. In contrast, low intake of arachidonic acid and high intake of total saturated fatty acids were associated with protection from development of asthma in offspring.[27] These studies intriguingly suggest that the type of fat exposure is important; however, systemic reviews of available studies demonstrate no consistent association.[28,29] In a randomized study involving 706 pregnant women (The DOMInO study, Docosahexaenoic acid to Optimize Mother Infant Outcome) given either a fish oil capsule (omega-3) or placebo supplement from 21 weeks' gestation until birth ,no significant difference was found in the development of food allergies in offspring at 1 year of life.[30]

Interestingly, increased maternal high-fat diet intake during lactation may also contribute to the offspring risk for development of allergies. A prospective cohort study examined the association between maternal fat intake during lactation (based on a food questionnaire) and offspring development of atopic sensitization at 12 months. The investigators found that infants who had a positive skin prick test to at least one antigen were more likely born to mothers with a higher intake of total fat.[31]

Several animal studies have also explored the association between maternal high-fat diet intake and allergy sensitization in offspring. Myles and colleagues showed that offspring of pregnant mice fed a high-fat (western) diet had increased allergic sensitization when compared with pups born to mothers on standard (low-fat) diet.[32] Similarly, MacDonald and colleagues showed that maternal high-fat diet exposure resulted in adult offspring that had increased airway hyperresponsiveness when compared with control offspring.[33]

Maternal Fiber Intake During Pregnancy and Allergy Development in Offspring

Thornburn and colleagues demonstrated that maternal high fiber intake throughout or during late pregnancy in mice protected adult offspring from developing allergic airway diseases, mediated by altered transcription of Foxp3 genes linked to asthma development.[34] Of note, high fiber intake during lactation did not similarly protect offspring. The investigators further showed that pregnant women who reported higher dietary fiber intake had higher levels of serum acetate with a decrease in their offspring presenting to their health care provider for cough or wheeze. This study demonstrated a potential association between maternal fiber intake and offspring susceptibility to development of asthma. Other animal studies have suggested that maternal high fiber intake can influence offspring T-cell differentiation,[35] increase proteins in the offspring intestine associated with immune and inflammatory responses,[36] and modify the

Table 1
Publications exploring association of maternal macronutrient intake with development of allergy in offspring

Maternal Macronutrient During Pregnancy	Allergy Development in offspring	Author
Dietary fat	High intake of margarine (aOR 1.49, 95% CI 1.08–2.04) and vegetable oils (aOR 1.48, 90% CI 1.14–1.91) positively associated with development of eczema in offspring up to 2 years old. High intake of fish (aOR 0.75, 95% CI 0.57–0.98) inversely associated with development of eczema up to 2 years old. High intake of deep-frying vegetable fat (aOR 1.61, 95% CI 1.02–2.54) associated with sensitization against inhalant allergens up to 2 years old. Low maternal linolenic acid (HR 1.67, 95% CI 1.12–2.48) and PUFA (HR 1.66, 95% CI 1.11–2.48) associated with increased risk of asthma in offspring up to 5 years old. High intake of total saturated fatty acids (HR 0.55, 95% CI 0.34–0.90) and palmitic acid (HR 0.51, 95% CI 0.31–0.83) associated with decreased risk of asthma up to 5 years old. Maternal supplementation with fish oil did not decrease food allergy susceptibility in offspring at 1 y (aRR 0.70, 95% CI 0.45–1.09). Meta-analyses show no consistent association between type of fat intake and susceptibility to offspring allergy development	German Birth Cohort LISA Study Lumia et al,[27] 2011 DOMInO study Venter et al, Garcia-Larsen et al,[29] 2018
High-fiber diet	High fiber intake throughout or during late pregnancy in mice protected adult offspring from asthma model Pregnant women who reported higher dietary fiber	Thorburn et al Thorburn et al

(continued on next page)

Table 1 (continued)		
Maternal Macronutrient During Pregnancy	Allergy Development in offspring	Author
	intake during pregnancy had decreased association of offspring presenting with cough or wheeze in first 12 mo of life	
Diabetic and cholestatic diet Vegan or elimination diet	Increased development of IgE-/IgG-mediated food hypersensitivity in offspring No association with offspring allergy development	Ogrodowczyk et al,[38] 2020 Ogrodowczyk et al,[38] 2020
Probiotic supplementation	Supplementation with Lactobacillus/Bifidobacterium/Propionibacterium from 36 wk and continued supplementation in infants up to 6 mo decreased allergic disease and eczema development *only in subgroup delivered via C-section at 13 years old.* Probiotic supplementation during pregnancy and lactation associated with reduced risk of eczema (RR 0.78, 95% CI 0.68–0.90)—meta-analysis Probiotic supplementation during pregnancy or infancy showed no association with protection from asthma (RR 0.99, 95% CI 0.81–1.21)—meta-analysis	Kallio et al,[39] 2019 Garcia-Larsen et al,[29] 2018 Azad et al,[40] 2013

Abbreviations: aOR, adjusted odds ratio; HR, hazard ratio; RR, risk ratio.

offspring microbiome[37] mechanisms that can potentially alter the offspring allergic march. Further investigation on the impact of maternal dietary fiber intake on offspring susceptibility to allergy development is needed.

Maternal Diabetic and Cholestatic Diet and Allergy Development in Offspring

Pregnancy complications such as gestational diabetes and cholestasis prompt mothers to modify their diet to reduce carbohydrate and fat consumption. In a study examining mothers who were on these specific gestational diets and association of development of allergies in offspring, the investigators used bioinformatic and multivariate analysis for complex data sets and found that gestational diabetic and cholestatic diets were associated with development of immunoglobulin E (IgE)-/IgG-mediated food hypersensitivity.[38] They found no association of a gestational vegan or elimination diet with offspring allergy development.

Probiotic Supplementation During Pregnancy: Does It Affect Offspring Allergy Development?

The potential promise of modifying the maternal microbiome and the offspring microbiome and reducing the risk of development of allergies with probiotic supplementation led to several large studies. Unfortunately, to date, the evidence has not consistently supported maternal probiotic supplementation to modify allergy risk in offspring. Kallio and colleagues randomized pregnant women to receive either supplementation with probiotics (*Lactobacillus/Bifidobacterium/Propionibacterium*) or placebo during later pregnancy (36 weeks until birth) and continued supplementation of infants until 6 months.[39] They followed-up offspring to 13 years old and found that the probiotics protected only that subgroup who were delivered via C-section from allergic disease and eczema development. A meta-analysis of studies examining probiotic supplementation during pregnancy and lactation found that it was associated with reduced risk of eczema (risk ration [RR] 0.78, 95% confidence interval 0.68–0.90).[29] Another meta-analysis examining association of probiotics during pregnancy or infancy with development of childhood asthma found no protective association.[40] A potential confounder is the heterogeneity in the literature with the use of a broad range of probiotics and with the majority continuing supplementation during infancy, making it difficult to tease out the role of supplementation during pregnancy alone.

Micronutrients Supplementation During Pregnancy and Offspring Susceptibility to Allergy Development

Allergic conditions are common among children. Various studies have postulated the association between micronutrient levels such as vitamin D, vitamin E, vitamin A, selenium, iron, copper, and iron during pregnancy and numerous allergic outcomes such as asthma, rhinitis, food sensitization as well as pulmonary function testing at differing stages of childhood. Complex relationships seem to exist between low and excessive vitamin D and folate levels and allergic outcomes, whereas there is no clear association between vitamin A and E levels and such outcomes. Several studies seem to show an association with low maternal iron status and allergic outcomes in offspring; however, in the largest maternal-child pair study this finding was not consistent.[41] Here the authors further examine a select group of micronutrient levels in pregnancy, cord blood, and allergic outcomes in offspring (**Table 2**).

Vitamin D: maternal supplementation and levels

Two vitamin D isoforms exist. One form (vitamin D3) can be made in the human dermis with exposure to ultraviolet B light. Vitamin D2 is synthesized in plants and fungi.[42] Although both isoforms are available as dietary supplements, vitamin D3 is more effective at increasing serum levels of 25(OH)D levels.[43] Insufficiency is defined by serum 25(OH)D concentrations of less than 10 to 30 ng/mL depending on which reference is used.[44] Options for improving vitamin D levels exist outside of supplementation via fortified foods such as cereals and milk.[45] Vitamin D deficiency remains common among pregnant women, with up to 60% of those in Asian countries meeting criteria for deficiency. Current recommendations for supplementation of 200 to 400 IU/day exist but it is not entirely clear if improved outcomes occur.[46] Vitamin D is potentially influential over many cellular mechanisms including those in the immune system affecting macrophages, monocytes, T cells, and B cells.[42] The vitamin D receptor is expressed on T cells, B cells, and antigen-presenting cells, and these cells can make the active form of vitamin D $(1,25 (OH)_2.D)$.[47] In addition, vitamin D has been shown to alter regulatory T cells and transforming growth factor β production.[42]

Table 2
Publications exploring association of maternal micronutrient intake with development of allergy in offspring

Maternal Micronutrient During Pregnancy	Allergy Development in Offspring	Author
Increasing maternal vitamin D intake	Decreased wheeze (Camargo et al.) and nonsignificant lower incidence of asthma/ recurrent wheeze at age 3 y Decreased asthma at 7 y, decreased admissions due to asthma, no difference in asthma at 18 mo, no difference in allergic rhinitis at 7 y Reduced rate of wheezing/ asthma, no change in atopic dermatitis or food allergy	Camargo et al,[48]2007 Li et al,[50]2019 Maslova et al,[49]2013 Litonjua et al
Maternal vitamin D levels	No association between level and any allergic outcome at 1 y of age Positive correlation between level and risk of food allergy by age 2 y	Woon et al,[54] 2020 Weisse et al,[55] 2013
Maternal folate supplementation	Increased risk of wheeze and URI up to 18 mo No association with wheezing/shortness of breath/atopic dermatitis, no association with asthma in childhood Supplementation with >500 mcg/ d increased eczema in offspring	Haberg et al,[60] 2009 Kiefte-de Jong et al,[60] 2012 Crider et al,[64] 2013
Maternal folate levels	Positive association with atopic dermatitis in highest quartile Folate level greater than the median resulted in decreased risk for lower respiratory tract infections at 6 mo of age and atopic dermatitis at 24 mo	Kiefte-de Jong et al,[61] 2012 Kim et al,[62] 2015
Cord blood folate levels	Levels 50–75 nmol/L were optimal to minimize sensitization	Dunstan et al,[63] 2012
Maternal vitamin E levels	No association with atopy, food allergy, wheezing up to age 2 y	Gromadzinska et al,[66] 2018

(continued on next page)

Table 2 (continued)		
Maternal Micronutrient During Pregnancy	Allergy Development in Offspring	Author
Maternal vitamin E intake	Positive association between low levels and childhood asthma Decreased asthma up to age 10 y with higher maternal intake	Hijazi et al,[67] 2000 Devereux et al,[68] 2019
Maternal vitamin A intake	Increased risk of asthma as intake becomes greater than recommended amount No association with asthma, rhinitis, or eczema Higher intake may be protective against development of eczema	Parr et al,[73] 2018 Nwaru et al,[83] 2014 Miyake et al,[76] 2010
Maternal vitamin A supplement	No difference in asthma/ wheeze in supplemented groups	Checkley et al,[74] 2011
Maternal hemoglobin	Lower values may be a risk factor for allergic sensitization; no association with asthma No association with allergic outcomes in childhood	Shaheen et al,[81]2004 Yang et al,[41] 2021
Maternal/Fetal iron status	Reduced iron status in mothers is adversely associated with childhood wheeze, lung function, and atopic sensitization Increased risk of inhalant allergy; no difference in lung function, asthma, or inhalant allergic sensitization Negative association with late-onset wheeze and eczema	Nwaru et al,[83] 2014 Quezada-Pinedo et al,[84] 2021 Shaheen et al.

Abbreviation: URI, upper respiratory illness.

Possible role in allergic disease

Several studies have assessed the association of vitamin D levels in pregnancy with allergic outcomes in offspring. Using questionnaires, Camargo and colleagues found that higher maternal vitamin D intake was associated with a lower risk of wheezing in children at age 3 years.[48] A large Danish study was conducted using questionnaires to assess the dietary intake of vitamin D during pregnancy at week 25 and outcomes such as a diagnosis of asthma at 18 months of age (via phone report from parent) and asthma or allergic rhinitis at age 7 years via record review. This study found a weak inverse relationship between total vitamin D and asthma outcomes in later childhood. The relationship did not hold true for early asthma. There was no association found with allergic rhinitis.[49] A meta-analysis conducted by Li and colleagues found an inverse relationship between the intake of vitamin D during pregnancy and wheezing or asthma in offspring. This analysis was primarily concerned with finding an optimal dose of vitamin D to prevent outcomes of wheezing or asthma, and their data suggest an optimal dose of 800 IU/day during pregnancy with a U-shaped association between vitamin D supplementation dosing and asthma outcomes.[50] The VDAART study, a randomized clinical trial, enrolled more than 400 pregnant women to receive either placebo plus 400 IU/day vitamin D or 4000 IU plus the standard 400 IU/day vitamin D. This group analyzed outcomes of physician-diagnosed asthma/wheezing by 3 years of age and third trimester vitamin D levels. Vitamin D levels in pregnant women were significantly higher in the supplemented group, and this study group did have a lower report of asthma in offspring; however, this did not reach significance.[51] A later 6-year follow-up study also did not show a difference in asthma or wheezing in this study group.[52] A meta-analysis by Venter and colleagues showed maternal supplementation with vitamin D may help prevent asthma in offspring, but there was no association with atopic dermatitis or food allergy.[28]

Other studies investigating maternal vitamin D levels in pregnancy and outcomes of food allergy, wheezing, or asthma have shown mixed results. Adams and colleagues concluded that the odds of wheezing/asthma decreased with increasing vitamin D levels in white mothers, but the odds of wheezing increased with increasing vitamin D levels in black mothers.[53] A study of maternal vitamin D levels in late pregnancy and risk of allergy in offspring showed that the nondeficient group did not have offspring with a significantly different amount of any type of allergic disease including food sensitization, inhalant allergen reaction, wheeze, or eczema.[54] The data are further confused by a study by Weisse and colleagues, which found that high maternal vitamin D levels and higher cord blood levels were associated with worsened outcomes with respect to food allergies.[55] It seems that normal vitamin D levels may lead to a protective effect, whereas either deficiency or excess vitamin D may incur increased risk of allergy or asthma.[56] Further studies are needed to fully elucidate the details of this complex relationship.

Folate (Vitamin B9): Maternal Levels, Supplementation, and Allergic Outcomes

Folate functions as a coenzyme necessary for multiple chemical reactions including purine synthesis.[57] The primary means of folate supplementation in pregnancy is via folic acid, the more stable and better-absorbed form. Dietary sources including fortified cereals, leafy greens, and liver are readily available in developed countries.[42] Current recommendations to consume 400mcg/d of folic acid remain in place due to known reduction of neural tube defects.[58] Increased folic acid intake can potentially influence gene expression involved in T-cell differentiation, which may affect allergic predisposition in an infant.[42]

Possible role in allergic disease

No randomized trials have been conducted to assess the role of folate levels during pregnancy and allergic outcomes in infants.[59] A large Norwegian study showed that folic acid supplementation in pregnancy seems to increase the risk of wheezing and upper respiratory infections in the first 18 months of life.[60] Similarly, a study conducted in the Netherlands found that a higher maternal folate level was associated with an increased risk of atopic dermatitis in children up to 4 years of age but there was no association seen with wheezing outcomes in this cohort.[61] Conversely, a study using maternal reporting of allergic and respiratory outcomes in comparison to folate levels in pregnancy found that a folate level greater than the median value in midpregnancy was associated with decreased risk of atopic dermatitis at age 2 years and lower respiratory tract infections by 6 months of age.[62] Dunstan and colleagues found that maternal folate supplementation greater than 500 mcg/d was associated with an increased presence of subsequent eczema in offspring. This study also investigated cord blood levels of folate and found a nonlinear relationship, showing a specific range of fetal levels (50–75 nmol/L) that seemed to optimize minimized sensitization.[63] Many of the studies conducted on this relationship are observational and require accurate maternal reporting of folic acid intake, dietary intake, and offspring outcomes. Overall study outcomes seem to be inconsistent with some displaying positive associations with increasing folate intake or maternal level with increasing allergic outcomes, whereas others seem to show no evidence of an association.[64]

Maternal vitamin E intake and offspring outcomes
Vitamin E acts as an antioxidant to aid in the decreased production of reactive oxygen species during fat oxidation. Maternal vitamin E intake may affect fetal growth and subsequently fetal lung growth and capacity and hence subsequent outcomes regarding lung health.[65] A Polish study of 252 mother-infant dyads aimed to assess the association of both vitamin A and vitamin E levels of pregnancy/cord blood and allergic outcomes. There was no association found for either vitamin with atopy, food allergy, or wheezing in the infants followed-up to age 2 years.[66] Hijazi and colleagues investigated the relationship between maternal vitamin E intake and asthma in offspring. This group found that childhood asthma was positively associated with a history of a maternal diet low in vitamin E.[67] A study conducted in the United Kingdom by Devereux and colleagues measured vitamin E intake during pregnancy and found decreased rates of asthma in children up to age 10 years who were born to women with higher intake of the vitamin. The decreased asthma outcome seemed to be lost by age 15 years.[68] There is unclear and insufficient evidence to suggest an association between vitamin E intake or maternal levels and outcomes of allergy/asthma.

Vitamin A–rich diets and supplementation: an unclear effect
Vitamin A and other retinoids are likely relevant to immune response by affecting the Th1/Th2 responses and maintaining mucosal immune homeostasis.[69,70] Lower levels of vitamin A are observed in both children and adults with asthma versus healthy controls.[71,72] Parr and colleagues studied the role of maternal intake of vitamin A on the presence of asthma in children at age 7 years. This large Norwegian cohort showed an increased rate of asthma, as the vitamin A intake increased to greater than the recommended quantity during pregnancy.[73] Several other studies have failed to show an association between either maternal vitamin A supplementation or diets shown to be higher in vitamin A with an outcome of asthma or allergic rhinitis.[74,75] Confounding evidence from other sources showed a lowered risk of eczema and wheezing in offspring with diets higher in ß-carotene.[76,77] It remains unclear if allergy, wheeze, or asthma can be truly correlated with vitamin A levels and vitamin A–rich diets during pregnancy.

Iron status in mothers and offspring may affect allergic outcomes
Iron is essential for normal immune development.[78,79] In addition, low iron status at birth is associated with eosinophilia, a marker of allergic disease. Weigert and colleagues conducted a prospective study of healthy newborns at risk for iron deficiency anemia. This study showed that infants who developed eosinophilia had lower cord ferritin values.[80] In addition, cord blood iron concentrations were shown to be negatively associated with the development of wheezing and eczema.[81] Shaheen and

colleagues also showed that lower maternal hemoglobin during pregnancy may be a risk factor for allergic sensitization, higher IgE levels, and lower forced vital capacity during childhood. There was no association shown for childhood asthma or other allergic diseases.[82] A large birth cohort in Japan, The Japan Environment and Children's Study (JECS), examined the relationship between maternal iron status and allergy in early childhood. More than 90,000 mother-child pairs took part in this study, which showed low maternal hemoglobin and hematocrit were not associated with allergic outcomes.[41] An additional maternal-child pair study conducted in the United Kingdom involved 157 pairs assessed for maternal iron status using hemoglobin concentrations and serum iron status at 11 weeks gestation and at delivery. As first trimester iron status decreased, an increased risk of wheezing was shown, and increased serum ferritin concentration was associated with increased pulmonary function measures in offspring. Increased maternal transferrin receptor–ferritin index was associated with increased risk of offspring with atopic sensitization.[83] Finally, a cohort study conducted in the Netherlands with more than 3800 mother-child pairs examined the relationship between maternal ferritin, transferrin concentrations, and transferrin saturation in early pregnancy and childhood lung function, asthma, allergic sensitization, and diagnosed inhalant allergy. Higher maternal transferrin concentrations during pregnancy and lower serum iron levels were associated with higher likelihood of childhood allergy as diagnosed by physicians. There was no difference in pulmonary outcomes.[84]

SUMMARY

In conclusion, there is some overall evidence that maternal macro- and micronutrient intake during pregnancy can affect allergic susceptibility in offspring, but specific recommendations based on the studies are difficult to conclude; this is due to multiple challenges with the studies evaluated here, including the use of food questionnaires and necessity for maternal recall, heterogeneity of the studies, timing of initiation of the supplement, continuation of supplementation in offspring after birth, and varied age of assessment of development of allergy in offspring ranging from 1 to 13 years. Based on the current evidence, advice to the pregnant woman would include avoiding a high-fat diet, increasing fiber intake, and maintaining normal micronutrient levels, as some studies suggest higher intake of certain vitamins can increase risk of allergies in offspring (see **Table 2**). Further studies are needed that are focused on both the micro- and macronutrient intake during pregnancy, as well as interaction with the maternal microbial and metabolic environment. This combined approach would help guide nutrition advice to pregnant women in the future to avoid allergic susceptibility in their offspring.

CLINICS CARE POINTS

- Maternal diet is potentially relevant to allergic outcomes in offspring.
- Maternal high-fat diet may lead to increased risk of allergic outcomes, although current supporting data are not conclusive.
- There is some evidence that probiotic supplementation or high-fiber diet during pregnancy may offer a protective effect against allergy development in offspring.
- Excess or depletion of vitamin D during pregnancy may impart higher risk of allergic outcomes in offspring.

- Supplementation of vitamin A and vitamin E during pregnancy do not seem to clearly affect offspring allergy risk.
- Specific recommendations for micronutrient or macronutrient supplementation are limited given the current heterogeneity of study outcomes.

FUNDING SUPPORT STATEMENT

This work was supported in part by the National Institutes of Health NIDDK R01 DK121975.

DISCLOSURE

The authors have nothing to disclose.

REFERENCES

1. Loh W, Tang MLK. The Epidemiology of Food Allergy in the Global Context. Int J Environ Res Public Health 2018;15(9).
2. Nutten S. Atopic dermatitis: global epidemiology and risk factors. Ann Nutr Metab 2015;66(Suppl 1):8–16.
3. Barker DJ. The developmental origins of adult disease. J Am Coll Nutr 2004;23(6 Suppl):588S–95S.
4. Gluckman PD, Hanson MA, Cooper C, et al. Effect of in utero and early-life conditions on adult health and disease. N Engl J Med 2008;359(1):61–73.
5. Kolodziejczyk AA, Zheng D, Elinav E. Diet-microbiota interactions and personalized nutrition. Nat Rev Microbiol 2019;17(12):742–53.
6. Zmora N, Suez J, Elinav E. You are what you eat: diet, health and the gut microbiota. Nat Rev Gastroenterol Hepatol 2019;16(1):35–56.
7. Leeming ER, Johnson AJ, Spector TD, et al. Effect of Diet on the Gut Microbiota: Rethinking Intervention Duration. Nutrients 2019;11(12).
8. Chen T, Qin Y, Chen M, et al. Gestational diabetes mellitus is associated with the neonatal gut microbiota and metabolome. BMC Med 2021;19(1):120.
9. Wang J, Zheng J, Shi W, et al. Dysbiosis of maternal and neonatal microbiota associated with gestational diabetes mellitus. Gut 2018;67(9):1614–25.
10. Crusell MKW, Hansen TH, Nielsen T, et al. Gestational diabetes is associated with change in the gut microbiota composition in third trimester of pregnancy and postpartum. Microbiome 2018;6(1):89.
11. Dominguez-Bello MG, Godoy-Vitorino F, Knight R, et al. Role of the microbiome in human development. Gut 2019;68(6):1108–14.
12. Stephen-Victor E, Chatila TA. Regulation of oral immune tolerance by the microbiome in food allergy. Curr Opin Immunol 2019;60:141–7.
13. Mendez CS, Bueno SM, Kalergis AM. Contribution of Gut Microbiota to Immune Tolerance in Infants. J Immunol Res 2021;2021:7823316.
14. Mirpuri J. Evidence for maternal diet-mediated effects on the offspring microbiome and immunity: implications for public health initiatives. Pediatr Res 2021; 89(2):301–6.
15. Grindstaff JL, Brodie ED 3rd, Ketterson ED. Immune function across generations: integrating mechanism and evolutionary process in maternal antibody transmission. Proc Biol Sci 2003;270(1531):2309–19.

16. van de Pavert SA, Ferreira M, Domingues RG, et al. Maternal retinoids control type 3 innate lymphoid cells and set the offspring immunity. Nature 2014; 508(7494):123–7.
17. Vuong HE, Pronovost GN, Williams DW, et al. The maternal microbiome modulates fetal neurodevelopment in mice. Nature 2020;586(7828):281–6.
18. Lu Z, Chan YT, Lo KK, et al. Levels of polyphenols and phenolic metabolites in breast milk and their association with plant-based food intake in Hong Kong lactating women. Food Funct 2021;12(24):12683–95.
19. Poulsen KO, Sundekilde UK. The Metabolomic Analysis of Human Milk Offers Unique Insights into Potential Child Health Benefits. Curr Nutr Rep 2021;10(1): 12–29.
20. Bardanzellu F, Puddu M, Peroni DG, et al. The Human Breast Milk Metabolome in Overweight and Obese Mothers. Front Immunol 2020;11:1533.
21. Peral-Sanchez I, Hojeij B, Ojeda DA, et al. Epigenetics in the Uterine Environment: How Maternal Diet and ART May Influence the Epigenome in the Offspring with Long-Term Health Consequences. Genes (Basel) 2021;13(1):31.
22. Canas JA, Nunez R, Cruz-Amaya A, et al. Epigenetics in Food Allergy and Immunomodulation. Nutrients 2021;13(12):4345.
23. Neeland MR, Martino DJ, Allen KJ. The role of gene-environment interactions in the development of food allergy. Expert Rev Gastroenterol Hepatol 2015;9(11): 1371–8.
24. Venter C, Palumbo MP, Glueck DH, et al. The maternal diet index in pregnancy is associated with offspring allergic diseases: the Healthy Start study. Allergy 2022; 77(1):162–72.
25. Chatzi L, Torrent M, Romieu I, et al. Mediterranean diet in pregnancy is protective for wheeze and atopy in childhood. Thorax 2008;63(6):507–13.
26. Sausenthaler S, Koletzko S, Schaaf B, et al. Maternal diet during pregnancy in relation to eczema and allergic sensitization in the offspring at 2 y of age. Am J Clin Nutr 2007;85(2):530–7.
27. Lumia M, Luukkainen P, Tapanainen H, et al. Dietary fatty acid composition during pregnancy and the risk of asthma in the offspring. Pediatr Allergy Immunol 2011; 22(8):827–35.
28. Venter C, Agostoni C, Arshad SH, et al. Dietary factors during pregnancy and atopic outcomes in childhood: A systematic review from the European Academy of Allergy and Clinical Immunology. Pediatr Allergy Immunol 2020;31(8):889–912.
29. Garcia-Larsen V, Ierodiakonou D, Jarrold K, et al. Diet during pregnancy and infancy and risk of allergic or autoimmune disease: A systematic review and meta-analysis. Plos Med 2018;15(2):e1002507.
30. Palmer DJ, Sullivan T, Gold MS, et al. Effect of n-3 long chain polyunsaturated fatty acid supplementation in pregnancy on infants' allergies in first year of life: randomised controlled trial. BMJ 2012;344:e184.
31. Hoppu U, Kalliomaki M, Isolauri E. Maternal diet rich in saturated fat during breastfeeding is associated with atopic sensitization of the infant. Eur J Clin Nutr 2000;54(9):702–5.
32. Myles IA, Fontecilla NM, Janelsins BM, et al. Parental dietary fat intake alters offspring microbiome and immunity. J Immunol 2013;191(6):3200–9.
33. MacDonald KD, Moran AR, Scherman AJ, et al. Maternal high-fat diet in mice leads to innate airway hyperresponsiveness in the adult offspring. Physiol Rep 2017;5(5):e13082.

34. Thorburn AN, McKenzie CI, Shen S, et al. Evidence that asthma is a developmental origin disease influenced by maternal diet and bacterial metabolites. Nat Commun 2015;6:7320.
35. Nakajima A, Kaga N, Nakanishi Y, et al. Maternal High Fiber Diet during Pregnancy and Lactation Influences Regulatory T Cell Differentiation in Offspring in Mice. J Immunol 2017;199(10):3516–24.
36. He Y, Peng X, Liu Y, et al. Effects of Maternal Fiber Intake on Intestinal Morphology, Bacterial Profile and Proteome of Newborns Using Pig as Model. Nutrients 2020;13(1).
37. Maher SE, O'Brien EC, Moore RL, et al. The association between the maternal diet and the maternal and infant gut microbiome: a systematic review. Br J Nutr 2020;1–29.
38. Ogrodowczyk AM, Zakrzewska M, Romaszko E, et al. Gestational Dysfunction-Driven Diets and Probiotic Supplementation Correlate with the Profile of Allergen-Specific Antibodies in the Serum of Allergy Sufferers. Nutrients 2020;12(8).
39. Kallio S, Kukkonen AK, Savilahti E, et al. Perinatal probiotic intervention prevented allergic disease in a Caesarean-delivered subgroup at 13-year follow-up. Clin Exp Allergy 2019;49(4):506–15.
40. Azad MB, Coneys JG, Kozyrskyj AL, et al. Probiotic supplementation during pregnancy or infancy for the prevention of asthma and wheeze: systematic review and meta-analysis. BMJ 2013;347:f6471.
41. Yang L, Sato M, Saito-Abe M, et al. Association of Hemoglobin and Hematocrit Levels during Pregnancy and Maternal Dietary Iron Intake with Allergic Diseases in Children: The Japan Environment and Children's Study (JECS). Nutrients 2021; 13(3):810.
42. Miles EA, Calder PC. Maternal diet and its influence on the development of allergic disease. Clin Exp Allergy 2015;45(1):63–74.
43. Tripkovic L, Lambert H, Hart K, et al. Comparison of vitamin D2 and vitamin D3 supplementation in raising serum 25-hydroxyvitamin D status: a systematic review and meta-analysis. Am J Clin Nutr 2012;95(6):1357–64.
44. Holick MF. The vitamin D deficiency pandemic: Approaches for diagnosis, treatment and prevention. Rev Endocr Metab Disord 2017;18(2):153–65.
45. Cashman KD. Vitamin D Deficiency: Defining, Prevalence, Causes, and Strategies of Addressing. Calcif Tissue Int 2020;106(1):14–29.
46. Palacios C, De-Regil LM, Lombardo LK, et al. Vitamin D supplementation during pregnancy: Updated meta-analysis on maternal outcomes. J Steroid Biochem Mol Biol 2016;164:148–55.
47. Aranow C. Vitamin D and the immune system. J Investig Med 2011;59(6):881–6.
48. Camargo CA Jr, Rifas-Shiman SL, Litonjua AA, et al. Maternal intake of vitamin D during pregnancy and risk of recurrent wheeze in children at 3 y of age. Am J Clin Nutr 2007;85(3):788–95.
49. Maslova E, Hansen S, Jensen CB, et al. Vitamin D intake in mid-pregnancy and child allergic disease - a prospective study in 44,825 Danish mother-child pairs. BMC Pregnancy Childbirth 2013;13:199.
50. Li W, Qin Z, Gao J, et al. Vitamin D supplementation during pregnancy and the risk of wheezing in offspring: a systematic review and dose-response meta-analysis. J Asthma 2019;56(12):1266–73.
51. Litonjua AA, Carey VJ, Laranjo N, et al. Effect of Prenatal Supplementation With Vitamin D on Asthma or Recurrent Wheezing in Offspring by Age 3 Years: The VDAART Randomized Clinical Trial. JAMA 2016;315(4):362–70.

52. Litonjua AA, Carey VJ, Laranjo N, et al. Six-Year Follow-up of a Trial of Antenatal Vitamin D for Asthma Reduction. N Engl J Med 2020;382(6):525–33.
53. Adams SN, Adgent MA, Gebretsadik T, et al. Prenatal vitamin D levels and child wheeze and asthma. J Matern Fetal Neonatal Med 2021;34(3):323–31.
54. Woon FC, Chin YS, Ismail IH, et al. Maternal Vitamin D Levels during Late Pregnancy and Risk of Allergic Diseases and Sensitization during the First Year of Life-A Birth Cohort Study. Nutrients 2020;12(8).
55. Weisse K, Winkler S, Hirche F, et al. Maternal and newborn vitamin D status and its impact on food allergy development in the German LINA cohort study. Allergy 2013;68(2):220–8.
56. Heine RG. Food Allergy Prevention and Treatment by Targeted Nutrition. Ann Nutr Metab 2018;72(Suppl 3):33–45.
57. Ebara S. Nutritional role of folate. Congenit Anom (Kyoto) 2017;57(5):138–41.
58. van Gool JD, Hirche H, Lax H, et al. Folic acid and primary prevention of neural tube defects: A review. Reprod Toxicol 2018;80:73–84.
59. McStay CL, Prescott SL, Bower C, et al. Maternal Folic Acid Supplementation during Pregnancy and Childhood Allergic Disease Outcomes: A Question of Timing? Nutrients 2017;9(2).
60. Haberg SE, London SJ, Stigum H, et al. Folic acid supplements in pregnancy and early childhood respiratory health. Arch Dis Child 2009;94(3):180–4.
61. Kiefte-de Jong JC, Timmermans S, Jaddoe VW, et al. High circulating folate and vitamin B-12 concentrations in women during pregnancy are associated with increased prevalence of atopic dermatitis in their offspring. J Nutr 2012;142(4):731–8.
62. Kim JH, Jeong KS, Ha EH, et al. Relationship between prenatal and postnatal exposures to folate and risks of allergic and respiratory diseases in early childhood. Pediatr Pulmonol 2015;50(2):155–63.
63. Dunstan JA, West C, McCarthy S, et al. The relationship between maternal folate status in pregnancy, cord blood folate levels, and allergic outcomes in early childhood. Allergy 2012;67(1):50–7.
64. Crider KS, Cordero AM, Qi YP, et al. Prenatal folic acid and risk of asthma in children: a systematic review and meta-analysis. Am J Clin Nutr 2013;98(5):1272–81.
65. Yong SB, Wu CC, Wang L, et al. Influence and mechanisms of maternal and infant diets on the development of childhood asthma. Pediatr Neonatol 2013;54(1):5–11.
66. Gromadzinska J, Polanska K, Kozlowska L, et al. Vitamins A and E during Pregnancy and Allergy Symptoms in an Early Childhood-Lack of Association with Tobacco Smoke Exposure. Int J Environ Res Public Health 2018;15(6).
67. Hijazi N, Abalkhail B, Seaton A. Diet and childhood asthma in a society in transition: a study in urban and rural Saudi Arabia. Thorax 2000;55(9):775–9.
68. Devereux G, Craig L, Seaton A, et al. Maternal vitamin D and E intakes in pregnancy and asthma to age 15 years: A cohort study. Pediatr Pulmonol 2019;54(1):11–9.
69. Hufnagl K, Jensen-Jarolim E. Does a carrot a day keep the allergy away? Immunol Lett 2019;206:54–8.
70. Ruhl R, Hanel A, Garcia AL, et al. Role of vitamin A elimination or supplementation diets during postnatal development on the allergic sensitisation in mice. Mol Nutr Food Res 2007;51(9):1173–81.
71. Al Senaidy AM. Serum vitamin A and beta-carotene levels in children with asthma. J Asthma 2009;46(7):699–702.

72. Riccioni G, Bucciarelli T, Mancini B, et al. Plasma lycopene and antioxidant vitamins in asthma: the PLAVA study. J Asthma 2007;44(6):429–32.
73. Parr CL, Magnus MC, Karlstad O, et al. Vitamin A and D intake in pregnancy, infant supplementation, and asthma development: the Norwegian Mother and Child Cohort. Am J Clin Nutr 2018;107(5):789–98.
74. Checkley W, West KP Jr, Wise RA, et al. Supplementation with vitamin A early in life and subsequent risk of asthma. Eur Respir J 2011;38(6):1310–9.
75. Nwaru BI, Erkkola M, Ahonen S, et al. Intake of antioxidants during pregnancy and the risk of allergies and asthma in the offspring. Eur J Clin Nutr 2011; 65(8):937–43.
76. Miyake Y, Sasaki S, Tanaka K, et al. Consumption of vegetables, fruit, and antioxidants during pregnancy and wheeze and eczema in infants. Allergy 2010;65(6): 758–65.
77. Litonjua AA, Rifas-Shiman SL, Ly NP, et al. Maternal antioxidant intake in pregnancy and wheezing illnesses in children at 2 y of age. Am J Clin Nutr 2006; 84(4):903–11.
78. Spencer SJ, Galic MA, Pittman QJ. Neonatal programming of innate immune function. Am J Physiol Endocrinol Metab 2011;300(1):E11–8.
79. Jason J, Archibald LK, Nwanyanwu OC, et al. The effects of iron deficiency on lymphocyte cytokine production and activation: preservation of hepatic iron but not at all cost. Clin Exp Immunol 2001;126(3):466–73.
80. Weigert R, Dosch NC, Bacsik-Campbell ME, et al. Maternal pregnancy weight gain and cord blood iron status are associated with eosinophilia in infancy. J Perinatol 2015;35(8):621–6.
81. Shaheen SO, Newson RB, Henderson AJ, et al. Umbilical cord trace elements and minerals and risk of early childhood wheezing and eczema. Eur Respir J 2004;24(2):292–7.
82. Shaheen SO, Macdonald-Wallis C, Lawlor DA, et al. Haemoglobin concentrations in pregnancy and respiratory and allergic outcomes in childhood: Birth cohort study. Clin Exp Allergy 2017;47(12):1615–24.
83. Nwaru BI, Hayes H, Gambling L, et al. An exploratory study of the associations between maternal iron status in pregnancy and childhood wheeze and atopy. Br J Nutr 2014;112(12):2018–27.
84. Quezada-Pinedo HG, Mensink-Bout SM, Reiss IK, et al. Maternal iron status during early pregnancy and school-age, lung function, asthma, and allergy: The Generation R Study. Pediatr Pulmonol 2021;56(6):1771–8.

Advancing Exposomic Research in Prenatal Respiratory Disease Programming

Check for updates

Rosalind J. Wright, MD, MPH[a,b],*

KEYWORDS

- Prenatal • Environmental programming • Respiratory • Asthma • Placenta
- Exposome

KEY POINTS

- Multiple pathways with complex interdependencies must be considered when examining the integrative influence of social, chemical, and physical environmental factors on respiratory disease programming.
- Existing and emegring tools and methods enable our ability to characterize exposure to a range of chemical, nonchemical, nutritional, and physical external factors.
- Novel approaches to assessing and analyzing the internal biological response to environmental factors on an integrated 'omics' scale also continue to evolve.
- Together these scientific advances have positioned researchers to pursue an exposomics approach to respiratory disease programming.

BACKGROUND

The developmental origins of asthma, related allergic disorders, and lung growth begin in utero.[1–3] Recurrent wheeze is a precedent of asthma and reduced lung function in childhood. Early lung function impairments persist into adulthood and contribute to chronic obstructive pulmonary disease, the fourth leading cause of death globally. A critical step in identifying lifelong risk is characterizing exposures and mechanisms that lead to and maintain this early predisposition.

Our understanding of the environmental influences on respiratory disease programming is growing increasingly complex with a multitude of environmental and microbial exposures (eg, ambient pollutants, smoking, psychological stress, diet, indoor allergens, viral infections, chemical toxins) playing a role. The underlying pathogenesis of multifactorial diseases, such as asthma, with variable onset, severity, and natural history, reflects development-specific exposures and individual response to these

[a] Department of Environmental Medicine and Public Health, New York, NY, USA; [b] Institute for Exposomic Research, New York, NY, USA
* Icahn School of Medicine at Mount Sinai, 1236 Park Avenue, New York, NY 10056.
E-mail address: rosalind.wright@mssm.edu

Immunol Allergy Clin N Am 43 (2023) 43–52
https://doi.org/10.1016/j.iac.2022.07.008
0889-8561/23/© 2022 Elsevier Inc. All rights reserved.
immunology.theclinics.com

exposures.[4] Programming effects result from toxin-induced shifts in a host of integrated molecular, cellular, and physiologic states and their interacting systems against a genetic background. Innumerable social[5] and chemical environmental,[6-9] nutritional,[10,11] and microbial[12] exposures modulate these mechanisms with few, if any, exposures impacting a single system. Although the availability of high-throughput technologies enabling profiling of the genome, transcriptome, and microbiome on a system-wide (omics) scale has revealed genetic factors and networks that advance our understanding to some extent,[13] disease causation reflects interactions between an individual's genetic susceptibility and his/her environment. Unlike the genome, which is static, relevant exposures as well as our response to ongoing exposures change over time. In light of these complexities, a National Heart Lung and Blood Institute Workshop highlighted the need to design studies that address both the relevant developmental windows and the importance of coincident exposures to elucidate disease cause.[14] This workshop underscored the need to leverage emerging technologies to assess environmental factors on a comparable omics scale (termed *the exposome*) to further the understanding of disease programming. A subsequent National Institute of Environmental Health Sciences (NIEHS) Workshop identified a need for traditional targeted environmental biomonitoring coupled with untargeted discovery of unknown exposures as critical tools in exposomic research.[15] We need to begin to implement an exposomic framework in respiratory health research starting in utero where environmental risk is rooted.

CONCEPTUALIZING THE PREGNANCY EXPOSOME

The exposome is ideally defined as the totality of environmental exposure from conception to death complementing the genome.[16,17] The pregnancy period is a key starting point to describe the exposome, owing to heightened sensitivity and potential lifetime impact on respiratory health and disease in the developing fetus. New and emerging technologies make it increasingly possible to apply the exposome concept in cohort studies with the practical understanding that even a partial characterization will bring major advances to understanding disease cause and variability.[18] Many of the tools to measure environment on an "omics" scale already exist, and recent advances in analytical chemistry, geospatial statistics, and the scientific and cultural developments that made smart phones ubiquitous now make the goal of estimating the exposome increasingly possible.

The pregnancy exposome includes an external domain, measured by methods including standardized survey tools and geospatial modeling, whereas the internal domain can be assessed through targeted (eg, specific chemical exposures, such as toxic metals, organic chemicals) and untargeted biomonitoring of external exposures via molecular omics platforms, with examples depicted in **Fig. 1**. The internal domain reflects the biological response to the external factors.[19] New and emerging tools and methods (traditional environmental/response biomonitoring, omics-based approaches for untargeted discovery of environmental exposures, remote sensing and geographic information systems [GIS]-based spatial methods, personal exposure devices, mobile apps, statistical tools for combined exposures) to characterize early-life exposure to a wide range of chemical (using targeted and untargeted approaches), nonchemical (eg, social context and social stressors), nutritional, and physical external environmental factors as well as the internal environment, facilitate an "early-life exposome" approach. Moreover, new statistical frameworks required to integrate and assess exposome health effects are also emerging. A handful of studies have started to move toward an exposome approach in assessing the effects of

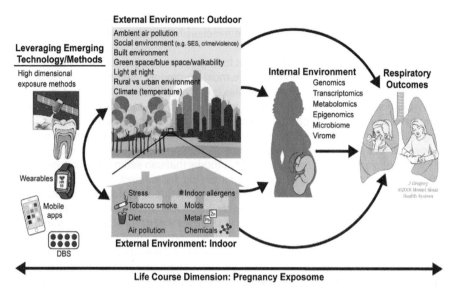

Fig. 1. Integrated approach to advancing exposomic research on respiratory outcomes. SES, socioeconomic status; DBS, dried blood spots.

multiple exposures during pregnancy on child development, primarily taking a targeted approach.[20–22]

Moving Exposure Research Toward Exposomic Approaches

Key concepts related to building an exposome framework are highlighted in later discussion.

Need to Address Susceptibility Windows in Exposure Assessment

Starting in utero, coordinated functioning of multiple networks of complex processes are necessary for optimal development and the maintenance of health. If the system is stressed, plasticity, the ability of the organism to respond to an insult and still maintain homeostasis, can be overwhelmed, and health impacts can arise as a consequence of environmental exposures. If environmental exposures occur during sensitive life periods, they can affect physiologic processes and regulatory systems that shape organ development and program later life health, a concept known as fetal programming.[19] The fetus is highly vulnerable, as differentiation is most active at this life stage, yet defense mechanisms against toxic environmental factors are underdeveloped. To produce programmed effects, environmental exposures must coincide with developmental changes that occur over timescales of weeks or even days, adding considerable complexity to research that seeks to understand these processes. Measuring exposure in the wrong susceptibility window may lead to missed or biased associations,[23] yet, the exact window of vulnerability is often unknown or varies depending on the outcome of interest or in the context of coincident exposures or other factors (eg, fetal sex). To advance the field, exposure assessment must operate at finer timescales than whole pregnancies. We cannot continue to rely on spot exposure assessments (ie, single blood/urine samples) in a discrete period of development (eg, trimesters). We must understand environmental exposure variability on a timescale that better approximates the rapidly occurring physiologic changes. Understanding the interplay between development and exposure timing would have an enormous impact on reducing random exposure misclassification and increasing statistical power, because random exposure misclassification tends to drive effects toward the null.

Biomonitoring is a commonly used tool for exposure assessment of environmental chemicals, with urine and blood being the most commonly used matrices. However, for children's studies, venous blood samples are often difficult to obtain, and minimally invasive options may be more desirable (eg, hair, teeth[24]). Moreover, methods have emerged to provide more highly temporally resolved exposure data (eg, daily, weekly) along with statistical methods to allow data-driven approaches to identify sensitive windows of effect. One exemplary approach involves air pollution modeling. This work leverages a satellite-based, daily $PM_{2.5}$ model that can estimate exposure dating back to conception on a daily basis, even if subjects are enrolled later in pregnancy.[25] Coupling highly temporally resolved exposure estimates with data-driven statistical techniques[23,26] allows researchers to identify susceptibility windows on a finer scale, removing subjectivity in determining the role of exposure timing in fetal programming. These methods have been implemented to link ambient air pollution, in particular, prenatal exposure to traffic-related pollutants found in urban environments, with asthma onset in children and lower lung function by age 7 years, identifying specific prenatal windows of vulnerability.[9,27–29] Objective identification of vulnerable windows can guide future research. For example, banking biological samples within more objectively delineated windows will allow investigators to use omics profiling to identify early biomarkers of risk as well as better inform mechanisms. Satellite remote sensing and GIS-based estimates of other environmental factors have also been linked to health, including climate (temperature), noise, walkability, green/blue space, and social experiences.[30–33]

Placenta as a Key Mediator of Fetal Programming

The placenta is the key regulator of the external environmental factors that affect the fetus.[34] During fetal life, cells differentiate and respond to signals induced by the maternal environment via the placenta, thereby setting a "program" that prepares the fetus for its ex utero life. Prenatal exposures leave signature changes in placental biomarkers, such as microRNAs (miRNAs), which are small noncoding RNA molecules that are critical regulators of numerous pathways and biological processes. Placental trophoblasts sort miRNAs into extracellular vesicles (EVs) that are then released into the extracellular environment and trafficked to distant maternal and fetal tissues where they repress gene expression via messenger RNA silencing. MiRNAs orchestrate complex signaling networks and play key roles in organogenesis,[35] including lung development.[36] EV-encapsulated placental miRNAs also regulate interrelated systems important in environmental programming of respiratory disorders, including immune and hypothalamic pituitary adrenal axis function and oxidative stress.

Although placenta cannot be sampled during pregnancy to measure biological changes induced by maternal environmental exposures, researchers can readily assess EV-encapsulated placental miRNAs via a minimally invasive blood draw in pregnant women and/or cord blood, a so-called *liquid biopsy*. In future research, investigators can leverage a range of environmental exposures to determine whether these predict profiles of signaling factors, such as EV-encapsulated placental miRNAs in maternal and cord plasma and placenta-specific miRNAs in placental tissue at birth, and importantly for possible clinical and diagnostic applications, whether these profile patterns precede subsequent alterations in child pulmonary phenotypes (**Fig. 2**).

In parallel, novel methods have also been developed to assess chemical mixtures in readily accessible tissues, which have quantifiable growth rates. For example, hair has

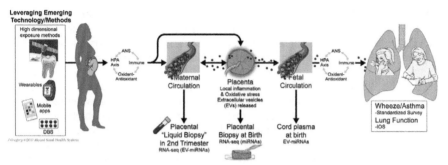

Fig. 2. Exposomic influences on placental-derived EV-associated miRNAs in maternal prenatal blood and/or cord blood in relation to early life respiratory phenotypes. ANS, autonomic nervous system; HPA, hypothalamic-pituitary-adrenal axis; IOS, impulse oscillometry system; DBS, dried blood spots; EV, extracellular vesicles.

daily growth rings allowing objective time measures. By sampling repeatedly along a hair shaft, one can see the time variable changes in toxin concentrations by coupling these data with known hair growth rates. By using maternal hair, researchers can leverage this property to reconstruct chemical exposures (eg, metals) from time of conception to delivery. One can reconstruct both a daily exposure diary for each chemical exposure (eg, metals) and aggregate levels to generate cumulative exposure data using described methods implemented with laser ablation-inductively coupled plasma-mass spectrometry to reconstruct past exposure timing.[37] Teeth also have identifiable growth rates starting in utero. A novel tooth-based biomarker can also be used to reconstruct chemical exposures in integrated weekly intervals from the second trimester through childhood.

Moving Toward Research on Multiple Pollutants

Although it is not possible to assess all environmental factors to which children are exposed in utero, the widespread methodologic interest in the exposome will increasingly make the study of multiple agents of broad interest.[38,39] Parallel to advances in exposure assessment to facilitate exposomic research, innovations have also been made in developing data analytics for an exposome framework.[40] For example, methods continue to evolve to assess mixtures of chemical exposures.[41] There is a range of relevant hypotheses in mixtures research, and certain methods are more suited for a particular question of interest than others, as reviewed in a NIEHS workshop on statistical methods for mixtures epidemiology.[42] Mixture methods have also been applied to consider multiple cooccurring social or psychological factors in programming children's disease risk.[43,44]

Need for Traditional and Nontraditional Biomonitoring

The following highlights the reasons traditional biomonitoring and nontraditional (exposomic) biomonitoring are critical in research aiming to capture the exposome.

High-Resolution Exposomics (Internal Dose)

Currently, more than 100,000 chemicals are registered for commercial use by the US Environmental Protection Agency with approximately 70,000 in common use. Exposure characterization on this magnitude far exceeds the abilities of traditional biomonitoring approaches. Future research can benefit from emerging hybrid targeted and untargeted high-resolution exposomics platform approaches that provide concentrations of known exposure biomarkers while enabling screening for other unanticipated and uncharacterized environmental pollutants.[45] Other emerging analytical methods allow characterization of multiclass biomarkers belonging to a range of chemical classes from a single small-volume urine sample.[46]

High-Resolution Metabolomics (Biological Response)

High-resolution metabolomics (HRM) provides an integrated measurement to link exposure to internal dose, biological response, and disease pathobiology.[47] Exposure to environmental chemicals can initiate local and global changes in gene transcription, enzyme activity, metabolite pathway alterations, and protein synthesis/folding. As a result, the microscale and macroscale interactions occur among these systems that can be characterized to study dose-response relationships. Measurements can provide information on both acute biological responses that occur at a biologically relevant dose and also on whether long-term alterations in physiology, that is, markers of exposure memory, have been detected from environmental stressors occurring years or decades before.[48] Current approaches, which are based on untargeted analyses using high-resolution mass spectrometry with advanced data extraction and annotation algorithms, allow measurement of greater than 20,000 chemical signals in biological samples, spanning endogenous metabolites, dietary chemicals, microbiome-derived metabolites, chemicals, commercial products, and drugs. HRM using liquid chromatography interfaced to ultra-high accuracy mass spectrometers is sufficiently developed to provide advanced clinical chemistry measures, environmental chemical surveillance, and bioeffect monitoring.[47,49]

Dried blood spots (DBS) represent a matrix for minimally invasive blood collection in children that can be used for biomonitoring.[50] Archived DBS following newborn screening are a particularly attractive resource for interrogating early-life biology using untargeted approaches.[51] For example, methods for metabolomics screening using DBS have been developed, including those archived for neonatal screening.[49,51] This is an important advance for studies examining programming in pregnancy and early childhood, as it lends itself more readily to repeated sampling.

SUMMARY

Existing and emerging tools and methods are available to characterize early-life exposure to a wide range of chemical, nonchemical, nutritional, and physical external environmental factors as well as the internal environment, constituting a "pregnancy exposome" approach. Moreover, novel statistical frameworks required to integrate and assess exposome health effects also continue to evolve. A commitment to understanding the interactions between our environment and genetic makeup on a comparable omics scale will elucidate mechanisms underlying disease cause and variability as well as identify novel biomarkers of early risk to inform prevention.

CLINICS CARE POINTS

- A commitment to understanding the interactions between our environment and genetic makeup on a comparable omics scale will better elucidate mechanisms underlying disease cause and variability as well as identify novel biomarkers of early risk to inform prevention.

ACKNOWLEDGMENTS

During preparation of this article, R.J. Wright was supported by National Institutes of Health (NIH) grants UH3OD0233337, P30ES023515, and U54TR004213.

REFERENCES

1. Zazara DE, Wegmann M, Giannou AD, et al. A prenatally disrupted airway epithelium orchestrates the fetal origin of asthma in mice. J Allergy Clin Immunol 2020; 145(6):1641–54.
2. Hui-Beckman J, Kim BE, Leung DY. Origin of allergy from in utero exposures to the postnatal environment. Allergy Asthma Immunol Res 2022;14(1):8–20.
3. Guerra S, Lombardi E, Stern DA, et al. Fetal origins of asthma: A longitudinal study from birth to age 36 years. Am J Respir Crit Care Med 2020;202(12): 1646–55.
4. Walker ML, Holt KE, Anderson GP, et al. Elucidation of pathways driving asthma pathogenesis: development of a systems-level analytic strategy. Review. Front Immunol 2014;5:447.
5. Rosa MJ, Lee A, Wright R. Evidence establishing a link between prenatal and early-life stress and asthma development. Curr Opin Allergy Clin Immunol 2018;18(2):148–58.
6. Chiu YM, Carroll KN, Coull BA, et al. Prenatal fine particulate matter, maternal micronutrient antioxidant intake, and early childhood repeated wheeze: Effect modification by race/ethnicity and sex. Antioxidants (Basel) 2022;(2):11. https://doi.org/10.3390/antiox11020366.
7. Rosa MJ, Tamayo-Ortiz M, Mercado Garcia A, et al. Prenatal lead exposure and childhood lung function: Influence of maternal cortisol and child sex. Environ Res 2022;205:112447. https://doi.org/10.1016/j.envres.2021.112447.
8. Adgent MA, Carroll KN, Hazlehurst MF, et al. A combined cohort analysis of prenatal exposure to phthalate mixtures and childhood asthma. Environ Int 2020; 143:105970. https://doi.org/10.1016/j.envint.2020.105970.
9. Wright RJ, Hsu HL, Chiu YM, et al. Prenatal ambient ultrafine particle exposure and childhood asthma in the northeastern united states. Am J Respir Crit Care Med 2021;204(7):788–96. https://doi.org/10.1164/rccm.202010-3743OC.
10. Warner JO, Warner JA. The foetal origins of allergy and potential nutritional interventions to prevent disease. Nutrients 2022;12(8):14. https://doi.org/10.3390/nu14081590.
11. Rosa MJ, Hartman TJ, Adgent M, et al. Prenatal polyunsaturated fatty acids and child asthma: Effect modification by maternal asthma and child sex. J Allergy Clin Immunol Mar 2020;145(3):800–7. https://doi.org/10.1016/j.jaci.2019.10.039, e4.
12. Burbank AJ, Sood AK, Kesic MJ, et al. Environmental determinants of allergy and asthma in early life. Review. J Allergy Clin Immunol 2017;140(1):1–12. https://doi.org/10.1016/j.jaci.2017.05.010.
13. Bunyavanich S, Schadt EE. Systems biology of asthma and allergic diseases: a multiscale approach. Review. J Allergy Clin Immunol 2015;135(1):31–42. https://doi.org/10.1016/j.jaci.2014.10.015.
14. Levy BD, Noel PJ, Freemer MM, et al. Future research directions in asthma. An NHLBI working group report. Am J Respir Crit Care Med 2015;192(11): 1366–72. https://doi.org/10.1164/rccm.201505-0963WS.
15. Dennis KK, Marder E, Balshaw DM, et al. Biomonitoring in the era of the exposome. Environ Health Perspect 2017;125(4):502–10. https://doi.org/10.1289/EHP474.

16. Miller GW, Jones DP. The nature of nurture: refining the definition of the exposome. Toxicol Sci 2014;137(1):1–2. https://doi.org/10.1093/toxsci/kft251.
17. Vineis P, Robinson O, Chadeau-Hyam M, et al. What is new in the exposome? Environ Int 2020;143:105887.
18. Wright RO. Environment, susceptibility windows, development, and child health. Review. *Current opinion in pediatrics* 2017;29(2):211–7.
19. Wright RO, Teitelbaum S, Thompson C, et al. The child health exposure analysis resource as a vehicle to measure environment in the environmental influences on child health outcomes program. Curr Opin Pediatr 2018;30(2):285–91.
20. Robinson O, Vrijheid M. The pregnancy exposome. research support, non-U.S. gov't review. Curr Environ Health Rep 2015;2(2):204–13.
21. Steckling N, Gotti A, Bose-O'Reilly S, et al. Biomarkers of exposure in environment-wide association studies - Opportunities to decode the exposome using human biomonitoring data. Rev *Environ Res* 2018;164:597–624.
22. Chen M, Guan Y, Huang R, et al. Associations between the maternal exposome and metabolome during pregnancy. Environ Health Perspect 2022;130(3):37003.
23. Wilson A, Chiu YM, Hsu HL, et al. Potential for bias when estimating critical windows for air pollution in children's health. Am J Epidemiol 2017;186(11):1281–9.
24. Petrick LM, Arora M, Niedzwiecki MM. Minimally invasive biospecimen collection for exposome research in children's health. Curr Environ Health Rep 2020;7(3):198–210.
25. Just AC, Arfer KB, Rush J, et al. Advancing methodologies for applying machine learning and evaluating spatiotemporal models of fine particulate matter (PM2.5) using satellite data over large regions. Atmos Environ (1994) 2020;239. https://doi.org/10.1016/j.atmosenv.2020.117649.
26. Wilson A, Chiu YM, Hsu HL, et al. Bayesian distributed lag interaction models to identify perinatal windows of vulnerability in children's health. Biostatistics 2017. https://doi.org/10.1093/biostatistics/kxx002.
27. Wright RJ, Brunst KJ. Programming of respiratory health in childhood: influence of outdoor air pollution. Research Support, N.I.H., Extramural Review. Curr Opin Pediatr 2013;25(2):232–9.
28. Hsu HH, Chiu YH, Coull BA, et al. Prenatal particulate air pollution and asthma onset in urban children. Identifying sensitive windows and sex differences. Am J Respir Crit Care Med 2015;192(9):1052–9.
29. Lee A, Leon Hsu HH, Mathilda Chiu YH, et al. Prenatal fine particulate exposure and early childhood asthma: Effect of maternal stress and fetal sex. J Allergy Clin Immunol 2017. https://doi.org/10.1016/j.jaci.2017.07.017.
30. Harouvi O, Ben-Elia E, Factor R, et al. Noise estimation model development using high-resolution transportation and land use regression. J Expo Sci Environ Epidemiol 2018. https://doi.org/10.1038/s41370-018-0035-z.
31. James P, Kioumourtzoglou MA, Hart JE, et al. Interrelationships between walkability, air pollution, greenness, and body mass index. Epidemiology 2017; 28(6):780–8.
32. Hartley K, Ryan PH, Gillespie GL, et al. Residential greenness, asthma, and lung function among children at high risk of allergic sensitization: a prospective cohort study. Environ Health 2022;21(1):52.
33. De Roos AJ, Kenyon CC, Yen YT, et al. Does living near trees and other vegetation affect the contemporaneous odds of asthma exacerbation among pediatric asthma patients? J Urban Health 2022;99(3):533–48.

34. Goldstein JA, Gallagher K, Beck C, et al. Maternal-fetal inflammation in the placenta and the developmental origins of health and disease. Front Immunol 2020;11:531543.

35. Salas-Huetos A, James ER, Aston KI, et al. The expression of miRNAs in human ovaries, oocytes, extracellular vesicles, and early embryos: A systematic review. Cells 2019;8(12). https://doi.org/10.3390/cells8121564.

36. Cushing L, Jiang Z, Kuang P, et al. The roles of microRNAs and protein components of the microRNA pathway in lung development and diseases. Am J Respir Cell Mol Biol 2015;52(4):397–408.

37. Stadlbauer C, Prohaska T, Reiter C, et al. Time-resolved monitoring of heavy-metal intoxication in single hair by laser ablation ICP-DRCMS. Anal Bioanal Chem 2005;383(3):500–8.

38. Rappaport SM, Barupal DK, Wishart D, et al. The blood exposome and its role in discovering causes of disease. Research support, N.I.H., extramural support, 2014 research support, non-U.S. gov't. Environ Health Perspect 2014;122(8): 769–74.

39. Vrijheid M. The exposome: a new paradigm to study the impact of environment on health. Thorax 2014;69(9):876–8.

40. Manrai AK, Cui Y, Bushel PR, et al. Informatics and data analytics to support exposome-based discovery for public Health. Review. Annu Rev Public Health 2017;38:279–94.

41. Carlin DJ, Rider CV, Woychik R, et al. Unraveling the health effects of environmental mixtures: an NIEHS priority. Environ Health Perspect 2013;121(1):A6–8.

42. Taylor KW, Joubert BR, Braun JM, et al. Statistical approaches for assessing health effects of environmental chemical mixtures in epidemiology: Lessons from an innovative workshop. Research support, N.I.H., extramural. Environ Health Perspect 2016;124(12):A227–9.

43. Brunst KJ, Sanchez Guerra M, Gennings C, et al. Maternal lifetime stress and prenatal psychological functioning and decreased placental mitochondrial DNA copy number in the PRISM study. Am J Epidemiol 2017;186(11):1227–36.

44. Campbell RK, Curtin P, Bosquet Enlow M, et al. Disentangling associations among maternal lifetime and prenatal stress, psychological functioning during pregnancy, maternal race/ethnicity, and infant negative affectivity at age 6 months: A mixtures approach. Health Equity 2020;4(1):489–99.

45. Go YM, Walker DI, Liang Y, et al. Reference standardization for mass spectrometry and high-resolution metabolomics applications to exposome research. Evaluation research support, 2015 research support, N.I.H. Extramural *Toxicol Sci* 2015;148(2):531–43.

46. Jagani R, Pulivarthi D, Patel D, et al. Validated single urinary assay designed for exposomic multi-class biomarkers of common environmental exposures. Anal Bioanal Chem 2022. https://doi.org/10.1007/s00216-022-04159-4.

47. Park YH, Lee K, Soltow QA, et al. High-performance metabolic profiling of plasma from seven mammalian species for simultaneous environmental chemical surveillance and bioeffect monitoring. Research support, N.I.H., extramural. Toxicology 2012;295(1–3):47–55.

48. Go YM, Jones DP. Exposure memory and lung regeneration. Review. Ann Am Thorac Soc 2016;13(Supplement_5):S452–61.

49. Petrick L, Edmands W, Schiffman C, et al. An untargeted metabolomics method for archived newborn dried blood spots in epidemiologic studies. Metabolomics 2017;13(3). https://doi.org/10.1007/s11306-016-1153-z.

50. Barr DB, Kannan K, Cui Y, et al. The use of dried blood spots for characterizing children's exposure to organic environmental chemicals. Environ Res 2021;195: 110796.
51. Yu M, Dolios G, Yong-Gonzalez V, et al. Untargeted metabolomics profiling and hemoglobin normalization for archived newborn dried blood spots from a refrigerated biorepository. J Pharm Biomed Anal 2020;191:113574.

Management of the Upper Airway Distress During Pregnancy

Jean Kim, MD, PhD[a,b,*], Michael Z. Cheng, MD[a],
Robert Naclerio, MD[a]

KEYWORDS

- Rhinitis of pregnancy • Pregnancy • Epidemiology • Management • Immunotherapy
- Corticosteroids • Antihistamines • Decongestants

KEY POINTS

- Rhinitis, which is highly prevalent during pregnancy, can manifest alone or with exacerbations of allergic rhinitis, acute bacterial rhinosinusitis, and upper respiratory tract infections.
- Sex hormones have been implicated in the pathophysiology of the rhinitis of pregnancy (ROP).
- There is limited efficacy of medical management in the control of symptoms of ROP.
- Initiation of new immunotherapy or escalating doses of immunotherapy are contraindicated during pregnancy.
- Evolving complications of rhinopathies during pregnancy need to be recognized and addressed expediently.

INTRODUCTION

A large proportion of women suffer symptoms of rhinitis during pregnancy, either as a new entity that arises over the course of pregnancy and resolves postpartum or as an exacerbation of previously existing symptoms. Here, the existing literature surrounding rhinitis of pregnancy (ROP) is reviewed with a summary of the evidence for the management of this disease.

Clinical Description of Rhinitis of Pregnancy

Pregnant women, like all patients, can be afflicted by any disease that occurs in the general population. ROP is a particular type of rhinitis that occurs only in pregnancy

[a] Department of Otolaryngology-Head and Neck Surgery, Johns Hopkins University School of Medicine, 601 North Caroline Street, Baltimore, MD 21287; [b] Department of Medicine, Division of Allergy and Clinical Immunology, Johns Hopkins University School of Medicine, Johns Hopkins Bayview Medical Center, 4940 Eastern Avenue, Suite A102B, Baltimore, MD 21224, USA
* Corresponding author. Department of Otolaryngology-Head and Neck Surgery, Division of Rhinology.
E-mail address: jeankim@jhmi.edu

Immunol Allergy Clin N Am 43 (2023) 53–64
https://doi.org/10.1016/j.iac.2022.05.010
0889-8561/23/© 2022 Elsevier Inc. All rights reserved.

and is defined as nasal congestion and other symptoms of rhinitis that initially manifest during pregnancy and resolve shortly after delivery, usually within 2 weeks. As a distinct entity from other forms of rhinitis, ROP is by definition not allergic, infectious, or cholinergic in etiology.[1] However, in terms of symptomatology it is similar to other forms of rhinitis and is characterized by nasal congestion, rhinorrhea, postnasal drip, nasal itching, sneezing, and hyposmia.[2] ROP seems to increase in prevalence as pregnancy progresses.[2,3] Additionally, the symptom severity of rhinitis and its negative impact to the quality of life also tends to increase as the pregnancy progresses.[4]

Rhinitis understandably decreases the quality of life with a particular impact on sleep, with 61% of women with ROP reporting difficulty sleeping.[2,5] In asthmatic women, rhinitis was associated with poor asthma control as well as higher incidence of anxiety symptoms, but was not associated with a greater rate of asthma exacerbation.[4] Rhinitis is postulated to increase the rates of snoring and obstructive sleep apnea, both of which are individually associated with adverse birth outcomes.[6–10] However, a direct association between rhinitis and adverse birth outcomes has not been demonstrated.[4,11]

Epidemiology of Rhinitis of Pregnancy

Rhinitis of pregnancy is a common entity, although studies vary on the exact prevalence. A large retrospective cohort study of 2264 women found that 65% of women had nasal congestion at some point during their pregnancy.[3] This same study demonstrated an increase in nasal congestion as pregnancy progressed, from 27% at 12 weeks of gestation to 42% at 36 weeks of gestation.[3] As this study focused on the single symptom of nasal congestion, it is an underestimate of the prevalence of ROP, which can also manifest without nasal congestion. The reported prevalence of symptoms of nasal congestion during pregnancy varies widely in the literature from 9% to 42%, likely due to heterogeneity in the strict clinical definition[2,12,13] Pregnancy has also been associated with worsening of rhinitis symptoms in 10% to 30% of women who had symptoms of other rhinopathies before pregnancy.[14]

Smoking increases the prevalence of rhinitis with an odds ratio of 1.7 compared with nonsmokers in one prospective study of 599 women.[12] Another study of 165 women evaluating allergen sensitivity demonstrated an association between sensitivity to dust mites and smoking with ROP.[15] However, sensitivities to other common allergens including timothy grass, animal dander, and Alternaria, showed no association with ROP.[15]

Pathophysiology of Rhinitis of Pregnancy

There is conflicting evidence for the role of sex hormones in the pathogenesis of ROP. Early electron microscopy studies of nasal mucosal biopsies obtained from pregnant women found ultrastructural and histochemical changes that were postulated to be due to rising estrogen and progesterone levels during pregnancy.[16] These changes included variations in succinic dehydrogenase, acid phosphatase, alkaline phosphate enzyme activity and increase acid mucopolysaccharide staining of mucous acini and goblet cells. Similar changes were found in mucosal specimens of symptomatic women who were taking estrogen/progestin oral contraceptive medications.[17] In vitro studies of cultured nasal epithelial cells found that estrogen and progesterone increased the expression of histamine H1 receptors.[18] Interestingly, in vivo immunohistochemical studies of receptors for these hormones found that only estrogen-beta receptors were present in nasal mucosal specimens, with estrogen-alpha and progesterone receptors being absent in all evaluated samples. The average number of estrogen receptor-positive cells in a cohort of pregnant and nonpregnant women and men correlated with worse rhinitis quality of life.[19] In contrast, there is contrasting evidence for negative correlations of the estrogen and progesterone receptors in ROP. The peak in rhinitis and nasal congestion occurs during the nadir of estrogen levels in the course of the normal menstrual cycle.[20] Also, the presence of rhinitis symptoms during pregnancy is not associated with higher estrogen or progesterone levels.[21] Finally, while estrogen elevation is universal during pregnancy, rhinitis symptoms are only present in 65% of women at any time during their pregnancy[3] .[22] Thus, more studies are needed to elucidate the role of sex hormones and their receptors in ROP.

Diagnostic Evaluation of Rhinitis in Pregnancy

The approach to the diagnosis of a pregnant patient clinically presenting with symptoms of ROP should differentiate ROP from other rhinopathies such as viral upper respiratory infections, nonallergic and allergic rhinitis, acute bacterial rhinosinusitis, and exacerbation of chronic rhinosinusitis (CRS). In addition to symptoms of ROP, careful attention to the onset of symptoms, environmental triggers, history of underlying rhinopathies such as allergic rhinitis and rhinosinusitis should be undertaken. Acute rhinosinusitis and exacerbations of CRS may present with symptoms of midface pain, facial pressure/congestion, facial pain, post nasal drip, rhinorrhea, cough, and decreased sense of smell[23] .[24] Worrisome physical exam findings indicating evolving complications of sinusitis such as facial numbness, eye swelling, severe headache, limited extraocular movements, and predisposing dental caries should elicit concern. Diagnostic nasal endoscopy, a routine part of a comprehensive rhinologic examination is considered safe (**Fig. 1**). Nasal endoscopy can document evidence of acute bacterial sinusitis or pyogenic granulomas. The latter can present during pregnancy and are benign granulomas of the nasal cavity that may cause acute epistaxis or nasal obstruction[25] .[26] In vitro allergy testing such as ImmunoCAP or RAST testing is considered safe and preferred over skin/puncture testing or food or drug challenges.[27]

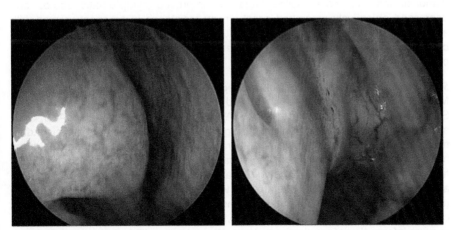

Fig. 1. Diagnostic nasal endoscopy: Left panel shows hypertrophic inferior turbinate and clear rhinorrhea of patients with ROP. Right panel shows mucopurulence in the sphenoethmoidal recess draining into the nasal cavity and nasopharynx in patients with acute bacterial rhinosinusitis.

Imaging studies may be needed to differentiate ROP from other sinonasal processes, especially if there are signs of symptoms of developing complications of sinusitis. According to the American College of Obstetricians and Gynecologists (ACOG), nonradiation inducing tests such as ultrasound or MRI without contrast is recommended over radiation modalities, such as radiography, nuclear medicine scans, or CT scans[28] .[29] The use of gadolinium contrast should be avoided if possible.[28] However, CT scans may be required in an emergent presentation of sinusitis complications. The use of intravenous iodinated CT contrast carries low adverse effects and animal studies have reported no teratogenic, mutagenic, or adverse effects of free iodine on the fetus[30] .[31] Thus, ACOG recommends that the use of CT and associated contrast material should not be withheld if clinically indicated, but a thorough discussion of risks and benefits should take place. As the pelvis is typically shielded from the radiation portal in a sinus CT scan, the fetal radiation doses are within the very low dose (<0.1 mGy) examination range of 0.001 to 0.01 mGy. In the evaluation of acute processes such as intracranial, intraorbital, or periorbital abscesses, the pregnant patient will benefit from early and accurate diagnosis which may outweigh the theoretic risks to the fetal.

Discussion: Treatment of Rhinitis and Sinonasal Complications During Pregnancy

There is little data on the effectiveness of any medication in the ROP.[32,33] Thus, once the diagnosis is established, physicians often try treatments used for allergic rhinitis, noting the potential adverse effects of these treatments on the fetus.[34] In general, the management of ROP is no different than the other forms of rhinitis that may occur in pregnancy. There should be a consideration for the fact that accurately identified ROP will be expected to resolve in the postpartum period. Nonetheless, given the impact of symptoms on the pregnant woman's quality of life, the symptoms of ROP warrant treatment. As with the general population, conservative treatment measures that do not include medications or alternative interventions can be very helpful in controlling symptoms with minimal side effects or risk to pregnant women with ROP. Nasal saline has no side effect profile and is recommended for all patients with allergic rhinitis, including pregnant women.[35] Additionally, a small randomized, control trial demonstrated that nasal saline irrigations improved symptomatic scores and decreased objectively measured nasal airway resistance in pregnant women with allergic rhinitis.[36] Physical exercise can induce a sympathomimetic response of vasoconstriction of nasal erectile tissue, thereby improving symptoms of nasal airway obstruction in the pregnant patient.[37]

Safety concerns of medications during pregnancy

Medications have historically been labeled for safety in pregnancy using the United States Food and Drug Administration (FDA) pregnancy risk categories of A, B, C, D, and X, in ascending order of risk[38] .[39] Drugs are labeled category A if sufficient data from studies in humans do not demonstrate risks to the fetus. Category B drugs have data supported by animal studies that do not demonstrate risks to the animal fetus, with the lack of corresponding human data. Category C drugs have data from animal studies that demonstrate fetal risk with no corresponding human data. Category D and X drugs have data that demonstrate risk to the human fetus.[38] The FDA changed its labeling system in 2015, moving away from simple risk categorization to more information of medication risks on (1) pregnancy, (2) lactation, and (3) reproductive potential.[40] However, this change does not pertain to generic drugs and drugs approved before 2001 which were not required to change their original classification of risk category.[41] As such, it is important for the clinician prescribing these drugs to be aware that most of the medications used for the treatment of ROP use the prior system of risk categorization (**Table 1**).

Medications used for the treatment of rhinitis of pregnancy
Corticosteroids play a significant role in the treatment of many forms of rhinitis with nasal steroids being a part of many first-line treatment regimens. In the general population, nasal topical steroids are preferred over oral steroids due to a lower amount of systemic absorption.[42] The data surrounding topical steroids generally indicate that they are safe to use during pregnancy with little to no effect on fetal outcomes.[43] A small placebo-controlled, randomized control trial showed no increase in adverse outcomes or defects with the use of nasal fluticasone during pregnancy.[32] Conversely, one large prospective study demonstrated an increase in the risk of respiratory system defects in children of women who used intranasal triamcinolone during pregnancy.[44] This increase was based on 6 out of 2498 observed cases of respiratory defects of malformations of the larynx, trachea, and bronchus and choanal atresia in the steroid-exposed group.

Table 1
Pregnancy risk categories of medications commonly used for rhinitis and sinusitis

Medication Class	Examples	FDA Risk Category[38,39]
Intranasal steroid	Fluticasone	B
	Budesonide	B
	Mometasone	C
Topical nasal antihistamine	Astelin	C
Topical nasal anticholinergic	Ipratropium bromide	B
Oral antihistamine	Cetirizine	B
	Loratadine	B
	Fexofenadine	C
Leukotriene antagonist	Montelukast	B
Oral steroid	Prednisolone	C

Antibiotics	Examples	FDA Risk Category
Penicillin	Penicillin	B
	Amoxicillin	B
	Amoxicillin clavulanate	B
Cephalosporin	Cefuroxime	B
	Cephalexin	B
	Cefadroxil	B
Macrolide	Azithromycin	B
	Clindamycin	B
	Vancomycin (IV)	B
	Clarithromycin	C
	Doxycycline	D
Aminoglycoside	Gentamicin (IV)	C
Sulfonamide	Sulfamethoxazole trimethoprim	C
Fluoroquinolone	Ciprofloxacin	C
	Levofloxacin	C

Most investigations on the effects of steroids during pregnancy studied inhaled steroids, which have higher systemic absorption than nasal sprays or irrigations. Most of the safety data is based on large retrospective studies of inhaled corticosteroids used in pregnant asthmatics, which demonstrate no increase in adverse birth outcomes or defects[45].[46] In general, oral steroids are contraindicated due to adverse effects on fetus, especially during the first trimester.[47] However, a short burst of oral steroids may be judiciously used in consultation with the patient's obstetrician to prevent impending complications of sinusitis.[47] A meta-analysis of 10 studies analyzing the association between oral steroids and adverse fetal outcomes was significant for an increased risk in cleft palate.[48] However, it should be noted that this analysis included studies evaluating steroids for all indications and dosages, including many disease processes that are treated with much higher steroid doses than is typically prescribed for rhinitis and rhinosinusitis exacerbations.

Antihistamines are commonly prescribed for rhinitis. Generally, oral antihistamines have been demonstrated to be safe in pregnancy when used for a variety of indications. A retrospective study of 17,776 pregnancies in women who used oral antihistamines found no increase in rates of fetal congenital anomalies or adverse birth outcomes for mother or fetus when compared with the general population.[49] A meta-analysis of 32 studies had similar findings for H1 antihistamine use.[50] Second-generation antihistamines with a lower side effect profile are preferable over first-generation antihistamines in pregnancy, similar to the general population. Multiple prospective cohort studies have found no increase in adverse birth outcomes or malformations with the use of loratadine[51].[52] In comparison to oral antihistamines, there is a relative lack of safety data on intranasal antihistamine sprays.

Topical nasal decongestants which provide rapid symptomatic relief of nasal congestion have fallen out of favor in the general population due to the known side effect of rhinitis medicamentosa that can occur with prolonged use.[53] Use of oral decongestants is not known to cause rhinitis medicamentosa, but there is mixed data surrounding their safety in pregnancy. A retrospective analysis of more than 4000 women who used oral decongestants both early and later in pregnancy found no increase in the risk of congenital malformations, lower rate of preterm births, and/or low birth weight compared with the general population.[54] In contrast, a retrospective case-control study of gastroschisis found the use of pseudoephedrine during pregnancy to be a significant risk factor.[55]

Nasal anticholinergic medications such as ipratropium are commonly prescribed for vasomotor rhinitis which presents with anterior watery rhinorrhea. There are no studies specifically evaluating the safety of nasal ipratropium in pregnancy. However, ipratropium is commonly used via the inhaled route for the treatment of asthma exacerbations during pregnancy and is considered FDA class B.[56]

Immunotherapy during pregnancy

Immunotherapy as it pertains to allergic rhinitis refers to exposing patients to immunologically verified allergens in a controlled and graded fashion to decrease the allergic response to those triggers. Continuing immunotherapy during pregnancy at the same dose as what the mother had been taking before pregnancy has been evaluated to be safe in multiple retrospective reviews.[57–59] However, initiating new immunotherapy or increasing the dose of ongoing immunotherapy carries a rare but possible risk of systemic allergic reactions including anaphylaxis. Therefore, escalating doses of allergen during pregnancy is contraindicated, given the greater risk to both mother and fetus.

Management of Complications of Rhinosinusitis During Pregnancy

Exacerbations of chronic rhinopathies during pregnancy that are poorly controlled can progress to rhinosinusitis, especially in those that have underlying CRS, CRS with nasal polyposis (CRSwNP), and aspirin-exacerbated respiratory disease (AERD). Acute bacterial rhinosinusitis can also occur. However, evidence-based management of exacerbations during pregnancy is not well studied. A systematic review was conducted by an expert panel of otolaryngologists from the US and Europe to make evidence-based recommendation for the management of rhinosinusitis. Of the 87 articles chosen for analysis after reviewing 3052 abstracts, the panel did not find "any level 1, 2, or 3 studies specific to the management of rhinosinusitis during pregnancy."[47] As a result, this review offered the following expert panel recommendations based on weighing the risks to fetus vs control of symptoms in the pregnant mother: 1. Penicillin and cephalosporins are considered safe and are recommended only with endoscopic evidence of purulence. 2. Tetracyclines, aminoglycosides, sulfa, and fluoroquinolones should be avoided. Long-term macrolide or doxycycline use for CRS is not recommended during pregnancy. 3. Only short bursts of oral corticosteroids to control acute exacerbations after the first trimester is justified, especially if patient has asthma exacerbated by CRS. 4. Off-label use of nasal steroid irrigations and steroid drops are not recommended. 5. Initiation or maintenance of antileukotrienes and oral decongestants for CRS is not recommended for control of exacerbations. 6. Discontinuation of aspirin therapy for pregnant patients with CRSwNP and AERD is advised. (n.b., Aspirin is category D). 7. Other medications for used for the treatment of ROP, including "modern" intranasal steroids are deemed safe as discussed above.

Management of Surgical Complications of Rhinosinusitis Requiring Surgery

Elective, nonemergent sinus surgery that is not for the treatment of a life-threatening process should be avoided. However, emergency surgery for the treatment of a complication of CRS demonstrating intracranial, intraorbital, or preseptal/periorbital extension may be performed safely with close anesthesia supervision (**Fig. 2**). Both

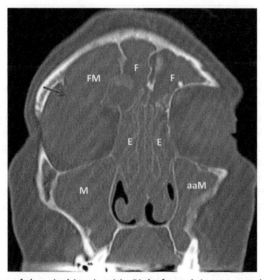

Fig. 2. Complication of chronic rhinosinusitis: Right frontal sinus mucocele (FM) erosion into right orbit (*arrow*) and chronic pansinusitis in pregnant patients with AERD exacerbation of CRSwNP. F (frontal sinus), M (maxillary sinus), and E (ethmoid sinus).

Table 2
Classification of Asthma control

Components of Control		Classification of Asthma Control (Youths ≥12 y of Age and Adults)		
		Well-Controlled	Not Well-Controlled	Very Poorly Controlled
Impairment	Symptoms	≤2 d/wk	>2 d/wk	Throughout the day
	Nighttime awakening	≤2x/month	1–3x/week	≥4x/week
	Interference with normal activity	None	Some limitation	Extremely limited
	Short-acting beta$_2$-agonist use for symptom control (not prevention of EIB)	≤ 2 d/wk	>2 d/wk	Several times per day
	FEV$_1$ or peak flow	>80% predicted/ personal best	60%–80% predicted/ personal best	<60% predicted/ personal best
	Validated Questionnaires			
	ATAQ	0	1–2	3–4
	ACQ	≤0.75%[a]	≥1.5	N/A
	ACT	≥20	16–19	≤15
Risk	Exacerbations	0–1/y	≥2/y (see note)	
		Consider severity and interval since last exacerbation		
	Progressive loss of lung function	Evaluation requires long-term followup care		
	Treatment-related adverse effects	Medication side effects can vary in intensity from none to very troublesome and worrisome. The level of intensity does not correlate to specific levels of control but should be considered in the overall assessment of risk		

Expert Panel Report 3: Guidelines for the Diagnosis and Management of Asthma, Full Report 2007. NIH Publication No. 07-4051.
Abbreviations: EIB, exercise-induced bronchospasm; FEV$_1$, forced expiratory volume in 1 s.
[a] ACQ values of 0.76–1.4 are indeterminate regarding well-controlled asthma.

the ACOG and the American Society of Anesthesiologists advise that a pregnant woman should never be denied medically necessary surgery or have that surgery delayed regardless of trimester because this can adversely affect the pregnant woman and her fetus.[60] There is no evidence to suggest that in utero human exposure to anesthetic or sedative drugs has any adverse effect on the developing fetal brain; and there are no animal data to support an effect with limited exposures less than 3 hours in duration. Screening and prophylaxis for venous thromboembolism should be instituted on all pregnant women undergoing surgery. In addition, surgery should be done at tertiary care institutions with neonatal services and obstetric care readily available.

SUMMARY

Rhinitis of pregnancy is well described as a highly prevalent disease with a significant impact on the quality of life of the patients it affects. Despite this, truly little is known about the pathophysiology of the disease. The treatments available for ROP are the same as the standard for rhinitis in nonpregnant patients; however, the efficacy of using currently prescribed medications is limited. The majority of studies evaluating treatments for ROP focus on safety outcomes of fetal and mother. However, there is a relative lack of data evaluating the efficacy of symptom reduction in the mother.. Early recognition of the progression of rhinitis into complications of the nasal and sinus cavities is key. Further investigation is necessary to elucidate the pathophysiology of ROP and to determine the efficacy of current treatment regimens on ROP for improved control of symptom outcomes (**Table 2**).

CLINICS CARE POINTS

- Medication treatment options for ROP are the same as treatment of standard rhinitis in nonpregnant patients.
- Immunotherapy may be continued at the same dose as established before pregnancy.
- Initiating new immunotherapy or escalating dose of ongoing immunotherapy is contraindicated during pregnancy.
- Early recognition and treatment of impending complications of sinusitis are important to prevent harm to both mother and fetus.

DISCLOSURE

M.z. Cheng: None. R. Naclerio is speaker for Sanofi and is part of the Advisory Board for Lyra, AstraZeneca, Sanofi, Regeneron, American Chemistry Council, Ismed and Celgene. J. Kim has been a consultant for ALK, GSK and Genentech and has received grant funding from Genentech.

REFERENCES

1. Ellegård E, Karlsson G. Nasal congestion during pregnancy. Clin Otolaryngol Allied Sci 1999;24(4):307–11.
2. Baudoin T, Šimunjak T, Bacan N, et al. Redefining pregnancy-induced rhinitis. Am J Rhinol Allergy 2021;35(3):315–22.
3. Bende M, Gredmark T. Nasal stuffiness during pregnancy. Laryngoscope 1999; 109(7):1108–10.
4. Powell H, Murphy VE, Hensley MJ, et al. Rhinitis in pregnant women with asthma is associated with poorer asthma control and quality of life. J Asthma 2015; 52(10):1023–30.
5. Gilbey P, McGruthers L, Morency A-M, et al. Rhinosinusitis-related quality of life during pregnancy. Am J Rhinol Allergy 2012;26(4):283–6.
6. Franklin KA, Åke Holmgren P, Jönsson F, et al. Snoring, pregnancy-induced hypertension, and growth retardation of the fetus. Chest 2000;117(1):137–41.
7. Chen Y-H, Kang J-H, Lin C-C, et al. Obstructive sleep apnea and the risk of adverse pregnancy outcomes. Am J Obstet Gynecol 2012;206(2):136.e131.
8. Ge X, Tao F, Huang K, et al. maternal snoring may predict adverse pregnancy outcomes: a cohort study in china. PLoS One 2016;11(2):e0148732.
9. Sharma SK, Nehra A, Sinha S, et al. Sleep disorders in pregnancy and their association with pregnancy outcomes: a prospective observational study. Sleep and Breathing 2016;20(1):87–93.

10. O'Brien LM, Bullough AS, Owusu JT, et al. Pregnancy-onset habitual snoring, gestational hypertension, and preeclampsia: prospective cohort study. Am J Obstet Gynecol 2012;207(6):e481–9.
11. Somoskövi Á, Bártfai Z, Tamási L, et al. Population-based case–control study of allergic rhinitis during pregnancy for birth outcomes. Eur J Obstet Gynecol Reprod Biol 2007;131(1):21–7.
12. Ellegård E, Hellgren M, Torén K, et al. the incidence of pregnancy rhinitis. Gynecol Obstet Invest 2000;49(2):98–101.
13. Shushan S, Sadan O, Lurie S, et al. Pregnancy-associated rhinitis. Am J Perinatol 2006;23(7):431–3.
14. Incaudo GA, Takach P. the diagnosis and treatment of allergic rhinitis during pregnancy and lactation. Immunol Allergy Clin N Am 2006;26(1):137–54.
15. Ellegård E, Karlsson G. IgE-mediated reactions and hyperreactivity in pregnancy rhinitis. Arch Otolaryngol Head Neck Surg 1999;125(10):1121–5.
16. Toppozada H, Michaels L, Toppozada M, et al. The human respiratory nasal mucosa in pregnancy: An electron microscopic and histochemical study. J Laryngol Otol 1982;96(7):613–26.
17. Toppozada H, Toppozada M, El-Ghazzawi I, et al. The human respiratory nasal mucosa in females using contraceptive pills: An ultramicroscopic and histochemical study. J Laryngol Otol 1984;98(1):43–51.
18. Hamano N, Terada N, Maesako K-i, et al. Expression of histamine receptors in nasal epithelial cells and endothelial cells – the effects of sex Hormones. Int Arch Allergy Immunol 1998;115(3):220–7.
19. Philpott CM, Robinson AM, Murty GE. Nasal pathophysiology and its relationship to the female ovarian hormones. J Otolaryngol Head Neck Surg 2008;37(4):540–6.
20. Ellegård E, Karlsson G. Nasal congestion during the menstrual cycle. Clin Otolaryngol 1994;19(5):400–3.
21. Ellegård E, Oscarsson J, Bougoussa M, et al. Serum level of placental growth hormone is raised in pregnancy rhinitis. Arch Otolaryngol Head Neck Surg 1998;124(4):439.
22. Ellegård EK. Clinical and pathogenetic characteristics of pregnancy rhinitis. Clin Rev Allergy Immunol 2004;26(3):149–60.
23. Rosenfeld RM, Piccirillo JF, Chandrasekhar SS, et al. Clinical practice guideline (update): adult sinusitis. Otolaryngology–Head Neck Surg 2015;152(2_suppl):S1–39.
24. Fokkens WJ, Lund VJ, Hopkins C, et al. european position paper on rhinosinusitis and nasal polyps 2020. Rhinology 2020;58(Suppl S29):1–464, 32077450.
25. Hsu IH, Shih J-C, Liao L-J, et al. Pyogenic Granuloma of the Nasal Cavity: An Unusual Complication of Pregnancy. Taiwanese J Obstet Gynecol 2005;44(1):101–4.
26. Mohd Yusof J, Abd Halim A, Wan Hamizan AK. Severe epistaxis in pregnancy due to nasal pyogenic granuloma: A case report. J Taibah Univ Med Sci 2020;15(4):334–7.
27. Pali-Schöll I, Namazy J, Jensen-Jarolim E. Allergic diseases and asthma in pregnancy, a secondary publication. World Allergy Organ J 2017;10(1):10.
28. Committee Opinion No. 723. Guidelines for diagnostic imaging during pregnancy and lactation. Obstet Gynecol 2017;130(4).
29. Tremblay E, Thérasse E, Thomassin-Naggara I, et al. Quality Initiatives: Guidelines for Use of Medical Imaging during Pregnancy and Lactation. RadioGraphics 2012;32(3):897–911.

30. Gjelsteen AC, Ching BH, Meyermann MW, et al. MRI, PET, PET/CT, and Ultrasound in the evaluation of obstetric and gynecologic patients. Surg Clin North America 2008;88(2):361–90.
31. Atwell TD, Lteif AN, Brown DL, et al. Neonatal thyroid function after administration of iv iodinated contrast agent to 21 pregnant patients. Am J Roentgenol 2008; 191(1):268–71.
32. Ellegård EK, Hellgren M, Karlsson NG. Fluticasone propionate aqueous nasal spray in pregnancy rhinitis. Clin Otolaryngol Allied Sci 2001;26(5):394–400.
33. Ellegård EK. Special considerations in the treatment of pregnancy rhinitis. Womens Health (Lond) 2005;1(1):105–14, 19803951.
34. Caparroz FA, Gregorio LL, Bongiovanni G, et al. Rhinitis and pregnancy: literature review. Braz J Otorhinolaryngol 2016;82:105–11.
35. Rabago D, Zgierska A. Saline Nasal Irrigation for Upper Respiratory Conditions. Am Fam Physician 2009;80(10):1117–9.
36. Garavello W, Somigliana E, Acaia B, et al. Nasal lavage in pregnant women with seasonal allergic rhinitis: a randomized study. Int Arch Allergy Immunol 2010; 151(2):137–41.
37. Eccles R. Nasal Airflow in Health and Disease. Acta Oto-Laryngol 2000;120(5): 580–95.
38. FDA Pregnancy Categories - CHEMM.
39. FDA Pregnancy Categories, F.a.D. Administration, Editor.
40. Food and A Drug. Pregnancy and lactation labeling (drugs) final rule. FDA; 2021.
41. Byrne JJ, Saucedo AM, Spong CY. Evaluation of Drug Labels Following the 2015 Pregnancy and Lactation Labeling Rule. JAMA Netw Open 2020;3(8):e2015094.
42. Benninger MS, Ahmad N, Marple BF. The safety of intranasal steroids. Otolaryngology–Head Neck Surg 2003;129(6):739–50.
43. Namazy J, Schatz M, Long L, et al. Use of inhaled steroids by pregnant asthmatic women does not reduce intrauterine growth. J Allergy Clin Immunol 2004;113(3): 427–32.
44. Bérard A, Sheehy O, Kurzinger M-L, et al. Intranasal triamcinolone use during pregnancy and the risk of adverse pregnancy outcomes. J Allergy Clin Immunol 2016;138(1):97–104.e107.
45. Norjavaara E, de Verdier MG. Normal pregnancy outcomes in a population-based study including 2968 pregnant women exposed to budesonide. J Allergy Clin Immunol 2003;111(4):736–42.
46. Källén B, Rydhstroem H, Aberg A. Congenital malformations after the use of inhaled budesonide in early pregnancy. Obstet Gynecol 1999;93(3):392–5.
47. Lal D, Jategaonkar AA, Borish L, et al. Management of rhinosinusitis during pregnancy: systematic review and expert panel recommendations. Rhinology 2016; 54(2):99–104, 26800862.
48. Park-Wyllie L, Mazzotta P, Pastuszak A, et al. Birth defects after maternal exposure to corticosteroids: Prospective cohort study and meta-analysis of epidemiological studies. Teratology 2000;62(6):385–92.
49. Källén B. Use of antihistamine drugs in early pregnancy and delivery outcome. J Matern Fetal Neonatal Med 2002;11(3):146–52.
50. Etwel F, Faught LH, Rieder MJ, et al. The risk of adverse pregnancy outcome after first trimester exposure to h1 antihistamines: a systematic review and meta-analysis. Drug Saf 2017;40(2):121–32.
51. Moretti ME, Caprara D, Coutinho CJ, et al. Fetal safety of loratadine use in the first trimester of pregnancy: a multicenter study. J Allergy Clin Immunol 2003;111(3): 479–83.

52. Diav-Citrin O, Shechtman S, Aharonovich A, et al. Pregnancy outcome after gestational exposure to loratadine or antihistamines: a prospective controlled cohort study. J Allergy Clin Immunol 2003;111(6):1239–43.
53. Zucker SM, Barton BM, McCoul ED. Management of rhinitis medicamentosa: a systematic review. Otolaryngol Head Neck Surg 2019;160(3):429–38.
54. Källén BAJ, Otterblad Olausson P. Use of oral decongestants during pregnancy and delivery outcome. Am J Obstet Gynecol 2006;194(2):480–5.
55. Werler MM, Mitchell AA, Shapiro S. First trimester maternal medication use in relation to gastroschisis. Teratology 1992;45(4):361–7.
56. Working Group Report on Managing Asthma During Pregnancy: Recommendations for Pharmacologic Treatment–Update 2004. p. 72.
57. Metzger WJ, Turner E, Patterson R. The safety of immunotherapy during pregnancy. J Allergy Clin Immunol 1978;61(4):268–72.
58. Oykhman P, Kim HL, Ellis AK. Allergen immunotherapy in pregnancy. Allergy Asthma Clin Immunol 2015;11(1):31.
59. Shaikh WA. A retrospective study on the safety of immunotherapy in pregnancy. Clin Exp Allergy 1993;23(10):857–60.
60. ACOG Committee Opinion No. 775. Nonobstetric surgery during pregnancy. Obstet Gynecol 2019;133(2):395–403.

Chronic Management of Asthma During Pregnancy

Jennifer A. Namazy, MD[a],*, Michael Schatz, MD[b]

KEYWORDS

- Asthma • Pregnancy • Perinatal outcomes • Pregnancy complications

KEY POINTS

- Asthma is one of the most common conditions that afflict pregnant women.
- The prevalence of asthma is also increasing in childbearing-aged women.
- Because uncontrolled asthma in pregnancy affects both maternal and offspring outcomes, careful attention to maintaining control of asthma symptoms throughout pregnancy is of critical importance.
- Suboptimal control of asthma or more severe asthma during pregnancy may be associated with an increased maternal or fetal risk.
- Physician reluctance to use medications during pregnancy and patient noncompliance remain important barriers to asthma control during pregnancy.
- There is a need for higher quality evidence human data regarding the safety of asthma medication during pregnancy that adequately accounts for the potential effect of uncontrolled asthma.

INTRODUCTION

Asthma during pregnancy has an estimated prevalence in the United States between 8.4% and 8.8%.[1] Between 2001 and 2007 prevalence was 5.5% in 2001 and increased to 7.8% in 2007.[2] It has been suggested that asthma may influence pregnancy outcomes, and that pregnancy may affect the course of asthma.

Effects of Pregnancy on Asthma

Pregnancy is associated with variable changes in asthma symptoms. In one recent study, 60% had asthma that stayed the same, 40% had asthma that worsened, and no subjects were observed to have asthma that improved.(3) Pregnancy itself can be associated with shortness of breath, and as a result, identification of accompanying symptoms of wheezing, chest tightness, and cough as well as lung function may be

[a] Department of Allergy and Immunology, Scripps Clinic, 7565 Mission Valley Road Suite 200, San Diego, CA 92108, USA; [b] Department of Allergy and Immunology, Kaiser Permanente, San Diego, CA, USA
* Corresponding author.
E-mail address: janamazy@me.com

Immunol Allergy Clin N Am 43 (2023) 65–85
https://doi.org/10.1016/j.iac.2022.09.001

important to distinguish changes in disease from pregnancy-induced dyspnea. Although lung volumes have been reported to change during pregnancy, measures of airway function such as forced expiratory volume in 1 second (FEV1) do not substantially change and can be used to monitor asthma during pregnancy as in nonpregnant patients.

One study found that maternal asthma worsened as pregnancy progressed in 50% of women reporting a loss of control, 16% having recurrent loss of control throughout pregnancy, and 20% experiencing at least one exacerbation during pregnancy.[3] One group reported that older maternal age, current smoking, baseline inhaled corticosteroid (ICS) use, and multiparity were risk factors for recurrent uncontrolled asthma.[4] Interestingly, having a written asthma action plan was also associated with an increased risk of exacerbation during pregnancy. An asthma plan may have been a marker for more severe disease in that study.[5]

Unfortunately, it has been difficult to design a study to examine the longitudinal changes in asthma control during pregnancy. In one study, a prospective cohort of women with and without asthma was followed from early pregnancy. Although 50% had asthma that stayed the "same"| as before pregnancy, 40% had asthma that worsened during pregnancy.[6] Airway responsiveness to mannitol and nonatopic status seem to characterize women at an increased risk of asthma exacerbations during pregnancy.[7] In contrast, characteristics of patients with a lower risk of asthma exacerbations during pregnancy were no history of prepregnancy exacerbations, no controller medication, and clinically stable asthma before pregnancy. This information could be considered helpful in discussions with pregnant asthmatic women undergoing prepregnancy counseling.

Very little is known about the potential mechanisms by which pregnancy affects asthma symptoms. The role of maternal hormones, such as cortisol, estradiol, or progesterone, has not been thoroughly investigated in the context of asthma control or exacerbations in pregnancy, with only one study investigating maternal serum progesterone and airway responsiveness in pregnancy but finding no significant relationship.[8] Other hypotheses have been put forward regarding the influence of fetal sex (with inconsistent results),[9–11] the role of beta-2-adrenoreceptor responsiveness,[12] or altered maternal immune function.[13–15]

Effects of Asthma on Pregnancy

A meta-analysis from Murphy and colleagues, derived from a substantial body of literature spanning several decades and including very large numbers of pregnant women (>1,000,000 for low birth weight and >250,000 for preterm labor), indicates that pregnant women with asthma are at a significantly increased risk of a range of adverse perinatal outcomes including low birth weight and preterm birth.[16]

This was supported by a study from Sweden, which reported an increased risk of preeclampsia, emergency caesarean section and small for gestational age, even when controlled for familial confounding factors.[17]

Data from 2 US health claims databases found increased risks of prematurity, small for gestational age, and neonatal intensive care unit (NICU) admissions among women with asthma. Women with uncontrolled asthma demonstrated increased risks of preterm birth and NICU admission. Those with more severe asthma had an increased risk of small for gestational age infants.[18]

Data from a case control study that investigated the relationship between maternal asthma, preeclampsia and preterm delivery, did not indicate a greater risk of preeclampsia among women with physician-diagnosed asthma.[19] However, there was a significant association between preeclampsia and asthma among a subgroup of women who experienced symptoms during pregnancy and had received their diagnosis more than 10 years earlier.[19]

Uncontrolled asthma can lead to hypoxia and other physiologic abnormalities that could lead to decreased fetal blood oxygen and result in abnormal growth and development of the fetus. For patients with persistent asthma, consideration should be made to begin fetal monitoring (usually nonstress testing) at 32 weeks gestation and during an asthma exacerbation if the fetus is potentially viable.

Exacerbations are a potential problem associated with asthma during pregnancy. Up to 45% of women have been reported to have an exacerbation of asthma requiring medical intervention during pregnancy.[20] A meta-analysis[16] sought to investigate if asthma exacerbations, oral corticosteroid use, or asthma severity, all related to poor asthma control, are associated with prematurity and intrauterine growth restriction. Data from this meta-analysis found a significantly increased risk of low-birth-weight infants of those subjects experiencing asthma exacerbation during pregnancy (relative risk (RR) 3.02[1.87,4.89]) and using oral corticosteroids during pregnancy (RR 1.41, 95%CI [1.04,1.93]). Overall, the risk of low birth weight or early preterm delivery was not increased in women with moderate/severe asthma compared with women with mild asthma.[21] Murphy and colleagues reported, in another meta-analysis, an increased risk of low birth weight in women who had an asthma exacerbation during pregnancy (RR 2.54, 95%CI 1.52–4.25) compared with women without asthma. This meta-analysis also reported a nonsignificant trend of increased preterm delivery in asthmatic women with exacerbations during pregnancy (RR 1.54[0.89,2.69]) and an increased relative risk of preterm delivery (RR 1.51, 95%CI [1.15,1.98]) in those asthmatic women using oral corticosteroids during pregnancy.[20] This group found that the combination of medium to high-dose oral corticosteroid use and exacerbation in the past 12 months was associated with an increased risk of severe asthma exacerbation during pregnancy (adjusted odds ration (aOR) 3.20; 95%CI, 1.85–5.53). Studies have shown that women with asthma exacerbations during pregnancy, a marker of poor control, had similar risk of preeclampsia to women with asthma who did not have exacerbations in pregnancy.[20,22] These data suggest that inherent asthma severity, rather than control or exacerbations, may be related to the increased risk of preeclampsia in asthmatic women.

Stenius-Aarniala and colleagues compared data from 47 patients with an attack of asthma during pregnancy to data from 457 asthmatics with no recorded acute exacerbation and 237 healthy subjects. The authors found no increased incidence of congenital malformations in the infants of asthma women with exacerbations during pregnancy.[23] However, a more recent cohort of more than 4000 pregnancies found an increased risk of total congenital malformations in the infants of pregnant asthmatic women who had an asthma exacerbation during pregnancy [1.48 (95%CI, 1.04–2.09) compared with infants of women who did not experience an exacerbation.[24] Stenius-Aarniala and colleagues did not find any increased risk of perinatal death in those women with an attack of asthma during pregnancy.[23] Similarly, a more recent study of 146 pregnant women with asthma exacerbations during pregnancy found that there was no increased risk of stillbirth in those women with severe exacerbations during pregnancy.[25] Two smaller retrospective studies also found that severe asthma was not associated with an increased risk of perinatal death compared with mild asthmatics and controls.[26,27] This was supported by a more recent prospective study conducted at 16 centers of the Maternal-Fetal Medicine Units Network of the National Institute of Child Health and Human Development in more than 2000 pregnant asthmatics. The authors found no increased risk of perinatal mortality when comparing moderate-to-severe asthmatics to those with milder disease.[28] In contrast, one of the largest retrospective database studies in a cohort of 13,100 and 28,042 single pregnancies in women with and without asthma found that there was an increased risk of perinatal mortality (odds ratio (OR) 1.35, 95%CI 1.08–1.67) in infants of asthmatic women.[29] In follow-up, the authors used a 2-stage sampling cohort design and found that the increased risk of perinatal mortality did not remain significant after adjusting for cigarette smoking (OR 1.12, 95%CI 0.87–1.45).[30]

A Korean study with a cohort of more than 500 women with asthma exacerbations during pregnancy compared with more than 9000 without exacerbations found that the groups were not different in regard to preterm birth, gestational diabetes or placenta previa. However, preeclampsia was more frequently seen in women with exacerbations.[31]

The prevalence of severe asthma in pregnant women in the United States has been difficult to establish but in a study looking at 2 large health-care claim databases, 19% of pregnant women with asthma had severe asthma.[32] Firoozi and colleagues investigated the effect of the severity of asthma during pregnancy on the risk of a small for gestational infants, low birth weight, and preterm birth. Their retrospective cohort study included more than 13,000 subjects and demonstrated an increased risk of small for gestational age infants in the moderate and severe asthmatic groups. There was no increased risk of low birth weight or preterm delivery in these groups.[33] Dombrowski and colleagues found no significant effect of mild asthma or moderate-severe asthma on preterm delivery (at either <32 weeks or <37 weeks gestation), compared with controls without asthma. However, when the subgroup of women with severe asthma (FEV_1 <60% predicted and/or used oral steroids in the 4 weeks before study enrollment) was compared with controls, there was a significantly increased risk of preterm delivery (adjusted OR 2.2, 95%CI 1.2, 4.2).[28] A large prospective cohort study that specifically examined the effect of asthma severity on preeclampsia found that women with moderate-to-severe symptoms during pregnancy were at increased risk of preeclampsia, suggesting a role of active maternal inflammation.[34] A study from Schatz and colleagues found a significant association between hypertension during pregnancy and lower FEV_1 after adjustment for covariates. The mean percent predicted FEV_1 was lower, and the proportion of women with FEV_1 less than 80% was higher, in women with hypertension during pregnancy compared with those without hypertension.[35] Mirzakhani and colleagues found an association of uncontrolled asthma during pregnancy with the risk of preeclampsia and reported that maternal vitamin D levels during early pregnancy could possibly affect this association.[36]

Nonpharmacologic Management of Asthma During Pregnancy

Assessment and monitoring

In a patient without a previous diagnosis of asthma, asthma must be differentiated from several other potential causes of respiratory symptoms during pregnancy. The most common differential diagnosis is dyspnea of pregnancy, which may occur in early pregnancy in approximately 70% of women. This dyspnea is usually differentiated from asthma by its lack of association with cough, wheezing, or airway obstruction. Other important masqueraders of asthma include vocal cord dysfunction, panic attacks, hyperventilation, and cough due to postnasal drip, laryngopharyngeal reflux, or angiotensin-converting enzyme inhibitor therapy. All of these can coexist with asthma. Even when these conditions coexist with asthma, their diagnosis and appropriate therapy usually reduce the patient's respiratory symptoms.

Wheezing, chest tightness, cough, and associated shortness of breath are common symptoms of asthma. The diagnosis is ideally confirmed by the demonstration of reversible airways obstruction, which most commonly is an increase in FEV1 by 12% or more and of at least 200 mL after an inhaled short-acting bronchodilator. In nonpregnant patients with normal pulmonary function, asthma can be confirmed by means of methacholine challenge testing. However, this type of testing is not recommended in pregnant patients.

Several biomarkers for asthma have been studied in the pregnant population as well. Hyaluronic acid, which has been shown to be a marker of systemic inflammation, was evaluated as a screening tool for asthma control during pregnancy.[37] In that study, hyaluronic acid values could discriminate patients with an Asthma Control Test (ACT) total score greater than 20 (controlled patients) and less than 20 (uncontrolled patient) (area under the curve (AUC) 0.78, 95%CI 0.65–0.92). Further studies are necessary to confirm these observations.

Although osteopontin increases during pregnancy irrespective of asthma severity, clusterin seems to correlate with lung function.[38] Recent studies suggest that an elevated fraction of exhaled nitric oxide (FeNO) can be used in pregnant women to follow asthma like its use in nonpregnant patients.[39] Thus, an elevated FeNO would likely support the diagnosis of nonoptimal asthma control in pregnant patients. If FeNO is normal or unavailable in patients with normal pulmonary function, therapeutic trials of asthma therapy, such as 2 to 4 weeks of regular ICSs, may be used during pregnancy in patients with possible but unconfirmed asthma.

FeNO may also be useful in the management of asthma during pregnancy. A double-blind, parallel-group, controlled study by Powell and colleagues tested the ability of measurement of FeNO to guide management of pregnant asthmatic women. The primary outcome was total asthma exacerbations. The authors found that the exacerbation rate was lower in the group using FeNO to adjust asthma therapies.[40]

Once the diagnosis of asthma is confirmed, the next step is the assessment of asthma severity (in patients not already on controller therapy) or assessment of control (in patients already on controller therapy; **Table 1**). Patients with intermittent asthma have short episodes and use rescue therapy 2 times or less per week, nocturnal symptoms 2 times or less a month, and normal pulmonary function between episodes. Patients with more frequent symptoms or who require daily asthma medications should be considered to have persistent asthma. Validated questionnaires are used in nonpregnant patients to assess asthma control, and the pregnancy ACT has recently been shown to be valid and reliable to monitor asthma control during pregnancy.[41] CARAT or "control of Allergic Rhinitis and Asthma Test" is a brief self-administered questionnaire to quantify the degree of control of allergic rhinitis and asthma. It was recently validated in a study of 42 pregnant asthmatic patients.[42] Although women with severe asthma are often followed more closely during pregnancy, women with milder symptoms may actually be more "at risk." One group found that women with mild asthma not requiring ICS prepregnancy had uncontrolled asthma during pregnancy and demonstrated the greatest alterations in placental function.[43]

Psychological considerations

Pregnancy represents a time of psychological vulnerability, even for healthy women. Changes in body image, the physical symptoms accompanying normal pregnancy, and various fears regarding the pregnancy and the developing infant cause additional stress. Anxiety and depression are common disorders that affect a large part of the population, and studies have indicated that the prevalence of depression is as high as 6% to 15% in pregnant women.[44] In a large population-based study, anxiety, depression, and asthma were associated with an increased risk of caesarean section.[17,44] In the pregnant woman with asthma or allergic disease, psychological stresses may be especially important. First, in women whose symptoms tend to worsen with stress, the stress of normal pregnancy may exacerbate symptoms.

Table 1
Classification of asthma severity in pregnant patients

Asthma Severity	Symptom Frequency	Nighttime Awakening	Interference with Normal Activity	FEV_1 or Peak Flow (Predicted Percentage of Personal Best)
Intermittent	2 d/wk or less	Twice per month or less	None	More than 80%
Mild persistent	More than 2 d/wk but not daily	More than twice per month	Minor limitation	More than 80%
Moderate persistent	Daily symptoms	More than once per week	Some limitation	60%–80%
Severe persistent	Throughout the day	For times per week or more	Extremely limited	<60%

From Dombrowski MP, Schatz M; ACOG Committee on Practice Bulletins-Obstetrics. ACOG practice bulletin: clinical management guidelines for obstetrician-gynecologists number 90, February 2008: asthma in pregnancy. *Obstet Gynecol.* 2008;111(2 Pt 1):457–464.

Furthermore, the morbidity associated with asthma or allergic symptoms, especially if the symptoms interfere with sleep, may add substantially to the stress of normal pregnancy. Even following delivery, women with asthma have an increased risk of postpartum depression compared with women without asthma (6.1% vs 2.9%).[45]

Although most patients have a social-familial support network, the physician managing the asthma or allergic disease should be an important additional source of support. Regular visits and easy accessibility to the physician for unanticipated problems should significantly reduce anxiety. One study reported anxiety and depression to be present in 45% of pregnant women with asthma and that women with anxiety and depression were more likely to have uncontrolled asthma.[46]

If the patient knows she can express her concerns to a knowledgeable and caring professional, if she understands the educational information presented, and if she has regular visits and easy accessibility to the physician, she will be reassured with a sense of confidence and security. In addition, the pregnant woman should be specifically reassured that the physicians will work with her as a team to optimize maternal and neonatal outcomes.

Although most pregnant women with asthma or allergic disease will require no additional psychological intervention, an occasional patient with unusual stress or impoverished coping mechanisms may require psychiatric consultation.

Patient education

Information should be given to the patient regarding asthma and allergies in general, effects of properly managed symptoms on pregnancy, possible effects of pregnancy on the symptoms, effects of carefully chosen medication on the baby, and anticipated course of labor and delivery.

Discussions may begin with a general overview of the effects pregnancy on asthma. Asthma course may worsen, improve, or remain unchanged during pregnancy, and the overall data suggest that these various courses occur with approximately equal frequency. The mechanisms responsible for the altered asthma course during pregnancy are unknown. The myriad of pregnancy-associated changes in levels of sex hormones, cortisol and prostaglandins, may contribute to changes in asthma course during pregnancy.

Uninformed decisions by pregnant asthmatic patients or those managing their asthma may lead to exacerbations of asthma during pregnancy and potentially lead to adverse perinatal outcomes. Therefore, asthma education is a critical component in the management of the pregnant asthmatic. One successful approach was recently reported in the multidisciplinary approach to the management of maternal asthma study or MAMMA. Subjects were randomized to either receive a pharmacist-led intervention (consisting of self-management strategies, such as proper inhaler technique, adherence support, monthly Asthma Control Questionnaire [ACQ] assessments, FEV1 and action plans) or usual care. There was communication between the pharmacist, family physician, midwife, and the patient. At the end of 6 months, there was a significant reduction in ACQ (improved asthma control) compared with the group that received usual care.[47] A recent prospective cohort study of more than 800 pregnant women with asthma found a high prevalence of nonadherence and poor self-management skills. After 3 educational sessions on medication knowledge, maximal improvements in adherence were seen.[48]

Potential confounders and barriers to control

Based on the available data, control of maternal asthma is essential to reduce the risk of perinatal complications. There are several factors that remain barriers to asthma control in this group of patients. They include smoking, obesity, adherence, physician undertreatment, and viral infections.

Genetic factors may also influence asthma during pregnancy and act as confounders when interpreting outcomes studies. Rejno and colleagues performed an analysis of perinatal outcomes in full cousin and sister pairs. They found that outcomes including preeclampsia, low birth weight, caesarean section, and gestational age were more common in women with asthma irrespective of heredity, suggesting that these associations are not confounded by genes but rather a true effect of asthma on pregnancy.[17]

It comes as no surprise that pregnant women are hesitant about continuing asthma medications during pregnancy for fear of causing untoward effects on their unborn baby. Medication nonadherence during pregnancy is a significant clinical problem. A cohort study of 115,169 pregnant asthmatics in South Korea reported that women tended to rapidly reduce their asthma medication use during the beginning of their pregnancy. This led to a greater number of exacerbations in a small proportion of the study population.[49] Kim and colleagues found that ICS-long-acting beta agonist (LABA), systemic steroids and short-acting beta agonist use was less likely in pregnant women.[31] Another study found that about one-third of pregnant asthmatics discontinued asthma medications during pregnancy, often without consulting their physicians.[50] Another study by Lim and colleagues[51] examined the reasons for nonadherence in this particular population of patients. Data were obtained from interviews with pregnant asthmatic women. Concerns about medication use, specifically steroid use, overshadowed concerns about the potential risks of uncontrolled asthma. Many women appeared content to rely on their reliever therapy, and many decreased their preventive therapy without consulting their doctors. Interestingly, most participants complained about the lack of information available regarding asthma during pregnancy. Lack of support was also a common complaint. Many women thought that the information they were receiving from their pharmacists, nurses and doctors was contradictory, leading them to make their own choices about medication management. As a result, many of the participants decreased or discontinued their asthma medications or withheld doses during pregnancy. According to the study's authors, it was clear from the interviews that women thought it would have been helpful if asthma had been discussed more by their health-care professionals, providing opportunities for pursuing more reliable information. Robijn and colleagues found that persistent nonadherence to ICS was associated with lower maternal age, higher parity and no prescribed ICS at baseline.[52]

A disappointing fact is that medical professionals can provide incorrect information. A recent study found that more than a quarter of family physicians would instruct their patients to decrease or discontinue asthma medication during pregnancy when asthma was well controlled by current therapy.[53] Another study by Cimbollek and colleagues surveyed 1000 physicians, almost half of whom were respiratory medicine specialists/allergy specialists and the other half were primary care physicians. Almost 30% of physicians would not perform spirometry in pregnant asthmatic patients, and only 64% reported that they followed the asthma guidelines in the management of pregnant asthmatic patients.[54]

Physician reluctance to treat may also affect the course of asthma during pregnancy. One study identified 51 pregnant women and 500 nonpregnant women presenting to the emergency department with acute asthma. Although asthma severity appeared to be similar in the 2 groups based on peak flow rates, pregnant women were significantly less likely to be discharged on oral corticosteroids (38% vs 64%). Presumably related to this undertreatment, pregnant women were 3 times more likely than nonpregnant women to report an ongoing exacerbation 2 weeks later.[55,56]

Obesity has been shown to be an inflammatory state that may play an important role in asthma initiation and control. Obesity during pregnancy has been associated with adverse perinatal outcomes including gestational diabetes, preeclampsia, thromboembolic disorders, postpartum hemorrhage, large for gestational age, fetal death, and congenital anomalies. The mechanisms leading to these outcomes are thought to be due to a heightened inflammatory response. It has been shown that airway macrophages from obese adults have impaired function in clearing apoptotic inflammatory cells.[16] This was associated with inflammation measured by increased oxidant levels and decreased corticosteroid responsiveness. Higher BMI has been associated with an increased risk for asthma exacerbations in both nonpregnant and pregnant women. In one study, 30.7% of participants were obese (BMI $\geq$30 kg/m^2) compared with controls, and obesity was associated with an increase in asthma exacerbations (OR 1.3, 95%CI, 1.1–1.7) compared with nonobese pregnant asthmatic women.[17] Another study reported that women with asthma exacerbations had a larger gestational weight gain in the first trimester of pregnancy and increased total gestational weight gain compared with women without exacerbation. In fact, more than 5 kg first-trimester weight gain was associated with an increased risk of asthma exacerbation (OR 9.35; 95%CI, 6.39–13.68, $P < .01$).[57]

Population-based studies have shown a relationship between smoking and airway hyperresponsiveness (11), implying that smoking is a risk factor for asthma. Tobacco smoke is also a common airway irritant. It has been reported that up to 20% of pregnant asthmatics smoke during pregnancy. Although asthma and smoking during pregnancy have been separately linked to adverse perinatal outcomes such as low birth weight and preterm birth, the combination of asthma and smoking greatly increases the risk of these complications.[58] Women with asthma who smoke may also be at an increased risk of caesarean section.[59] Even passive smoke exposure has been associated with an increased risk of uncontrolled asthma during pregnancy.[60,61]

An increased risk of preterm birth has been linked to exposure to traffic-related air pollutants. There were significant interactions with exposure to nitrogen oxides especially at 35 weeks gestation. Studies have shown increased risk of wheeze in pregnant women exposed to nitrogen oxide, irrespective of continuing or stopping asthma maintenance therapy.[13,62,63]

Infections during pregnancy can certainly affect the course of gestational asthma and be a barrier to asthma control. Some degree of decrease in cell-mediated immunity may make the pregnant patient more susceptible to viral infection, and upper respiratory tract infections have been reported to be the most common precipitants of asthma exacerbations during pregnancy.[25] Sinusitis, a known asthma trigger, has been reported to be 6 times more common in pregnant compared with nonpregnant women.[64] In addition, pneumonia has been reported to be greater than 5 times more common in asthmatic than nonasthmatic women during pregnancy.[65]

Pregnant women are at an increased risk for respiratory viral infections including influenza A (H1N1)[66] and rhinovirus.[15] These infections may be complicated by bronchitis, bacterial pneumonia, and bacterial sinusitis, all of which may have adverse effects on both mother and baby. Therefore, vaccination for influenza for the pregnant asthmatic is an important part of management.

Updated guidelines for the pharmacologic management of asthma during pregnancy
Because pregnant women are generally excluded from clinical trials, there is a lack of adequate prospective efficacy or safety information for most medications taken during pregnancy, especially newer medications, including asthma biologics. Moreover, the existing observational data are often limited by small sample size, and important

confounding information is not always captured. Drug pregnancy registries are limited by the difficulty in raising awareness among clinicians and patients. Even if they meet sample size goals, they may not be adequate in providing definitive evidence of risk or safety. A multiproduct, disease-based approach may help overcome this limitation.[67]

Once the diagnosis of asthma is confirmed, the next step is the assessment of asthma severity (in patients not already on controller therapy) or assessment of control (in patients already on controller therapy; see **Tables 1** and **2**). Patients with intermittent asthma have short episodes and use rescue therapy 2 times or less per week, nocturnal symptoms 2 times or less a month, and normal pulmonary function between episodes. Patients with more frequent symptoms or who require daily asthma medications should be considered to have persistent asthma.

Asthma medications generally are divided into long-term control medications and rescue therapy. Long-term control medications are used for maintenance therapy to prevent asthma manifestations and include ICSs, long-acting beta-agonists, and leukotriene receptor antagonists. Rescue therapy, most commonly inhaled short-acting beta-agonists, provides immediate relief of symptoms. Oral corticosteroids can either be used as a form of rescue therapy or as chronic therapy for severe persistent asthma.

The steps in therapy for patients with asthma during pregnancy are similar to those for the nonpregnant patients with asthma (**Table 3**). Short-acting beta agonists, preferably albuterol, are typically used in Step 1 for intermittent and as rescue therapy. For more persistent symptoms, ICSs are the mainstay of controller therapy during pregnancy.

Commonly prescribed asthma medications
A summary of the gestational safety data for asthma medications is presented in **Table 4**.

Inhaled corticosteroids
The prevalence of ICS use among pregnant women in the United States was recently reported to be around 34%.[48] Many studies have shown no increased perinatal risks (including preeclampsia, preterm birth, low birth weight, and congenital malformations) associated with ICSs.[68–74] Specific safety data is found in **Table 4**.

Budesonide and fluticasone have the most safety data and are considered preferred ICSs for use during pregnancy. That is not to say that the other ICS preparations are unsafe. Therefore, ICSs other than budesonide and fluticasone may be continued in patients who were well controlled by these agents before pregnancy, especially if it is thought that changing formulations may jeopardize asthma control.

Inhaled short-acting beta-agonists
First patented in 1972, albuterol is one of the most commonly used asthma medications. Although there are a lot of reassuring data, there is still some question regarding its safety. Specific safety data is available in **Table 4**. However, the observations in both studies may be a result of confounding since asthma exacerbations may be associated with both increased use of bronchodilators and congenital malformations.

Long-acting beta-agonists
The use of LABA is the preferred add-on controller therapy for asthma during pregnancy. The prevalence of the use of combination ICS and LABA therapy was estimated to be about 45% of pregnant patients with persistent asthma in the United States from a recent report.[75] Because long-acting and short-acting inhaled beta-agonists have similar pharmacology and toxicology, LABAs are expected to have a safety profile similar to that of albuterol. Two LABAs that are available in the United

Table 2
Assessment of asthma control in pregnant women

Variable	Well-Controlled Asthma	Asthma Not Well Controlled	Very Poorly Controlled Asthma
Frequency of symptoms	≤2 d/wk	>2 d/wk	Throughout the day
Frequency of nighttime awakening	≤2 times per month	1–3 times per week	≥ 4 times per week
Interference with normal activity	None	Some	Extreme
Use of short-acting β-agonist for symptoms control	≤2 d/wk	>2 d/wk	Several times per day
FEV_1 or peak flow (% of the predicted or personal best value)	>80	60–80	<60
Exacerbation requiring use of systemic corticosteroid (no.)	0–1 in the past 12 mo	≥2 in the past 12 mo	≥2 in the past 12 mo

From Schatz M, Dombrowski MP. Clinical practice. Asthma in pregnancy. *N Engl J Med.* 2009;360(18):1862-1869.

Table 3
Steps of asthma therapy during pregnancy

Step	Preferred Controller Medication	Alternative Controller Medication
1	None	–
2	Low-dose ICS	LTRA, theophylline ICS + albuterol PRN[a] ICS/formoterol PRN[a]
3	Medium-dose ICS	Low-dose ICS + either LABA, LTRA or theophylline ICS/formoterol PRN[a]
4	Medium-dose ICS + LABA	Medium-dose ICS + LTRA or theophylline
5	High-dose ICS + LABA	• Omalizumab
6	High-dose ICS + LABA + oral prednisone	• Omalizumab

Abbreviations: LTRA, leukotriene-receptor antagonists.
[a] Updated recommendations on asthma therapy from the 2020 Global Initiative for Asthma (GINA) report; however, these recommendations have not been studied specifically during pregnancy.
Modified from Schatz M, Dombrowski MP. Clinical practice. Asthma in pregnancy. N Engl J Med. 2009;360(18):1862-1869.

States have been studied during pregnancy, salmeterol, and formoterol, although the data are limited. Specific safety data is available in **Table 4**. Expert panels suggest that the benefits of the use of LABAs appear to outweigh the risks if they are used concurrently with ICSs.

Leukotriene modifiers
Both zafirlukast and montelukast are selective leukotriene receptor antagonists indicated for the maintenance treatment of asthma. Data on the use of leukotriene receptor antagonists during pregnancy are more limited than for ICSs. Specific safety data is included in **Table 4**. Although the data that are available are reassuring, more data are needed. Leukotriene modifiers are considered alternate add-on therapy for pregnant asthmatic patients with persistent asthma not controlled by ICS.

Anticholinergics
Although there is no available human safety data currently available for inhaled anticholinergic medications such as tiotropium, you may consider for patients uncontrolled on medium-dose or high-dose combination ICS/LABA therapy.

Oral corticosteroids
Some patients with severe asthma may require regular oral corticosteroid use to achieve adequate asthma control. Oral corticosteroids are also typically part of the discharge regimen after an acute asthma episode. Prednisone doses are typically 40 to 60 mg in a single dose or 2 divided doses for 3 to 10 days. Specific safety data may be found in **Table 4**. Because these risks would be less than the potential risks of a severe asthma exacerbation, which include maternal or fetal mortality, oral corticosteroids are still recommended when indicated for the management of severe asthma during pregnancy.

Asthma biologics
Safety of asthma biologics during pregnancy will be covered in another article of this monograph.

Table 4
Safety of commonly used medications for the treatment of asthma during pregnancy

Medication	Major Birth Defects	Other Birth Outcomes
Systemic corticosteroids	Meta-analysis of cohort studies showed no overall increased risk of major birth defects in pooled 535 exposed pregnancies; meta-analysis of 4 case control studies showed an increased risk of ~3-fold for oral clefts.[76] However, most recent and largest case control study from US National Birth Defects Prevention Study showed no increased risk for oral clefts with first trimester systemic steroid use for any indication in 2372 cases and 5922 controls[77]	Preterm delivery, low birth weight or reduced birth weight, preeclampsia and gestational diabetes have all been reported to occur more frequently in women treated with systemic steroids in pregnancy; however, studies that attempted to control for underlying maternal disease and disease activity typically find the associated risks for these outcomes reduced or eliminated[78]
Any ICSs including beclomethasone, budesonide, flunisolide, fluticasone, triamcinolone	No increased risk for major birth defects in 396 exposed compared with the general population.[79] A meta-analysis of studies of inhaled steroids did not find increased risk of major birth defects overall[80]	No increased risks for preterm delivery, low birth weight, or pregnancy-induced hypertension in 396 exposed or in meta-analysis[79]
Budesonide	No increased risk for major birth defects overall or oral clefts among 2014 exposed in population-based Scandinavian register[73]	No increased risks for preterm birth, reduced birth weight or length, or stillbirths in 2968 exposed in population-based Scandinavian register[70]
Fluticasone	No increased risk of major congenital malformations overall in a cohort study of 1602 mother–infant pairs exposed to fluticasone compared with 3678 exposed to other ICS, stratified by severity[81]	No increased risk of low birth weight, preterm birth, or small for gestational age in retrospective database study of infants of 3190 mothers exposed to fluticasone compared with 608 mothers exposed to budesonide[82]
Cromolyn Nedocromil	No increase in major birth defects overall in 296 pregnancies exposed throughout pregnancy[83] No increase in major birth defects overall in 151	No increased risk for premature delivery or spontaneous abortion/stillbirth in 296 pregnancies exposed throughout pregnancy.[83]

(*continued on next page*)

Table 4 (continued)		
Medication	**Major Birth Defects**	**Other Birth Outcomes**
	exposed pregnancies.[69] No overall increase in major birth defects in case control study of 5124 malformed compared with 30,053 controls; 9 cases exposed to cromones; some suggestion of an increased risk for musculoskeletal malformations among the 9 cases but no specific pattern noted[22]	No increased risk for premature delivery, preeclampsia, or low birth weight in 243 women exposed anytime in pregnancy[69]
Montelukast	No increased risk of major birth defects overall in 74 and 180 exposed pregnancies.[84,85] No increased risk in major birth defects overall or specific birth defects in 1164 exposed pregnancies in claims study.[86] No increased risk in major birth defects in 1827 exposed pregnancies in Danish register study[87]	No increased risk for reduced birth weight or shortened gestational age in 180 exposed when compared with other asthmatics[84] No increased risk for preterm delivery, low birth weight or preeclampsia in 1827 exposed compared with other treated asthmatics[87]
Omalizumab	No increased risk compared with general population for major birth defects overall in 169 exposed pregnancies (156 live births) enrolled in a registry[88]	
Short-acting beta-agonists (Primarily albuterol)	No increase in major birth defects over expected among 1090 albuterol-exposed pregnancies in a claims database[89] No increase in major birth defects in 1753 albuterol-exposed pregnancies compared with other asthmatic pregnancies[68] Modest increased risk in isolated cleft lip or cleft palate (odds ratios from 1.65 to 1.79) in albuterol-exposed pregnancies in case control study of 2711 cases of oral clefts	No increase in preterm delivery, low birth weight, or small for gestational age infants in 1828 pregnancies exposed to short-acting beta-agonists compared with other asthmatic pregnancies[68]

(continued on next page)

Table 4 *(continued)*		
Medication	**Major Birth Defects**	**Other Birth Outcomes**
	and 6482 controls[90] Several additional studies have suggested modest increased risks (odds ratios <3) for specific birth defects such as any cardiac or gastroschisis, esophageal atresia, omphalocele[91–93]	
Short-acting beta-agonists (Others)	Ephedrine: No increased risk in major birth defects in 373 exposed[94] Epinephrine: Increased risk for major and minor birth defects overall and specifically for inguinal hernia in 189 exposed[94] Metaproterenol: No excess in major birth defects noted in 361 exposed pregnancies from a database[89] Terbutaline: No increased risk for major birth defects in 149 exposed[89]	
Long-acting beta-agonists	No evidence of increased risk in major birth defects in 65 salmeterol-exposed pregnancies.[95] In one analysis of a database, increased risks for major cardiac and major "other" birth defects were seen with first trimester exposure in 165 pregnancies.[96] However, in a later study from the same database, 841 pregnancies exposed to long-acting beta-agonists with low-dose or medium-dose ICSs showed no increased risk of major birth defects overall compared with pregnancies exposed to medium-dose to high-dose ICSs alone[97]	No difference in low birth weight, preterm birth or small for gestational age was noted in infants of mothers exposed to salmeterol vs formoterol in a retrospective database study[82]
Theophylline	No increase in major birth defects overall in 212, 292 and 273 pregnancies.[68,69,98] Three	

(continued on next page)

Table 4 (continued)		
Medication	**Major Birth Defects**	**Other Birth Outcomes**
	case reports of severe cardiac defects in exposed[99]	
Anticholinergics	No available human safety data	

Modified from Chambers C. Chapter 2: Safety of Asthma and Allergy Medications During Pregnancy. In: Namazy JA, Schatz M, eds. Asthma, Allergic and Immunologic Diseases During Pregnancy: A Guide to Management. 1st ed. Springer Link; 2019: 15-27.

SUMMARY

Asthma is a common medical problem that may worsen during pregnancy. In addition to affecting maternal quality of life, uncontrolled asthma may lead to adverse perinatal outcomes. Awareness of proper treatment options for asthma during pregnancy is important for clinicians who care for pregnant patients to optimize maternal and infant health. One of the most important needs for the future is the availability of additional safety information for asthma medications used during pregnancy that can also account for asthma control.

CLINICS CARE POINTS

- Discussions regarding asthma management should start in the prepregnancy planning period.
- Pregnant patients with asthma should be followed on a monthly basis throughout their pregnancy.
- Enroll patients into pregnancy registries when applicable particularly for asthma biologics.
- Review asthma plan, inhaler technique, medication use at each visit and promote self-management skills.

DISCLOSURE

The authors have nothing to disclose.

REFERENCES

1. Kwon HL, Triche E, Belanger K, et al. The epidemiology of asthma during pregnancy : Prevalence, diagnosis, and symptoms. Immunol Allergy Clin North Am 2006;26(1):29–62.
2. Hansen C, Joski P, Freiman H, et al. Medication exposure in pregnancy risk evaluation program: the prevalence of asthma medication use during pregnancy. Research Support, N.I.H., Extramural Research Support, Non-U.S. Gov'tResearch Support, U.S. Gov't, P.H.S. Matern Child Health J 2013;17(9):1611–21.
3. Williamson G, O'Connor A, Kayleigh E. Women's experiences of personlised support for asthma care during pregnancy: a systematic review of the literature. BMC Pregnancy Childbirth 2017;17:69.

4. Grzeskowia LE, Smith B, Roy A, et al. Patterns,predictors and outcomes of asthma control and exacerbations during pregnancy: a prospective cohort study. Eur Respir J 2016;18(2):00054–2015.

5. Bokem MP, Robijn AL, Jensen ME, et al. Factors associated with asthma exacerbations during pregnancy. J Allergy Cin Immunol Pract 2021;9(12):4343–52.

6. Stevens DR, Perkins N, Chen Z, et al. Determining the clinical course of asthma in pregnancy. J Allergy Cin Immunol Pract 2021;21:01125–9.

7. Ali Z, Nilas L, Ulrik CS. Postpartum airway responsiveness and exacerbation of asthm during pregnancy-a pilot study. J Asthma Allergy 2017;10:261–7.

8. Juniper E, Daniel E, Roberts R, et al. Improvement in airway hyperresponsiveness and asthma severity during pregnancy. a prospective study. Am Rev Respir Dis 1989;140:924–31.

9. Murphy VE, Gibson PG, Giles WB, et al. Maternal asthma is associated with reduced female fetal growth. Am J Respir Crit Care Med 2003;168(11):1317–23.

10. Firoozi F, Ducharme FM, Lemiere C, et al. Effect of fetal gender on maternal asthma exacerbations in pregnant asthmatic women. Respir Med 2009;103(1):144–51.

11. Bakhireva LN, SChatz M, Jones KL, et al. Fetal sex and maternal asthma control in pregnancy. J Asthma 2008;45(5):403–7.

12. Tan KS, McFarlane LC, Lipworth BJ. Paradoxical down-regulation and desensitization of beta2-adrenoceptors by exogenous progesterone in female asthmatics. Chest 1997;111(4):847–51.

13. Murphy VE, Gibson PG, Smith R, et al. Asthma during pregnancy: mechanisms and treatment implications. Eur Respir J 2005;25(4):731–50.

14. Forbes RL, Gibson PG, Murphy VE, et al. Impaired type I and III interferon response to rhinovirus infection during pregnancy and asthma. Thorax 2012;67(3):209–14.

15. Forbes RL, Wark PA, Murphy VE, et al. Pregnant women have attenuated innate interferon responses to the 2009 pandemic influenza A virus subtype H1N1. J Infect Dis 2012;206(5):646–53.

16. Murphy V, Namazy J, Powell H, et al. A meta-analysis of adverse perinatal outcomes in women with asthma. Br J Obstet Gynaecol 2011;118(11):1314–23.

17. Rejno G, lundholm C, Larsson K, et al. Adverse pregnancy outcomes in asthmatic women: a population=based family design study. J Allergy Cin Immunol Pract 2017;6(3):916–22.

18. Yland J, Bateman B, Huybrecht K, et al. Perinatal outcomes associated with maternal asthma and its severity and control during pregnancy. J Allergy Clin Immunol In Pract 2020;8(6):1928–37.e3 (In Press).

19. Rudra CB, Williams MA, Frederick IO, et al. Maternal asthma and risk of preeclampsia: a case-control study. J Reprod Med 2006;51(2):94–100.

20. Murphy VE, Clifton VL, Gibson PG. Asthma exacerbations during pregnancy: incidence and association with adverse pregnancy outcomes. Thorax 2006;61(2):169–76.

21. Namazy J, Murphy V, Powell H, et al. Effects of asthma severity,exacerbations and oral corticosteroids on perinatal outcomes. Eur Respir J 2012;41(5):1082–90.

22. Tata LJ, Lewis SA, McKeever TM, et al. A comprehensive analysis of adverse obstetric and pediatric complications in women with asthma. Am J Respir Crit Care Med 2007;175(10):991–7.

23. Stenius-Aarniala BS, Hedman J, Teramo KA. Acute asthma during pregnancy. Thorax 1996;51(4):411–4.

24. Blais L, Forget A. Asthma exacerbations during the first trimester of pregnancy and the risk of congenital malformations among asthmatic women. J Allergy Clin Immunol 2008;121(6):1379–84.

25. Murphy VE, Gibson P, Talbot PI, et al. Severe asthma exacerbations during pregnancy. Obstet Gynecol 2005;106(5 Pt 1):1046–54.

26. Jana N, Vasishta K, Saha SC, et al. Effect of bronchial asthma on the course of pregnancy, labour and perinatal outcome. J Obstet Gynaecol (Tokyo 1995 1995;21(3):227–32.

27. Greenberger PA, Patterson R. The outcome of pregnancy complicated by severe asthma. Allergy Proc 1988;9(5):539–43.

28. Dombrowski MP, Schatz M, Wise R, et al. Asthma during pregnancy. Obstet Gynecol 2004;103(1):5–12.

29. Breton M-C, Beauchesne M-F, Lemiere C, et al. Risk of perinatal mortality associated with asthma during pregnancy. Thorax 2009;64(2):101–6.

30. Breton M, Beauchesne MF, Lemiere C, et al. Risk of perinatal mortality associated with asthma durng pregnancy: 2-stage sampling cohort study. Ann Allergy Asthma Immunol 2010;105(3):211–7.

31. Kim S, Kim J, Park SY, et al. Effect of pregnancy in asthma on health care use and perinatal outcomes. J Allergy Clin Immunol 2015;136(5):1215–23.

32. Cohen J M, Bateman BT, Huybrechts KF, et al. Poorly controlled asthma during pregnancy remains common in the united states. J Allergy Clin Immunology-In Pract 2019;7(8):2672–80.

33. Firoozi F, Lemiere C, Ducharme FM, et al. Effect of maternal moderate to severe asthma on perinatal outcomes. Respir Med 2010;104(9):1278–87.

34. Triche EW, Saftlas AF, Belanger K, et al. Association of asthma diagnosis, severity, symptoms, and treatment with risk of preeclampsia. Obstet Gynecol 2004;104(3):585–93.

35. Schatz M, Dombrowski MP, Wise R, et al. Spirometry is related to perinatal outcomes in pregnant women with asthma. Am J Obstet Gynecol 2006;194(1):120–6.

36. Mirzakhani H, Carey VJ, McElrath TF, et al. The association of maternal asthma and early pregnnacy vitamin D with risk of Preeclampsia: an observation fro viatmin D antenatal asthma reduction trial. J Allergy Cin Immunol Pract 2017;6:600–8.

37. Eszes N, Toldi G, Bohacs A, et al. Relationship of circulating hyaluronic acid levels to disease control in asthma and asthmatic pregnancy. PLoS One 2014;15(9).

38. Dombai B, Ivancso I, Bikov A, et al. Circulating clusterin and osteopontin levels in asthma and asthmatic pregnancy. Can Respir J 2017;2017:1602039.

39. Tamasi L, Somoskovi A, Muller V, et al. A population-based case-control study on the effect of bronchial asthma during pregnancy for congenital abnormalities of the offspring. J Asthma 2006;43(1):81–6.

40. Powell H, Murphy VE, Taylor DR, et al. Management of asthma in pregnancy guided by measurement of fraction of exhaled nitric oxide: a double-blind, randomised controlled trial. Lancet 2011;378(9795):983–90.

41. Palmsten K, Schatz M, Chan PH, et al. Validation of the Pregnancy Asthma Control Test. J Allergy Clin Immunol 2016;4(2):310–5.e1, in press.

42. Amaral L, Martins C, Coimbra A. Use of the control of allergic rhinitis and asthma test and pulmonary function tests to assess asthma control in pregnancy. Aust N Z J Obstet Gynaecol 2017;58:1–5.

43. Meakin AS, Saif Z, Seedat N, et al. The impact of maternal asthma during pregnancy on fetal growth and development: a review. Expert Rev Resp Med 2020; 14(12):1207–16.
44. Rejno G, Lundholm C, Oberg S, et al. Maternal anxiety,depression and asthma and adverse pregnancy outcomes - a population based study. Sci Rep 2019; 9(1):13101.
45. L Blais, Ahmed SIS, Beauchesne MF, et al. Risk of postpartum depression among women with asthma. J Allergy Cin Immunol Pract 2019;7:925–33.
46. Grzeskowiak LE, Smith B, Roy A. Impact of a history of maternal depression and anxiety on asthma control during pregnancy. J Asthma 2017;54(7):706–13.
47. Lim AS, Stewart K, Abramson MJ, et al. Multidisciplinary Approach to Management of MAternal ASthma (MAMMA): a randomized controlled trial. Chest 2014;145(5):1046–54.
48. Robijn AL, Jensen ME, Gibson PG, et al. Trends in asthma self-management skills and inhaled corticosteroid use during pregnancy and postpartum from 2004-2017. J Asthma 2018;56(6):594–602.
49. Koo YH, Kim Y, Park GW, et al. Effect of pregnancy on quantitative medication use and relation to exacerbations in asthma. Biomed Res Int 2017;2017:8276190.
50. Sawicki E, Stewart K, Wong S, et al. Management of asthma by pregnant women attending an Australian maternity hospital. Aust N Z J Obstet Gynaecol 2012; 52(2):183–8.
51. Lim AS, Stewart K, Abramson MJ, et al. Asthma during pregnancy: the experiences, concerns and views of pregnant women with asthma. J Asthma 2012; 49(5):474–9.
52. Robijn AL, Barker D, Gibson P, et al. Factors associated with nonadherence to inhaled corticosteroids for asthma during pregnancy. J Allergy Cin Immunol Pract 2020;9(3):1242–52.
53. Lim A, Stewart K, Abramson M, et al. Management of pregnant women with asthma by Australian general practitioners. BMC Fam Pract 2011;12:121.
54. Cimbollek S, Plaza V, Quirce S, et al. Knowledge, attitude and adherence of Spanish healthcare professionals to asthma management recommendations during pregnancy. Allergol Immunopathol (Madr) 2012;41(2):114–20.
55. Cydulka R, Emerman C, Schreiber D, et al. Acute asthma among pregnant women presenting to thw emergency department. Am J Respir Crit Care Med 1999;160:887–92.
56. McCallister J, Benninger C, Frey H, et al. Pregnancy related treatement disparities of acute asthma exacerbations in the emergency department. Respir Med 2011;105(10):1434–40.
57. Ali Z, Ulrik CS. Incidence and risk factors for exacerbations of asthma during pregnancy. J Asthma Allergy 2013;6:53–60.
58. Hodyl NA, Stark MJ, Schell W, et al. Perinatal outcomes following maternal asthma and cigarette smokin during pregnancy. Eur Respir J 2014;43(3):704–16.
59. Fazel N, Kundi M, Kazemzadeh A, et al. Environmnetal tobacco smoke exposure during pregnancy affects complications and birth outcomes in women with and without asthma. BMC Pregnancy Childbirth 2020;20(1):314.
60. Murphy VE, Clifton VL, Gibson PG. The effect of cigarette smoking on asthma control during exacerbations in pregnant women. Thorax 2010;65(8):739–44.
61. Grarup PA, Janner JH, Ulrik CS. Passive smoking is associated with poor asthma control during pregnancy: a prospective study of 500 pregnancies. PLoS One 2014;9(11):e112435.

62. Gent JF, Kezik JM, Hill ME. Asthma medication use during pregnancy, wheeze and estimated exposure to ambient nitrogen dioxide. Eur Respir J 2015;45(2): 538–40.

63. Mendola P, Wallace M, Hwang BS. Preterm birth and air pollution: critical windows of exposure for women with asthma. J Allergy Cin Immunol 2016;138(2): 432–40.

64. Sorri M, Hartikainen A, Karja I. Rhinitis during pregnancy. Rhinology 1980; 18(2):83–6.

65. Munn M, Groome L, Atterbury J. Pneumonia as a complication of pregnancy. J Matern Fetal Med 1999;8:151–4.

66. Cox S, Posner SF, McPheeters M, et al. Hospitalizations with respiratory illness among pregnant women during influenza season. J Obstet Gynecol 2006;107: 1315–22.

67. Chambers C, Krishnan JA, Alba L, et al. The safety of asthma medications during pregnancy and lactation:clinical management and research priorities. J Allergy Cin Immunol 2021;147(6):2009–20.

68. Schatz M, Dombrowski MP, Wise R, et al. The relationship of asthma medication use to perinatal outcomes. J Allergy Clin Immunol 2004;113(6):1040–5.

69. Schatz M, Zeiger RS, Harden K, et al. The safety of asthma and allergy medications during pregnancy. J Allergy Clin Immunol 1997;100(3):301–6.

70. Norjavaara E, de Verdier MG. Normal pregnancy outcomes in a population-based study including 2,968 pregnant women exposed to budesonide. J Allergy Clin Immunol 2003;111(4):736–42.

71. Bracken MB, Triche EW, Belanger K, et al. Asthma symptoms, severity, and drug therapy: a prospective study of effects on 2205 pregnancies. Obstet Gynecol 2003;102(4):739–52.

72. Martel MJ, Rey E, Beauchesne MF, et al. Use of inhaled corticosteroids during pregnancy and risk of pregnancy induced hypertension: nested case-control study. BMJ 2005;330(7485):230.

73. Kallen B, Rydhstroem H, Aberg A. Congenital malformations after the use of inhaled budesonide in early pregnancy. Obstet Gynecol 1999;93(3):392–5.

74. Bakhireva LN, Jones KL, Schatz M, et al. Asthma medication use in pregnancy and fetal growth. J Allergy Clin Immunol 2005;116(3):503–9.

75. Murphy VE, Jensen JS, Gibson P. Asthma during pregnancy: exacerbations, management, and health outcomes for mother and infant. Semin Respir Crit Care Med 2017;38:160–73.

76. Park-Wyllie LMP, Pastuszak A, et al. Birth defects after maternal exposure to corticosteroids: Prospective cohort study and meta-analysis of epidemiologic studies. Teratology 2000;62:385–92.

77. Skuladottir H, Wilcox AJ, Ma C, et al. Corticosteroid use and risk of orofacial clefts. Birth Defects Res A Clin Mol Teratol 2014;100(6):499–506.

78. Palmsten K, Bandoli G, Watkins J, et al. Oral corticosteroids and risk of preterm borth in the california medicaid program. J Allergy Cin Immunol Pract 2021;9: 375–84.

79. Namazy J, Schatz M, Long L, et al. Use of inhaled steroids by pregnant asthmatic women does not reduce intrauterine growth. J Allergy Clin Immunol 2004;113(3): 427–32.

80. Rahimi R, Nikfar S, Abdollahi M. Meta-analysis finds use of inhaled corticosteroids during pregnancy safe: a systematic meta-analysis review. Hum Exp Toxicol 2006;25(8):447–52.

81. Charlton RA, Hutchison A, Davis KJ, et al. Asthma management in pregnancy. Research Support, Non-U.S. Gov't. PLoS One 2013;8(4):e60247.
82. Cossette B, Beauchesne MF, Forget A, et al. Relative perinatal safety of salmeterol vs formoterol and fluticasone vs budesonide use during pregnancy. Comparative Study Research Support, Non-U.S. Gov't. Ann Allergy Asthma Immunol 2014;112(5):459–64.
83. Wilson J. Use of sodium cromoglycate during pregnancy: results on 296 asthmatic women. Acta Therap 1982;8(Suppl):45–51.
84. Sarkar M, Koren G, Kalra S, et al. Montelukast use during pregnancy;a multicentre,prospective,comparative study of infant outcomes. Eur J Clin Pharmacol 2009;65(12):1259–64.
85. Bakhireva LN, Jones KL, Schatz M, et al. Safety of leukotriene receptor antagonists in pregnancy. J Allergy Clin Immunol 2007;119(3):618–25.
86. Nelsen LM, Shields KE, Cunningham ML, et al. Congenital malformationsamong infants born to women receiving montelukast, inhlaed corticosteroids, and other asthma medications. J Allergy Clin Immunol 2012;129(1):251–4, e6.
87. Cavero-Carbonell C, Vinketl-Hansen A, Rabanque-Hernandez MJ, et al. Fetal exposure to montelukast and congenital anomalies: a population based study in Denmark. Birth Defects Original Res 2017;109:452–9.
88. Namazy J, Cabana M, Scheuerle A, et al. The Xolair pregnancy registry(EXPECT):An observational study of Omalizumab during pregnancy in women with asthma. Am J Respir Crit Care Med 2012;185:A4221.
89. Briggs GG, Freeman RK, Towers CV, et al. Drugs in pregnancy and lactation : a reference guide to fetal and neonatal risk. 11th edition. Wolters Kluwer; 2017. p. 1646, xiii.
90. Munsie JP SL, Browne ML, et al. Maternal bronchodilator use and the risk of orofacial clefts. Hum Reprod 2011;26:3147–54.
91. Lin S, Herdt-Losavio M, Gensburg L, et al. Maternal, asthma medication use, and the risk of congenital heart defects. Borth Defects Res A Clin Mol Teratol 2009; 85(2):161–8.
92. Garne E, Hansen AV, Morris J, et al. Use of asthma medicaiton during pregnancy adn risk of specific congenital anomalies:A European case-malformed control study. J Allergy Clin Immunol 2015;136:1496–502.
93. Lin S, Munsie JPW, Herdt-Losavio ML, et al. Maternal asthma medication use and the risk of selected birth defects. Pediatrics 2012;129:e317–24.
94. Heinonen OP, Slone D, Shapiro S. Birth defects and drugs in pregnancy Massachusetts: Publishing Sciences Group; 1977. p. 516, xi.
95. Wilton LV, Pearce GL, Martin RM, et al. The outcomes of pregnancy in women exposed to newly marketed drugs in general practice in England. Br J Obstet Gynaecol 1998;105(8):882–9.
96. Eltonsy S, Forget A, Blais L. Beta2-agonists use during pregnancy and the risk of congenital malformations. Birth Defects Res A Clin Mol Teratol 2011;91(11): 937–47.
97. Eltonsy S, Forget A, Beauchesne MF, et al. Risk of congenital malformations for asthmatic pregnant women using long-acting beta-agonist and inhaled corticosteroid combination versus higher-dose inhlaed corticosteroid monotherapy. J Allergy Clin Immunol 2015;135(1):123–30.
98. Stenius-Aarniala B, Riikonen S, Teramo K. Slow-release theophylline in pregnant asthmatics. Chest 1995;107(3):642–7.
99. Park JM, Schmer V, Myers TL. Cardiovascular anomalies associated with prenatal exposure to theophylline. South Med J 1990;83:487–8.

Status Asthmaticus Gravidus

Emergency and Critical Care Management of Acute Severe Asthma During Pregnancy

Charles B. Cairns, MD[a],*, Monica Kraft, MD[b]

KEYWORDS

- Acute asthma • Pregnancy • Emergency department • ED • Critical care • ICU
- Treatment • Critical asthma syndrome

KEY POINTS

- One-third of women with asthma have deterioration of their asthma during pregnancy and one-fourth of pregnant women with asthma will have acute exacerbations requiring emergency department (ED) visits or hospitalizations. The highest risk for acute exacerbations is during the second and third trimesters with a peak incidence around 6 months gestation.
- Nearly one-half of women with asthma will reduce asthma medication use during pregnancy. Acute asthma exacerbations in pregnancy can result from undertreated disease, recent exposure to viruses and environmental triggers, physiological changes due to pregnancy or a combination of all these factors.
- Prompt recognition of acute severe asthma is critical. Consensus recommendations for the initial acute management strategies in the ED and intensive care unit settings are similar for pregnant and nonpregnant patients and include immediate β2-agonists, systemic corticosteroids, and anticholinergic agents. Patients with severe distress or unresponsive to repeated β2-agonist therapy are in status asthmaticus (critical asthma syndrome).
- Additional guideline-based treatment options to enhance maternal and fetal oxygenation during status asthmaticus gravidus (status asthmaticus in pregnancy) include magnesium, heliox, leukotriene antagonists, xanthines, intravenous β-agonists, antibiotics, anesthetics, and noninvasive positive pressure ventilation. In the rare cases of impending respiratory failure or arrest, invasive mechanical ventilation and even extracorporeal membrane oxygenation should be considered.

---

[a] College of Medicine, Medical Affairs, Drexel University, 245 N. 15th Street, 19th Floor, Philadelphia, PA 19102, USA; [b] Samuel Bronfman Department of Medicine, Icahn School of Medicine at Mount Sinai, Mount. One Gustav Levy Place, PO Box 1118, Annenberg 5-02, New York, NY 10029, USA
* Corresponding author.
E-mail address: cbc77@drexel.edu

Immunol Allergy Clin N Am 43 (2023) 87–102
https://doi.org/10.1016/j.iac.2022.07.010
0889-8561/23/© 2022 Elsevier Inc. All rights reserved.
immunology.theclinics.com

INTRODUCTION

Asthma is a common disease that is more common in women and that effects 4% to 12% of all pregnancies.[1–6] One-third of women with asthma have deterioration of their asthma during pregnancy, and one-fourth of pregnant women with asthma will experience severe exacerbations, necessitating emergency department (ED) visits or hospitalizations.[1,7]

Asthma-related morbidity and mortality is generally high during pregnancy, although variable across patients.[1,6] Generally, a third of pregnant patients experience worse asthma control, a third will have clinical improvement, and a third will experience no change.[8] In addition, nearly half of pregnant women experience exacerbations.[6] Acute asthma exacerbations remain a common reason why pregnant patients seek emergency care.[9–11]

Reasons for these asthma exacerbations include undertreated disease (including medication noncompliance), exposure to triggers (viruses and allergens), and physiological changes due to pregnancy.[6,12] Pregnant women are at particular risk for undertreatment given that half of women with asthma discontinue bronchodilator medications during pregnancy.[13] This undertreatment is thought to be due to the lack of understanding about asthma and to the concern that medical treatment can affect the health of the fetus.[6] One study found that despite dedicated educational interventions, pregnant asthma patients demonstrated reductions in the use of key asthma medications including inhaled corticosteroids (23%), short-acting beta-agonists (13%), and oral corticosteroids (54%).[14]

In addition, asthma is more common in women and can result in more frequent hospitalizations and serious complications, especially during the gestational ages of women from 20 to 50 years.[6] Asthma disease severity is related to estrogen levels during menstruation and that asthma exacerbations occur at a higher rate before pregnancy.[6] The asthma disease course during pregnancy may be due to the variable balance between the protective effects of cortisol and progesterone levels versus deleterious effects of increased levels of bronchoconstrictors during pregnancy, such as prostaglandin F2α.[6]

The purpose of this review is to describe an approach to the management of acute severe asthma in pregnancy, including status asthmaticus, in the ED and intensive care unit (ICU). Per consensus recommendations, early and aggressive interventions are necessary to treat severe acute asthma exacerbations in pregnant women and to minimize the risk for maternal and fetal hypoxia. Acute asthma exacerbations importantly affect not only fetal morbidity and mortality during pregnancy but also maternal, including an increased risk of preeclampsia, gestational diabetes, placental abruption, and placenta previa.[6,15,16] There is also a significant association between severe asthma exacerbations in the first trimester of pregnancy and congenital malformations.[6]

Characteristics of Pregnant Patients with Acute Asthma Exacerbations

Asthma is clinically characterized by recurrent episodes of wheezing, shortness of breath, and cough secondary to reversible airflow obstruction.[6,12,17] A key pathophysiological aspect of asthma is airways hyperresponsiveness, especially in response to factors and environmental conditions that provoke airway inflammation such as viral infections and allergens.[6,12,17]

This airways hyperresponsiveness and inflammation can lead to asthma exacerbations during pregnancy, most commonly in the second and third trimesters of gestation.[1] Reasons for these asthma exacerbations include undertreated disease, exposure to triggers (viral infections, allergens) and physiological changes due to pregnancy.[6,12] Pregnant women are at particular risk for undertreatment given that half of women with asthma discontinue bronchodilator medications during pregnancy.[13] As discussed above, undertreatment is thought to be due to the lack of understanding about asthma, the importance of anti-inflammatory therapy even during pregnancy, and the concern that medical treatment can affect the health of the fetus.[6,14]

Physiological respiratory, hormonal, immune system changes during pregnancy also have the potential adversely affect the course of asthma, resulting in exacerbations.[4,18,19] Indeed, pregnancy results in multiple complex mechanical, biochemical and physiologic changes in the respiratory system. Yet key pulmonary physiological parameters relevant to asthma do not change during pregnancy.[4,19] Importantly, there are no significant change in respiratory rate, arterial oxygen saturation (SaO_2), vital capacity, lung compliance, and diffusion capacity (DLCO) measurements during pregnancy.[4,19] Importantly, in the nonasthma pregnancy state, measures of forced vital capacity (FVC), forced expiratory volume in one second (FEV_1), the ratio of FEV_1 to FVC, and peak expiratory flow rate (PEFR) do not change significantly.[4,19] Thus, any changes in FEV_1 or PEFR during pregnancy can be related to asthma-related airflow obstruction.

Acute exacerbations requiring emergency visits and hospitalization are more common in patients who have severe persistent asthma.[20] In addition, African American women experience more asthma morbidity than do white women, including increased rates of rescue corticosteroids, ED visits, and hospitalizations during pregnancy.[21]

Risk factors for acute asthma exacerbations during pregnancy have been identified from multiple cohort series. These risk factors include comorbidities (obesity), behaviors (smoking), disease states (gastrointestinal reflux), multiparity, inadequate prenatal care, weight increase in the first trimester, noncompliance, and greater prepregnancy asthma severity.[1,4,19,22–24] A summary of the risk factors for acute asthma exacerbations in pregnant patients are listed in **Box 1**.

MANAGEMENT OF ACUTE EXACERBATIONS DURING PREGNANCY

The management of acute asthma exacerbations during pregnancy includes physiologic assessment, including maternal and fetal monitoring, and immediate pharmacologic

---

Box 1
Risk factors for worsening asthma during pregnancy

Smoking

Obesity

Gastrointestinal reflux

Multiparity

Inadequate prenatal care

Weight increase in the first trimester

Inappropriate medication use (inhaled corticosteroids)

Greater prepregnancy asthma severity
- History of asthma exacerbations in the year preceding pregnancy
- Medium to high doses (>500 µg daily) of inhaled corticosteroids
- Written asthma action plan (with potential medication nonadherence)
- Worse asthma control measured by standard tools (Asthma Control Questionnaire)

Data from References[1,4,22–24,80]

treatment. The goals of emergency treatment are to maintain maternal oxygen saturation at 94% to 98% to prevent fetal hypoxia[10,18,25] and to relieve airflow obstruction.[26]

Recommended primary pharmacologic treatment is similar per consensus guidelines for both pregnant and general adult populations.[1,12,23,26] Early recognition of acute severe asthma, including life-threatening status asthmaticus, and aggressive medical interventions with β2-agonists, anticholinergic agents, and systemic corticosteroids are necessary to treat maternal exacerbations, to support maternal and fetal oxygenation, and to avoid adverse fetal outcomes.[1,4,6]

Assessment

Per the Global Initiative for Asthma (GINA) guidelines, emergency interventions for asthma should be guided by pulmonary function tests, FEV_1, PEFR, vital signs, chest and heart examinations, and the patient's subjective assessment of dyspnea.[17,26]

Status Asthmaticus

Status asthmaticus is an acute severe asthma condition that can directly lead to respiratory exhaustion and death. Status asthmaticus is defined as an acute severe asthma exacerbation that does not respond to aggressive use of repeated courses of β-agonist therapy.[27] Status asthmaticus can be considered a *critical asthma syndrome*, a term that also includes acute severe asthma, refractory asthma, and near fatal asthma, all of these conditions can lead to respiratory arrest.[27,28]

Airway function

Per the GINA guidelines, spirometry is recommended in confirming the diagnosis of asthma and peak flow measurements are recommended in the assessment of patients with acute asthma exacerbations.[1,17] Spirometry provides more information regarding the pattern of respiratory disease and is more sensitive in measuring airflow obstruction. *In acute severe asthma exacerbations, early treatment with oxygen, β2-agonists and steroids take precedence over spirometry.*[1,12,17]

Physical examination

A focused physical examination (airway, lungs, heart) should be performed rapidly with particular attention to vital signs, maternal oxygen saturation, and the work of breathing.[26] If feasible, fetal monitoring should be performed to help detect fetal distress.[26] Further assessment of the severity of the asthma exacerbation is accomplished by reviewing speech, physical signs, peak flow measurements, and maternal pulse oximetry as outlined in **Table 1**.[12,17]

Ancillary studies

Blood tests are rarely helpful in the assessment of asthma exacerbations. Arterial blood gas measurements need to be obtained only in pregnant patients who

Table 1 Initial clinical assessment of severity in acute asthma in pregnancy		
Findings	**Mild/Moderate**	**Severe**
Speaking in	Sentences or phrases	Words or unresponsive
Respiratory rate	18–29/min	>30/min
Heart rate	100–120 beats/min	>120 beats/min
Peak Flow/FEV_1 (% predicted)	50%–75%	<50%
Pulse oximetry (room air)	90%–95%	<90%

Data from References[12,17]

experience severe or prolonged asthma attacks.[26] As gestation progresses, the normal arterial partial pressure of carbon dioxide ($PaCO_2$) decreases to between 27 and 32 mm of mercury (mm Hg).[8] Thus, a $PaCO_2$ greater than 35 mm Hg during an asthma exacerbation in pregnancy indicates severe airway obstruction with impending ventilatory failure.[26]

Similarly, chest X-rays are needed only for suspected pulmonary pathologic condition (pneumonia, pneumothorax, pneumomediastinum) or if there is minimal response to aggressive bronchodilator therapy.[1,17,29,30] Generally, electrocardiography is unlikely to help guide acute management, except to rule out suspected cardiac issues (arrhythmias, ischemia).[26]

Importantly, blood glucose should be monitored closely because high doses of β2-agonists can result in maternal hyperglycemia with significant effects on the fetus.[18] The risk of paradoxical neonatal hypoglycemia is greater if high doses of β-agonists have been administered within 48 hours before delivery, especially in preterm infants.[10,18]

Pharmacologic Treatment

As noted above, pharmacologic treatments for acute asthma exacerbations are similar per consensus guidelines for both pregnant and general adult populations.[1,12,17,23,26] Robust evidence from clinical interventional trials in acute severe asthma are few and even less so in pregnant patients with severe asthma.[17]

Aggressive treatment with repeated doses of β2-agonists and early systemic corticosteroids are the primary treatment of patients with acute severe asthma in pregnancy. Oxygen is recommended for use to maintain arterial oxygen saturation between 94% and 98%.[10,18] Pregnancy treatment options for acute asthma adapted from the GINA,[17] National Asthma Education and Prevention Program (NAEPP),[23] British,[25] and Australian[31] guidelines are presented as a stepwise approach in **Fig. 1**. An overview of specific medications is summarized in **Table 2**.

Inhaled β2-agonists

Beta-adrenergic agonists used in asthma activate the β2-adrenergic receptor to inhibit bronchial smooth muscle contractility, leading to bronchodilation and reduced airway hyperresponsiveness.[19] Inhaled albuterol is the primary β2-agonist used for bronchodilation in acute asthma management.[17] Although both multidose inhalers and nebulized routes are similar in efficacy in acute asthma exacerbations, nebulized administration is preferred for ED patients due to the simplicity of delivery and use in severely ill patients.[1,32,33]

Continuous administration of albuterol (defined as 2.5–5 mg albuterol every 15 minutes or 4 or greater albuterol nebulizations per hour) has been shown to improve pulmonary function compared with intermittent albuterol nebulization in acute severe asthma exacerbations.[1,34]

Systemic corticosteroids

Corticosteroids suppress both airway and systemic type 2 inflammation in acute severe asthma mainly by inhibiting eosinophils.[19] Early administration of systemic corticosteroids (within 1 hour) speeds resolution of exacerbations and reduces the need for hospital admission.[1,12,17,35–37] Double-blind, randomized trials have clearly demonstrated that IV and oral corticosteroids have comparable efficacy.[17] For acute severe asthma exacerbations, intravenous corticosteroids are recommended given the challenges of severe dyspnea, vomiting, and ventilatory support.[17]

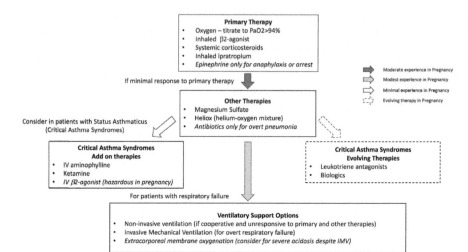

Fig. 1. *Stepwise approach to therapeutic options in pregnant patients with acute severe asthma.* Stepwise approach to therapy in pregnant patients with severe asthma. Moderate experience for use in pregnancy includes asthma therapies published multiple clinical studies in pregnant patients, modest experience consists of multiple published asthma cohort studies in pregnant patients, minimal experience consists of published asthma case reports and case series in pregnant patients, evolving therapies for pregnant patients with acute asthma are described further in the text. (*Abbreviation:* IMV, invasive mechanical ventilation); IV, intravenous; SaO₂, arterial oxygen saturation.

Table 2
Guideline recommended pharmacologic options in acute severe asthma

PRIMARY MEDICATIONS	
Oxygen	Initially 100%, titrate to SaO_2 >94%
β-agonists	Inhaled albuterol 0.5 mg every 20 min × 3
Corticosteroids	Prednisone 60 mg orally ×1 per day (up to 5 days)
	Consider 2 mg/kg methylprednisolone IV load in patients unable to tolerate oral medications
Anticholinergics	Inhaled ipratropium 0.5 mg every 30 min × 3
OTHER OPTIONS FOR STATUS ASTHMATICUS GRAVIDUS (Critical Asthma Syndromes)	
Epinephrine (anaphylaxis)	0.3–0.5 mg intramuscular injection every 5 to 15 min
	Consider 0.1 mcg/kg/min IV in near arrest states
Magnesium sulfate	Adults—2 g IV infusion over 20 min
Heliox	80%helium/20% oxygen, titrate up to 50%helium/50%oxygen to maintain SaO_2 >94%.
Aminophylline	Loading dose 5 mg/kg IV, followed by infusion of 0.5 mg/kg/h
IV Albuterol	Loading dose 200 μg IV over 1 min, then 5 μg/min (can increase to 10 μg/min, then up to 20 μg/min every 15–30 min according to response)
Ketamine	Loading dose 0.2 mg/kg IV followed by 0.5 mg/kg per hour × 2 h

Abbreviations: IV, intravenous; SaO₂, arterial oxygen saturation.
  Data from References[17,23,25,31]

Ipratropium bromide

Ipratropium bromide is an anticholinergic agent that antagonizes muscarinic receptors to inhibit vagal nerve tone to the airways resulting in bronchodilation.[19] Addition of multiple doses of inhaled ipratropium bromide to early β2-agonist treatments improve expiratory flow measurements (FEV_1, PEFR) and reduces hospital admissions, especially for severe asthma exacerbations.[17] Thus, the anticholinergic ipratropium bromide should be added to β2-agonists for patients with moderate-to-severe exacerbations of asthma in the emergency and critical care settings.[1,12]

Epinephrine

Epinephrine is both an α-adrenergic and β2-adrenergic receptor agonist. Although routine use of epinephrine is not endorsed in asthma, epinephrine is recommended for acute severe asthma associated with allergic anaphylaxis.[17] However, systemic epinephrine should be avoided in pregnancy due to placental and uterine vasoconstriction.[38]

Other Treatments

Most pregnant patients with acute severe asthma respond to aggressive therapy with inhaled β2-agonists, anticholinergics, and early systematic steroids.[1,39] For those patients that do not respond to this initial therapy, including those with status asthmaticus and other critical asthma syndromes, international consensus guideline recommend consideration of additional therapies such as magnesium.[17] Please note that the evidence base from clinical interventional trials in acute severe asthma is limited. In particular, the data on these interventions are truly minimal in pregnant patients with acute severe asthma.

Magnesium

Magnesium has been shown to inhibit extracellular calcium influx resulting in both bronchial smooth muscle relaxation and inhibition of inflammatory cell responses.[1,12,40,41] Magnesium is considered safe in pregnancy and is frequently used during pregnancy for multiple conditions, including neuroprotection for prematurity.[42] Evidence from systematic reviews indicates that intravenous magnesium sulfate provides benefits in acute asthma, especially in patients with acute severe asthma exacerbations.[1,12,17,43,44] Nebulized inhaled magnesium sulfate, in addition to β-agonist in the treatment of an acute asthma exacerbation, also seems to have benefit with respect to improved pulmonary function and reduced rates of hospital admission from the ED.[1,12,17,45,46]

Furthermore, magnesium has been studied in pregnant patients with acute asthma. In a study of 60 pregnant patients with acute asthma in the ED, inhaled magnesium sulfate resulted in improved lung function and reduced exacerbations.[47]

Heliox (helium-oxygen)

Helium oxygen mixtures (heliox) have lower densities than air and have been used to improve laminar airflow in emergency and critical care settings.[1] A systemic review suggests that the benefit of heliox on airway function in acute asthma may be limited to patients with severe exacerbations.[1,48,49] Some guidelines suggest using nebulized albuterol with heliox (starting with 80% helium/20% oxygen and titrating oxygen concentration as needed to keep SaO_2 >94%) in patients with life-threatening acute severe exacerbations or in those with no improvement with recommended therapies after 1 hour.[1,12,50] Recent expert opinion suggests discontinuing heliox if no effect is seen within 15 minutes of use.[39,51]

Leukotriene antagonists

Leukotriene receptor antagonists (LTRAs) can improve symptoms in asthma and enhance both proximal and distal lung functions.[52] There are additional anti-inflammatory effects of LTRAs beyond those provided by corticosteroids,[53] particularly in severe asthma.[54] Some studies have shown improvement in lung function with LTRA in acute asthma but the impact on hospital admission and other clinical parameters is unclear and requires more study.[1,17,55,56] Current international consensus guidelines conclude that there is only limited evidence to support a role for oral or intravenous LTRAs in acute asthma.[1,17]

Antibiotics

International consensus guidelines recommend the use of antibiotics in patients with acute asthma only for patients with strong evidence of lung infection (fever, purulent sputum or X-ray findings of pneumonia).[1,17] Although a meta-analysis suggested that antibiotics may improve symptoms of asthma patients without obvious signs or symptoms,[57] a recent large-scale cohort study in children admitted for acute asthma exacerbations found that routine antibiotic use was associated with an increased length of hospitalization and no clinical benefit.[58]

Intravenous aminophylline

Methylxanthines, such as aminophylline and theophylline, are nonselective phosphodiesterase inhibitors, adenosine receptor antagonists, and histone deacetylase activators.[59] These actions can result in airway smooth muscle relaxation, bronchodilation and reduced inflammatory gene activation.[59] The GINA guidelines do not recommend the use of aminophylline in the acute treatment of asthma, even in acute severe exacerbations.[1,17] Indeed, intravenous aminophylline (theophylline) has been shown to add little bronchodilation to the use of β2-agonists and increases adverse effects.[60] The Australian national guidelines suggest the use of intravenous aminophylline as a third-line agent for patients unresponsive to continuous inhaled β2-agonists and intravenous magnesium.[31]

Intravenous β-agonists

Although the GINA guidelines do not recommend the use of intravenous β2-agonists in the acute treatment of asthma, there may be a role in patients with life-threatening acute severe exacerbations, including status asthmaticus and other critical asthma syndromes.[1,31] The Australian national guidelines suggest the use of intravenous salbutamol (albuterol) for patients unresponsive to continuous inhaled β2-agonists and intravenous magnesium.[31] Furthermore, the Australian clinical guidelines also suggest the use of intramuscular or subcutaneous injection of terbutaline or epinephrine in the critically ill or rapidly deteriorating patient with acute severe asthma exacerbations.[1,31] However, intravenous β2-agonists can be particularly hazardous in pregnancy. Systemic β2-agonists can cause placental and uterine vasoconstriction as well as paradoxical hypoglycemia in the fetus, especially if given within 48 hours of delivery.[10,18,38]

Biologics

Recently, biological agents have been used to rapidly reduce eosinophil counts in patients with asthma. Benralizumab, a biologic that binds to the IL-5 receptor, has been shown to reduce blood eosinophils after a single dose.[39] In one study of ED patients with acute asthma, single-dose benralizumab therapy given up to 7 days after a qualifying exacerbation, reduced the rate and severity of subsequent exacerbations over the next 12 weeks.[61] Omalizumab, a humanized recombinant monoclonal anti-IgE antibody, has been used recently for rescue treatment in acute severe asthma refractory to β2-agonists, ipratropium, and corticosteroids.[62,63] However, none of these biologics is approved for the treatment of acute asthma exacerbations.[39,62] Data on the use of these biologics in pregnancy are sparse.

Ketamine

Ketamine and other anesthetic agents have been proposed as adjuncts for the treatment of acute severe asthma exacerbations refractory to other therapies. Ketamine is an N-methyl-D-aspartate receptor antagonist that can have dosing-related bronchodilatory effects without causing respiratory depression.[39] A meta-analysis of ketamine use in acute asthma in children demonstrated minimal additional benefit of ketamine.[64] The British acute asthma guidelines note the potential value of bronchodilation but conclude that evidence is insufficient to recommend.[25] Ketamine is classified as category B for safety in pregnancy by the United States Food and Drug Administration (FDA).[38] Expert opinion suggests that ketamine may be useful in patients with critical asthma states, including status asthmaticus in pregnant patients, to facilitate noninvasive ventilation (NIV) and as an induction agent for intubation.[1,38,39]

Ventilatory Support

The mainstay of therapy in acute severe asthma exacerbations in pregnancy is aggressive pharmacologic therapy with inhaled β2-agonists, ipratropium, and early systemic corticosteroids. In patients are unresponsive to this, then use of the alternative other pharmacological options is reasonable. Only if a patient has signs of impending respiratory failure should assisted ventilation be considered.

Assisted ventilation can include NIV, invasive mechanical ventilation (IMV), and extracorporeal membrane oxygenation (ECMO). A trial of NIV may be beneficial for pregnant patients with acute severe asthma unresponsive to initial medical therapy.[1,27,38,39,62,65] Endotracheal intubation and IMV may be needed if the respiratory failure is progressing despite aggressive pharmacological therapy.[38,39,62,65] ECMO should be considered in patients who remain severely acidotic and hypercapnic despite conventional critical care therapy.[39,62,65]

Noninvasive ventilation

Noninvasive positive pressure ventilation has the advantage that it can be applied intermittently for short periods, which may be sufficient to reverse the breathing problems experienced by patients during severe acute asthma.[1,12] However, the effectiveness of NIV in acute severe asthma exacerbations remains unclear.[1,12,39] International consensus asthma guidelines state that there is insufficient data regarding the use of NIV in the acute treatment of asthma for it to be recommended.[17] A systematic review concluded that there was insufficient evidence that NIV in acute asthma had significant impact on the clinical outcomes but only 2 small studies even qualified for review.[66,67] A recent large cohort study in nonpregnant patients suggests that NIV is associated with improved outcomes, including reduced need for mechanical ventilation, reduced hospitalizations and improved respiratory rate and lung function measurements.[68]

There are few studies of the use of NIV in severe acute asthma in pregnancy, mainly case reports.[69,70] There are some concerns about using NIV in pregnant patients given the risk of aspiration due to pregnancy-induced increased abdominal pressure and reduced esophageal sphincter tone.[71] In these cases, NIV was successfully used in patients who were fully conscious, cooperative, and able to maintain an upright position.[69–71]

Thus, a trial of NIV in alert, cooperative, upright sitting patients may be reasonable in care centers with expertise and experience in NIV therapy using inspiratory pressure of 10 to 15 cm H_2O and an expiratory pressure of 4 to 8 cm H_2O to start, and with a fraction of inspired oxygen titrated for arterial oxygen saturation of 94% to 98%.[39,69–71] Garner and colleagues[39] recommend intubation if no improvement occurs within 30 to 60 minutes of NIV initiation.

Invasive mechanical ventilation

Patients with overt respiratory distress, unconsciousness, hemodynamic instability, and inadequate oxygenation (or who fail a trial of NIV) should be intubated and mechanically ventilated.[1,39,71] The goals of IMV are to improve the delivery of inhaled bronchodilators, minimize the work of breathing, provide sufficient oxygenation, and improve gas exchange while minimizing the risk of dynamic hyperinflation.[1,39,71] Dynamic hyperinflation occurs when the inhaled tidal volume exceeds the volume that can be exhaled due to airflow limitation and alveolar air trapping.[71,72]

Intubation and IMV is a particular challenge in pregnant patients with intubation failure rates more than 8 times that in nonpregnant patients.[71,73,74] Anatomic changes during pregnancy can result in smaller upper airway caliber (due to mucosal edema and capillary engorgement), increased thoracic weight (due to breast enlargement) and increased risk of aspiration (due to increased abdominal pressure and decreased lower esophageal sphincter tone).[65,71,74] Thus, one should prepare for a difficult intubation with the heads-up position at a 20° to 30° degree angle.[74] Some authors recommend using an endotracheal tube 0.5 cm smaller than recommended for a similarly sized nonpregnant women with 7.0 cm endotracheal tube fitting most patients.[65] Suggested initial ventilator settings include: tidal volume of 6 to 8 mL/kg ideal weight, respiratory rate of 10 to 12 breaths/min, inspiratory flow of 60 to 75 L/min, positive end-expiratory pressure (PEEP) at 5 cm H_2O.[1,39,74] The goal is to keep the plateau pressure less than 30 cm H_2O by titrating tidal volume or respiratory rate and keeping intrinsic PEEP less than 10 cm H_2O.[1,39,74] Although permissive hypercapnia as a ventilator strategy is recommended in asthma, hypercarbia can reduce uterine blood flow and reduce fetal oxygen availability by unfavorably shifting the fetal oxyhemoglobin curve toward the right.[74] Thus, it is recommended in pregnant patients, to try to keep $PaCO_2$ less than 50 to 60 mm Hg.[65,71]

There are few data on prolonged sedation in pregnancy. Chan and colleagues[38] recommended propofol as the preferred sedative in pregnancy given its safe FDA designation (category B) and potential for bronchodilation. In addition, they suggested the avoidance of benzodiazepines in pregnant asthmatic patients given its unfavorable FDA designation (category D) and potential for late-term effects (neonatal withdrawal syndrome).[38] If short-term neuromuscular paralysis is needed in the intubated pregnant asthmatic patients, cisatracurium (FDA category B) is the recommended agent.[38]

Extracorporeal membrane oxygenation

ECMO allows for the external control of gas exchange and support of systemic oxygenation by removing venous blood from a large cannula in a central vein, oxygenating and removing carbon dioxide with a membrane lung, and returning that oxygenated blood back to the circulation.[72]

Acute severe asthma exacerbations rarely require consideration of ECMO but may be considered for IMV patients with persistent severe respiratory acidosis (pH < 7.2) with hemodynamically unstable dynamic hyperinflation.[39] Multiple retrospective case series have suggested a benefit of ECMO in acute severe asthma, and there are reports of ECMO being beneficial in pregnant patients with acute severe asthma.[39,75–78] Nonetheless, ECMO is a complex procedure, carries significant risks and should be performed in centers with appropriate experience and expertise.[39,65]

COVID-19 considerations

Pregnant women seem to be more susceptible to SARS-CoV2 infection and have higher rates of ICU admission for COVID-19.[79] Yet, asthma does not seem to be a risk factor for COVID-19 infection, and there is some evidence that asthma in those who are not pregnant may be protective against COVID-19.[80,81] However, whether asthma may increase susceptibility or severity of SARS-CoV-2 infection in pregnancy is not known. Current guidance is to not alter asthma medications or management plans for pregnant patients with mild-to-moderate disease during the COVID-19 pandemic.[18,80]

For patients with concomitant COVID-19-related pneumonia, prone positioning for ventilation may be required.[82] In pregnant patients with prone positioning, chest and hip support are necessary to reduce abdominal pressure.[65,82,83]

Discussion of Disease Variation and Treatment Evidence Gaps

Asthma is a common chronic disease in pregnancy, affecting up to 12% of pregnant patients. As noted above, there is wide variation in the disease course. A better understanding of the pathobiological factors underlying this variation seems warranted. Although medication nonadherence has been well documented, there remain key questions regarding the pathobiology of asthma during pregnancy, especially those potentially modifiable by specific anti-inflammatory biologics. Identifying asthma patient phenotypes may facilitate this, even during acute episodes.[12]

The evidence basis for the primary pharmacologic treatments in acute severe asthma, including corticosteroids, β2-agonists and ipratropium, are well established in nonpregnant patients.[1] Although it seems reasonable to extrapolate these results to pregnant patients, the variation in disease course suggests that there may be additional variation in response to these medications during pregnancy.

Status asthmaticus, and other critical asthma syndromes, are characterized by reduced or nonresponsiveness to these primary pharmacologic interventions. Yet there is a marked paucity of evidence for other treatments for acute severe asthma exacerbations in nonpregnant patients, including magnesium, leukotriene antagonists, heliox, antibiotics, ketamine, aminophylline and intravenous β2-agonists. The applicable international guidelines are inconsistent in their recommendations on aminophylline and intravenous β2-agonists. Importantly, data of these other treatments in pregnant patients is extremely limited or nonexistent (beyond case reports). Given the number of acute severe asthma exacerbations, the high morbidity and mortality of critical asthma syndromes on the mother and the short-term and long-term consequences for the fetus, higher levels of evidence for these interventions are required.

The evidence for evolving therapies, including biologics, is interesting, especially given the rapid onset of anti-inflammatory effects (eg, benralizumab). Further trials of these agents in acute severe asthma seem warranted. The evidence for ECMO is too limited to be widely applied. Nonetheless, in life-threatening situations, ECMO and advanced ventilatory support treatments are worthy of consideration.

SUMMARY

One-third of women with asthma will have deterioration of their asthma during pregnancy. Prompt recognition of acute severe asthma is critical and immediate treatment includes inhaled β2-agonists, anticholinergic agents, and systemic corticosteroids. Patients with severe distress or unresponsive to aggressive primary therapy are in status asthmaticus, a life-threatening critical asthma syndrome. Additional consensus-based treatment options to enhance maternal and fetal oxygenation includes magnesium and potentially heliox, leukotriene antagonists, xanthines, intravenous β-agonists, antibiotics, ketamine and noninvasive positive pressure ventilation. In the rare cases of impending respiratory failure or arrest, IMV, and ECMO may be considered.

CLINICS CARE POINTS

- "Treat the mother, not the baby." Supporting maternal ventilation and oxygenation is the key to maintaining fetal oxygenation. However, both maternal and fetal monitorings are important for ongoing care.
- "Treatment time is critical." Primary treatment includes immediate use of inhaled β2-agonists, inhaled ipratropium and timely (within 30–60 minutes) administration of systemic corticosteroids.
- Status asthmaticus gravidus is a critical asthma syndrome that may require additional therapy, most of which have limited efficacy data in pregnant patients.
- In patients with overt respiratory failure, be prepared for a complicated intubation and challenging course of mechanical ventilation due to pregnancy-induced changes in anatomy and function.

DISCLOSURE

Dr Cairns has no disclosures directly related to the topic of asthma. He has served as a consultant for bioMerieux for the development and use of biomarkers. He has received grant support from the National Institutes of Health (NIAID, NHLBI) and the Bill and Melinda Gates Foundation for COVID-19 studies and interventions.

Dr Kraft has received funds paid directly to the institution for research in asthma by the National Institutes of Health, American Lung Association, AstraZeneca, and Sanofi-Regeneron. She has served as a scientific consultant with funds paid to her to address pathobiology of asthma for AstraZeneca, Sanofi-Regeneron, Chiesi Pharmaceuticals, and Genentech. Dr Kraft is also cofounder and Chief Medical Officer for Rae-Sedo, Inc. created to develop peptidomimetics for the treatment of inflammatory lung disease. The company is currently in the preclinical phase of therapeutic development.

REFERENCES

1. Hasegawa K, Craig SS, Teach SJ, et al. Management of asthma exacerbations in the emergency department. J Allergy Clin Immunol Pract 2021;9:2599–610.
2. Charlton RA, Hutchison A, Davis KJ, et al. Asthma management in pregnancy. PLoS One 2013;8:e60247.
3. Kwon HL, Belanger K, Bracken MB. Asthma prevalence among pregnant and childbearing-aged women in the United States: estimates from national health surveys. Ann Epidemiol 2003;13:317–24.
4. Wang H, Li N, Huang H. Asthma in pregnancy: pathophysiology, diagnosis, whole-course management, and medication safety. Can Respir J 2020;2020: 9046842.
5. Australian Bureau of Statistics. National Health Survey, First results, 2014-15. Available at: http://www.abs.gov.au/AUSSTATS/abs@.nsf/Lookup/4364.0.55. 001Explanatory%20Notes12014-15?OpenDocument. Accessed July 20, 2022.
6. Labor S, Dalbello Tir AM, Plavec D, et al. What is safe enough - asthma in pregnancy - a review of current literature and recommendations. Asthma Res Pract 2018;4:11.

7. Enriquez R, Griffin MR, Carroll KN, et al. Effect of maternal asthma and asthma control on pregnancy and perinatal outcomes. J Allergy Clin Immunol 2007; 120:625–30.

8. Kircher S, Schatz M, Long L. Variables affecting asthma course during pregnancy. Ann Allergy Asthma Immunol 2002;89(5):463–6.

9. Guy ES, Kirumaki A, Hanania NA. Acute asthma in pregnancy. Crit Care Clin 2004;20(4):731–45.

10. Vatti RR, Teuber SS. Asthma and pregnancy. Clinic Rev Allerg Immunol 2012;43: 45–56.

11. Murphy VE, Clifton VL, Gibson PG. Asthma exacerbations during pregnancy: incidence and association with adverse pregnancy outcomes. Thorax 2006; 61(2):169–76.

12. Cairns CB. Acute asthma exacerbations: phenotypes and management. Clin Chest Med 2006;27(1):99–108.

13. Kwon HL, Triche EW, Belanger K, et al. The epidemiology of asthma during pregnancy: prevalence, diagnosis and symptoms. Immunol Allergy Clin N Am 2006; 26(1):29–62.

14. Enriquez R, Wu P, Griffin MR, et al. Cessation of asthma medication in early pregnancy. Am J Obstet Gynecol 2006;195:149–53.

15. Ali Z, Hansen AV, Ulrik CS. Exacerbations of asthma during pregnancy: impact on pregnancy complications and outcome. J Obstet Gynaecol 2016;36(4):455–61.

16. Grzeskowiak LE, Smith B, Roy A, et al. Patterns, predictors and outcomes of asthma control and exacerbations during pregnancy: a prospective cohort study. ERJ Open Res 2016;2(1):00054–2015.

17. Global Initiative for Asthma (GINA). Global Strategy for Asthma Management and Prevention. 2022. Available at. www.ginasthma.org. Accessed June 10, 2022.

18. Popa M, Peltecu G, Gica N, et al. Asthma in pregnancy: review of current literature and recommendations. Maedica 2021;16(1):80–7.

19. Couillard S, Connolly C, Borg C, et al. Asthma in pregnancy: an update. Obstet Med 2021;14(3):135–44.

20. Schatz M, Dombrowski MP, Wise R, et al. Asthma morbidity during pregnancy can be predicted by severity classification. J Allergy Clin Immunol 2003;112(2): 283–8.

21. Carroll KN, Griffin MR, Gebretsadik T, et al. Racial differences in asthma morbidity during pregnancy. Obstet Gynecol 2005;106(1):66–72.

22. Bokern MP, Robijn AL, Jensen MD, et al. Factors associated with asthma exacerbations during pregnancy. Allergy Clin Immunol Pract 2021;9(12):4343–52.

23. National heart, lung, and blood institute. national asthma education and prevention program asthma and pregnancy working group: NAEPP expert panel report. Managing asthma during pregnancy: recommendations for pharmacologic treatment—2004 update. J Allergy Clin Immunol 2005;115:34–46.

24. Belanger K, Hellenbrand ME, Holford TR, et al. Effect of pregnancy on maternal asthma symptoms and medication use. Obstet Gynecol 2010;115:559–67.

25. British SIGN. guideline on the management of asthma. Available at. https://www.sign.ac.uk/our-guidelines/british-guideline-on-the-management-of-asthma/. Accessed June 10, 2022.

26. Cydulka RK. Acute asthma during pregnancy. Immunol Allergy Clin N Am 2006; 26(1):103–17.

27. Kostakou E, Kaniaris E, Filiou E, et al. Acute severe asthma in adolescent and adult patients: current perspectives on assessment and management. J Clin Med 2019;8(9):1283.

28. Kenyon N, Zeki A, Albertson TE, et al. Definition of critical asthma syndromes. Clin Rev Allergy Immunol 2015;48:1–6.
29. Cousins L. Fetal oxygenation, assessment of fetal well-being, and obstetric management of the pregnant patient with asthma. J Allergy Clin Immunol 1999;103: S343–9.
30. Coutts II, White RJ. Asthma in pregnancy. J Asthma 1991;28(6):433–6.
31. National Asthma Council. Australian Asthma Handbook, Version 2.1. 2020. Available at: https://www.asthmahandbook.org.au/. Accessed June 12, 2022.
32. Cates CJ, Welsh EJ, Rowe BH. Holding chambers (spacers) versus nebulisers for beta-agonist treatment of acute asthma. Cochrane Database Syst Rev 2013;9: CD000052.
33. Press VG, Hasegawa K, Heidt J, et al. Missed opportunities to transition from nebulizers to inhalers during hospitalization for acute asthma: a multicenter observational study. J Asthma 2017;54:968–76.
34. Camargo CA Jr, Spooner CH, Rowe BH. Continuous versus intermittent beta agonists in the treatment of acute asthma. Cochrane Database Syst Rev 2003;4: CD001115.
35. Kirkland SW, Cross E, Campbell S, et al. Intramuscular versus oral corticosteroids to reduce relapses following discharge from the emergency department for acute asthma. Cochrane Database Syst Rev 2018;6(6):CD012629.
36. Rowe BH, Spooner CH, Ducharme FM, et al. Corticosteroids for preventing relapse following acute exacerbations of asthma. Cochrane Database Syst Rev 2007;3:CD000195.
37. Edmonds ML, Milan SJ, Camargo CA Jr, et al. Early use of inhaled corticosteroids in the emergency department treatment of acute asthma. Cochrane Database Syst Rev 2012;12(12):CD002308.
38. Chan AL, Juarez MM, Gidwani N, et al. Management of critical asthma syndrome during pregnancy. Clin Rev Allergy Immunol 2015;48(1):45–53.
39.. Garner O, Ramey JS, Hanania NA. Management of life-threatening asthma: severe asthma series. Chest 2022. https://doi.org/10.1016/j.chest.2022.02.029. S0012-3692(22)00395-00396.
40. Skobeloff EM, Spivey WH, McNamara RM, et al. Intravenous magnesium sulfate for the treatment of acute asthma in the emergency department. JAMA 1989;262: 1210–3.
41. Cairns CB, Kraft M. Magnesium attenuates the neutrophil respiratory burst in adult asthmatic patients. Acad Emerg Med 1996;3:1093–7.
42. Fanni D, Gerosa C, Nurchi VM, et al. The role of magnesium in pregnancy and in fetal programming of adult diseases. Biol Trace Elem Res 2021;199(10):3647–57.
43. Rowe BH, Bretzlaff JA, Bourdon C, et al. Intravenous magnesium sulfate treatment for acute asthma in the emergency department: a systematic review of the literature. Ann Emerg Med 2000;36(3):181–90.
44. FitzGerald J. Magnesium sulfate is effective for severe acute asthma treated in the emergency department. West J Med 2000;172(2):96.
45. Gallegos-Solórzano MC, Pérez-Padilla R, Hernández-Zenteno RJ. Usefulness of inhaled magnesium sulfate in the coadjuvant management of severe asthma crisis in an emergency department. Pulm Pharmacol Ther 2010;23(5):432–7.
46. Knightly R, Milan SJ, Hughes R, et al. Inhaled magnesium sulfate in the treatment of acute asthma. Cochrane Database Syst Rev 2017;11:CD003898.
47. Badawy MSH, Hassanin IMA. The value of magnesium sulfate nebulization in treatment of acute bronchial asthma during pregnancy. Egypt J Chest Dis Tuberc 2014;63:285–9.

48. Rodrigo GJ, Castro-Rodriguez JA. Heliox-driven beta2-agonists nebulization for children and adults with acute asthma: a systematic review with metaanalysis. Ann Allergy Asthma Immunol 2014;112:29–34.

49. Rodrigo GJ. Advances in acute asthma. Curr Opin Pulm Med 2015;21(1):22–6.

50. National Asthma Education and Prevention Program. Expert Panel Report 3: guidelines for the diagnosis and management of asthma. Full report 2007. Available at: https://www.nhlbi.nih.gov/health-topics/guidelines-for-diagnosis-management-of-asthma. Accessed June 10, 2022.

51. Anderson M, Svartengren M, Bylin G, et al. Deposition in asthmatics of particles inhaled in air or in helium and oxygen. Am Rev Respir Dis 1993;147(3):524–8.

52. Kraft M, Cairns CB, Ellison MC, et al. Improvements in distal lung function correlate with asthma symptoms after treatment with oral montelukast. Chest 2006; 130(6):1726–32.

53. O'Connor BJ, Löfdahl CG, Balter M, et al. Zileuton added to low-dose inhaled beclomethasone for the treatment of moderate to severe persistent asthma. Respir Med 2007;101(6):1088–96.

54. Berger W, De Chandt MT, Cairns CB. Zileuton: clinical implications of 5-Lipoxygenase inhibition in severe airway disease. Int J Clin Pract 2007;61(4):663–76.

55. Ramsay CF, Pearson D, Mildenhall S, et al. Oral montelukast in acute asthma exacerbations: a randomised, double-blind, placebo-controlled trial. Thorax 2011; 66(1):7–11.

56. Watts K, Chavasse RJ. Leukotriene receptor antagonists in addition to usual care for acute asthma in adults and children. Cochrane Database Syst Rev 2012;5: CD006100.

57. Normansell R, Sayer B, Waterson S, et al. Antibiotics for exacerbations of asthma. Cochrane Database Syst Rev 2018;6(6):CD002741.

58. Okubo Y, Horimukai K, Michihata N, et al. Association between early antibiotic treatment and clinical outcomes in children hospitalized for asthma exacerbation. J Allergy Clin Immunol 2021;147:114–22.

59. Zafar Gondal A, Zulfiqar H. Aminophylline. In: StatPearls. 2022. Available at: https://www.ncbi.nlm.nih.gov/books/NBK545175/. Accessed July 22, 2022.

60. Nair P, Milan SJ, Rowe BH. Addition of intravenous aminophylline to inhaled beta(2)-agonists in adults with acute asthma. Cochrane Database Syst Rev 2012;12:CD002742.

61. Nowak RM, Parker JM, Silverman RA, et al. A randomized trial of benralizumab, an antiinterleukin 5 receptor alpha monoclonal antibody, after acute asthma. Am J Emerg Med 2015;33(1):14–20.

62. Benes J, Skulec R, Jilek D, et al. Successful treatment of refractory status asthmaticus with omalizumab: a case report. Allergy Asthma Clin Immunol 2021; 17(1):128.

63. Milger K, Schroeder I, Behr J, et al. Omalizumab rescue therapy for refractory status asthmaticus. Ann Intern Med 2019;170(5):351–2.

64. Jat KR, Chawla D. Ketamine for management of acute exacerbations of asthma in children. Cochrane Database Syst Rev 2012;11:CD009293.

65. Pandya ST, Krishna SJ. Acute respiratory distress syndrome in pregnancy. Indian J Crit Care Med 2021;25:S241–7.

66. Lim WJ, Mohammed Akram R, Carson KV, et al. Non-invasive positive pressure ventilation for treatment of respiratory failure due to severe acute exacerbations of asthma. Cochrane Database Syst Rev 2012;12:CD004360.

67. Landry A, Foran M, Koyfman A. Does noninvasive positive-pressure ventilation improve outcomes in severe asthma exacerbations? Ann Emerg Med 2013; 62(6):594–6.
68. Althoff MD, Holguin F, Yang F, et al. Noninvasive ventilation use in critically ill patients with acute asthma exacerbations. Am J Respir Crit Care Med 2020;202(11): 1520–30.
69. Sekiguchi H, Kondo Y, Fukuda T, et al. Noninvasive positive pressure ventilation for treating acute asthmatic attacks in three pregnant women with dyspnea and hypoxemia. Clin Case Rep 2019;7(5):881–7.
70. Dalar L, Caner H, Eryuksel E, et al. Application of non-invasive mechanical ventilation in an asthmatic pregnant woman in respiratory failure: a case report. J Thorac Dis 2013;5(1):97–100.
71. Schwaiberger D, Karcz M, Menk M, et al. Respiratory failure and mechanical ventilation in the pregnant patient. Crit Care Clin 2016;32(1):85–95.
72. Mosier JM, Hypes C, Joshi R, et al. Ventilator strategies and rescue therapies for management of acute respiratory failure in the emergency department. Ann Emerg Med 2015;66(5):529–41.
73. Munnur U, de Boisblanc B, Suresh MS. Airway problems in pregnancy. Crit Care Med 2005;33:S259–68.
74. Mushambi MC, Kinsella SM, Popat M, et al. Obstetric Anaesthetists' Association and Difficult Airway Society guidelines for the management of difficult and failed tracheal intubation in obstetrics. Anaesthesia 2015;70(11):1286–306.
75. Maqsood U, Patel N. Extracorporeal membrane oxygenation (ECMO) for near-fatal asthma refractory to conventional ventilation. BMJ Case Rep 2018;2018. bcr2017223276.
76. Di Lascio G, Prifti E, Messai E, et al. Extracorporeal membrane oxygenation support for life-threatening acute severe status asthmaticus. Perfusion 2017;32(2): 157–63.
77. Mikkelsen ME, Woo YJ, Sager JS, et al. Outcomes using extracorporeal life support for adult respiratory failure due to status asthmaticus. ASAIO J 2009;55(1): 47–52.
78. Steinack C, Lenherr R, Hendra H, et al. The use of life-saving extracorporeal membrane oxygenation (ECMO) for pregnant woman with status asthmaticus. J Asthma 2017;54(1):84–8.
79. Gao YD, Ding M, Dong X, et al. Risk factors for severe and critically ill COVID-19 patients: a review. Allergy 2021;76(2):428–55.
80. Global Initiative for Asthma. GINA guidance about COVID-19 and asthma. Available at: https://ginasthma.org/wp-content/uploads/2022/05/COVID-19-and-asthma-GINA-22_04_30.pdf. Accessed July 22, 2022.
81. Adir Y, Saliba W, Beurnier A, et al. Asthma and COVID-19: an update. Eur Respir Rev 2021;30:210152.
82. Tolcher MC, McKinney JR, Eppes CS, et al. Prone positioning for pregnant women with hypoxemia due to coronavirus disease 2019 (COVID-19). Obstet Gynecol 2020;136:259–61.
83. Ghafoor H, Abdus Samad A, Bel Khair AOM, et al. Critical care management of severe COVID-19 in pregnant patients. Cureus 2022;14(5):e24885.

Anaphylaxis in Pregnancy

Margaret M. Kuder, MD, MPH[a],*, Rachael Baird, MD[b,1],
Maeve Hopkins, MD[b,2], David M. Lang, MD[a,1]

KEYWORDS

- Anaphylaxis • Pregnancy • Epinephrine • Cesarean delivery

KEY POINTS

- The inciting agents for anaphylaxis in the first trimester of pregnancy are similar to those observed in nonpregnant patients; causes for the second and third trimester generally reflect drug-induced anaphylaxis.
- Symptoms of anaphylaxis can mimic physiologic symptoms of pregnancy, including shortness of breath, nausea/vomiting, diarrhea, and low blood pressure.
- Cesarean delivery is the most frequently reported event associated with anaphylaxis in the pregnant population.
- Epinephrine is the first drug of choice for the treatment of anaphylaxis in the pregnant patient.

INTRODUCTION

Anaphylaxis is a potentially serious and life-threatening systemic hypersensitivity reaction, defined by a range of clinical characteristics. Anaphylaxis occurs suddenly and may involve multiple organ systems.[1] The reported frequency of anaphylaxis is 1.6% to 5.1%,[1,2] which is increasing, and is likely an underestimate.[3] Older age and comorbidities (eg, cardiac and lung disease) are associated with heightened risk for severe anaphylaxis.[4]

Anaphylaxis during pregnancy has both similarities and important differences from anaphylaxis in nonpregnant patients. The calamitous occurrence of severe anaphylaxis can entail the risk for maternal and fetal harm, including fatality and severe sequelae for the newborn.

Epidemiology

Anaphylaxis during pregnancy is fortunately a rare event, with an estimated frequency of 1.5 to 3.8 per 100,000 pregnancies.[5] Using a national surveillance system in France,

---

[a] Department of Allergy and Clinical Immunology, Respiratory Institute, Cleveland Clinic Foundation; [b] Women's Health Institute, Cleveland Clinic Foundation
[1] Present address: 9500 Euclid Avenue, Cleveland, OH 44195.
[2] Present address: 18101 Lorain Avenue, Cleveland, OH 44111.
* Corresponding author. 5001 Rockside Road. IN 80, Independence, OH 44131.
E-mail address: kuderm@ccf.org

Immunol Allergy Clin N Am 43 (2023) 103–116
https://doi.org/10.1016/j.iac.2022.07.004
0889-8561/23/© 2022 Elsevier Inc. All rights reserved.
immunology.theclinics.com

Tacquard and colleagues[6] identified 973 cases of maternal mortality over a 12-year period; 5 cases were attributed to anaphylaxis, leading to an estimated rate of anaphylaxis-related maternal mortality of 0.5 per 100,000 live births (95% confidence interval [CI], 0.02–0.19).

Fig. 1 describes the most common inciting agents for anaphylaxis observed in 730 cases of anaphylaxis seen at Cleveland Clinic from July 2002 to October 2013 across all populations.[7] The most commonly implicated causes were foods, hymenoptera venom, and medications. The frequency of these triggers varied by age: for adults medications and hymenoptera venom were more commonly observed; for children, foods and hymenoptera venom were common.

Although the causes for anaphylaxis in the first trimester of pregnancy may be somewhat similar to the pattern observed in nonpregnant patients illustrated in **Fig. 1**, the inciting agents for the second and third trimester generally reflect drug-induced anaphylaxis. Mulla and colleagues[8] examined the epidemiology of anaphylaxis in 2004 to 2005 among obstetric patients in Texas and identified 19 cases; of these 13 were caused by antibiotics of which 11 were due to β-lactams. McCall and colleagues[9] analyzed the United Kingdom Obstetrics Surveillance System from 2012 to 2015, and identified 37 cases, with an average age of 33 (± 7) years, which fulfilled their case definition. Two-thirds (67%) of these reactions occurred intrapartum or postdelivery. Half of the women had a suspected reaction to an antibiotic, with two-thirds of these cases related to a prophylactic antibiotic administered at the time of cesarean delivery. Of the 5 fatal cases described in France by Tacquard and colleagues,[6] anaphylaxis occurred in all cases after anesthesia induction, with neuromuscular blockers being the most common cause. In an analysis of hospitalizations of pregnant women in the United States from 2004 to 2014, McCall and colleagues[10] identified 3 risk factors associated with anaphylaxis: cesarean delivery (odds ratio [OR] = 4.19; 95% CI, 3.28–5.35), history of an allergic reaction (OR = 4.05; 95% CI, 2.64–6.23), and black (OR = 1.57; 95% CI, 1.15–2.15) and other races (OR = 1.69; 95% CI, 1.08–2.63) compared with white race. The investigators concluded that identification of such patients may aid in identifying those at increased risk, but they also speculated that these factors may be markers for pregnant women who may be more

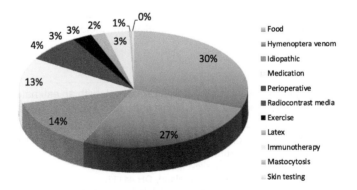

Fig. 1. The most common inciting agents for anaphylaxis in 730 cases. (*Data from* Gonzalez-Estrada A, Silvers SK, Klein A, et al. Epidemiology of anaphylaxis at a tertiary care center: a report of 730 cases. Ann Allergy Asthma Immunol 2017;118(1):80–5.)

likely to lack insurance coverage, present late for antenatal care, and be at increased risk for a complicated pregnancy.

In a systematic review of severe anaphylaxis in pregnancy, Simionescu and colleagues[11] assessed publications using PubMed, Web of Science, and Scopus databases from 1985 through April 2021 and identified 47 cases. The investigators reported that three-fourths of the events occurred peripartum, involving 22 allergens. β-Lactam antibiotics accounted for 21% of cases, anesthetic agents were responsible for 23%, and 20% were due to latex.

Carra and colleagues[5] performed a systematic review to identify publications related to anaphylaxis during pregnancy on August 1, 2020, using PubMed, Science Direct, SciELO, and LILACS Web sites and Cochrane database with no language restrictions. Twelve articles were identified that fulfilled inclusion criteria. The most common causes identified for anaphylaxis during pregnancy were β-lactam antibiotics (58%), latex (25%), and anesthetic agents (17%).

Signs and symptoms characterized by the 730 cases of anaphylaxis reported from Cleveland Clinic are displayed in **Fig. 2**.[7] Of note is that, similar to other large series of anaphylaxis cases,[12] cutaneous symptoms predominated to such an extent that the lack of cutaneous symptoms may be regarded as a navigational signal to consider another conditions (eg, vasovagal reaction) in the differential diagnosis of anaphylaxis.[13] However, cutaneous symptoms are absent in 35% of cases of anaphylaxis during pregnancy.[9] It is unclear whether the manifestations of anaphylaxis may indeed be altered by pregnancy, or whether the reduced rate of cutaneous symptoms, similar to what has been observed in cases of intraoperative anaphylaxis,[13] may reflect the predominance of cases during labor and delivery—which is also a time when patients are commonly draped.

Pregnancy Physiology and Its Relation to Anaphylaxis

To understand the special considerations of anaphylaxis in pregnant women, one must understand the unique physiology of pregnancy (**Table 1**). Owing to the increasing demands of a rapidly growing fetus and placenta, the maternal metabolic

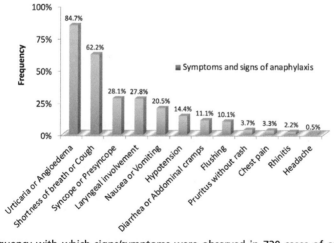

Fig. 2. Frequency with which signs/symptoms were observed in 730 cases of anaphylaxis. (*Data from* Gonzalez-Estrada A, Silvers SK, Klein A, et al. Epidemiology of anaphylaxis at a tertiary care center: a report of 730 cases. Ann Allergy Asthma Immunol 2017;118(1):80–5.)

Table 1
Physiologic adaptations of pregnancy by organ system and considerations in anaphylaxis

Organ System	Physiologic Adaptations in Pregnancy	Considerations in Anaphylaxis
Cardiac	↑Cardiac output 30%–50% ↓Arterial blood pressure until third trimester ↑Heart rate ↓Peripheral vascular resistance ↑Left ventricular mass	• Cardiovascular collapse or asystole can compromise placental blood flow • Standard ACLS algorithm should be used in the event of cardiac arrest, delivery should be performed if no ROSC[a] after 4 min
Pulmonary	↓Functional residual capacity 20%–30% ↑Inspiratory capacity 5%–10% ↑Tidal volume ↑Resting minute ventilation ↑Total oxygen-carrying capacity ↑Oxygen consumption 20% -Physiologic edema of the nasal cavities, larynx, pharynx, and trachea	• Differentiating physiologic dyspnea from pathologic dyspnea can be challenging. • Prepare for a difficult airway in all patients • Increased risk of pulmonary edema
Hematologic	↑Plasma volume 40%–50% ↑Clotting factors ↑Fibrinogen ↓Colloid oncotic pressure	• Increased risk of thromboembolism • Careful interpretation in laboratory test results for evaluation of disseminated intravascular coagulation
Immunologic	↓Th1-mediated immunity ↑Th2-mediated immunity ↑IL-4, IL-10, and IL-13 ↑Humoral immunity ↑Leukocyte count, leukocyte alkaline phosphatase, C-reactive protein, erythrocyte sedimentation rate	• Immune tolerance of pregnancy can make recognition and diagnosis of abnormalities more complex
Renal	↓Plasma bicarbonate level ↑Blood pH ↑Glomerular filtration rate 50% ↑Creatinine clearance 30% ↓Serum creatinine	• Must remember physiologic compensated respiratory alkalosis when interpreting blood gas • Potential for faster clearance of medications

Abbreviations: ↓, Decrease; ↑, increase; ACLS, advanced cardiac life support; ROSC, return of spontaneous circulation.
[a] Return of spontaneous circulation.

rate increases by 20%.[14] Plasma volume increases starting around 6 to 8 weeks of pregnancy, reaching 40% to 45% above nonpregnant levels,[15] accompanied by increased water retention via the resetting of osmotic thresholds for thirst and vasopressin secretion secondary to progesterone.[16] This increased water retention can result in edema, particularly in late pregnancy due to decreased interstitial colloid osmotic pressure and greater venous pressure below the level of the uterus.[17] This swelling differs from that of angioedema, in that it typically is persistent over days to weeks and responds to elevation.

Pregnancy also involves notable changes to the cardiovascular system. Cardiac output increases via reduced systemic vascular resistance and increased heart rate, which begins as early as the fifth week of gestation.[18] Brachial systolic and diastolic blood pressure decrease significantly by 6 to 7 weeks' gestation with a concomitant increase in resting heart rate of 10 beats/min.[19] Arterial blood pressure continues to decline during pregnancy to a nadir at 24 to 26 weeks followed by an increase to near prepregnancy levels at term. This decrease in blood pressure is more notable with diastolic pressures when compared with systolic.[20] These blood pressure changes are driven, at least partially, by an upregulation of the renin-angiotensin-aldosterone axis. Dysregulation of this axis may be involved in hypertensive disorders of pregnancy[20]; this is an important consideration when assessing blood pressure during suspected anaphylactic events. As discussed earlier, plasma volume expansion begins early in pregnancy, leading to increased preload and resulting in larger left atrial volumes and ejection fraction.[18] Cardiac output increases by 30% to 50% in pregnancy, mostly mediated by stroke volume in early pregnancy and near term due to increase in baseline heart rate.[21] Structurally, the increased blood volume also leads to increased concentric left ventricular mass beginning at 26 to 30 weeks that returns to prepregnancy state by 3 months postpartum.[22] However, despite this increasing mass, plasma brain natriuretic peptide levels are maintained in the nonpregnant range and an elevation should be considered abnormal.[23] Anatomically, as the gravid uterus grows it begins to compress the great veins and diminishes venous return from the lower body.[24] In approximately 10% of women, this compression by the uterus can cause significant arterial hypotension referred to as supine hypotensive syndrome.[25] Owing to this, gravid women are recommended to avoid supine positioning. This is relevant when considering positioning of pregnant women in the context of suspected anaphylactic events, because it is imperative to transition to a recumbent position with lower extremities elevated to maintain perfusion of vital organs; upright posture in the setting of hypoperfusion has been associated with fatal outcomes.[26] Secondary to these cardiac adaptions to pregnancy, normal cardiac sounds on physical examination are modified in pregnancy with an exaggerated splitting of the first heart sound and a notably loud third heart sound. Most pregnant women also have a systolic murmur.[20] In the peripartum and early postpartum period, cardiac output further increases secondary to autotransfusion of placental blood during contractions and the release of the great vein compression following delivery.[21]

During pregnancy, both coagulation and fibrinolysis are increased with a slight shift toward a procoagulant state, particularly at term.[27] There are increased concentrations of all clotting factors except factors XI and XIII, and the level and rate of thrombin generation increases throughout pregnancy. Notably, fibrinogen increases approximately 50% and averages 450 mg/dL in late pregnancy and therefore must be interpreted appropriately when assessing for possible disseminated intravascular coagulation (DIC).[28]

From a respiratory standpoint, the diaphragm rises 4 cm during pregnancy, but the subcostal angle widens and the chest wall circumference increases to maintain an unchanged total lung capacity. Functional residual capacity decreases by 20% to 30% due to a decrease in both expiratory reserve volume and residual volume. The inspiratory capacity increases by 5% to 10%.[29] The tidal volume and resting minute ventilation increase significantly, driven by enhanced respiratory drive from progesterone, resulting in compensated respiratory alkalosis.[30,31] These changes, combined with increased 2,3-diphosphoglyceric acid, leads to increased total oxygen-carrying capacity, which helps to compensate for the oxygen consumption that increases by 20% during pregnancy.[32] This increased tidal volume and minute ventilation often leads to a physiologic dyspnea.[33] This physiologic dyspnea needs to be carefully distinguished from pathologic dyspnea that may be a harbinger of poorly controlled asthma. Pregnancy also results in important airway changes including physiologic edema of the nasal cavities, larynx, pharynx, and trachea. Preparations should be made for a difficult airway, and supraglottic airway devices should be available. Given this baseline edema, early intubation should be considered if there is concern for serious angioedema leading to airway compromise.[34] Decreased colloid oncotic pressure also predisposes pregnant patients to pulmonary edema.[20]

To compensate for this respiratory alkalosis of pregnancy, plasma bicarbonate level decreases to 22 mmol/L, leading to a minimal increase in blood pH that shifts the maternal oxygen dissociation curve to the left to help facilitate oxygen and carbon dioxide exchange with the fetus.[20] The glomerular filtration rate increases by up to 25% within 4 weeks and up to 50% by the second trimester due to increased renal plasma flow and hypervolemia-induced hemodilution of pregnancy and results in a reduced serum creatinine level. Cr of 0.9 mg/dL or greater is considered abnormal in a normal pregnant woman, and creatinine clearance averages 30% higher.[35,36]

From an immunologic perspective, pregnancy is associated with suppression of humoral and cell-mediated immune function, allowing tolerance of the fetal allograft. On the maternal-fetal interface there is expression of special major histocompatibility complex molecules on trophoblasts that does not vary between individuals, namely, human leukocyte antigen class Ib, which includes HLA-E, HLA-F, and HLA-G.[37] In addition, there are changes in the CD4 T lymphocyte subpopulations with Th1-mediated immunity shifting to Th2-mediated immunity resulting in increased secretion of interleukin (IL)-4, IL-10, and IL-13[38]; this results in promotion of humoral immunity. Owing to changes in the immune system, typical inflammatory markers such as leukocyte count, leukocyte alkaline phosphatase, C-reactive protein, and erythrocyte sedimentation rate are increased in normal pregnancy.[20] During labor and the early puerperium, particularly, leukocyte counts can increase to as high as 25,000/μL, which may be a combination of stress response of the physical demands of labor and reappearance of leukocytes previously shunted out of the active circulation.[20] Tryptase levels should not be affected in pregnancy state; however, when completing serologic assessment for anaphylactic events, it is important to consider the physiologically normal increase in inflammatory markers that can occur.

The symptoms of anaphylaxis, shown in **Table 1**, can mimic physiologic symptoms of pregnancy, including shortness of breath, nausea/vomiting, diarrhea, and low blood pressure. A clinician must maintain high index of suspicion, particularly in the context of any recent triggering factors such as medication administration. When applying the physiologic changes of pregnancy to anaphylaxis, particularly with regard to fetal well-being, collapse of the respiratory and cardiovascular systems is of greatest concern. A relatively high uterine blood flow is required for normal fetal oxygenation (up to 942 mL/min at 36 weeks). Owing to inefficiencies of the placenta, the arterial Po_2 in the placenta is approximately one-third to one-fourth of the arterial Po_2 in the maternal bloodstream. Therefore, fetal oxygenation is directly compromised by maternal hypoxemia and indirectly compromised by maternal hypotension or vasoconstriction, which in turn leads to reduced uterine blood flow.[39,40] The fetus can compensate for a period to the stress of reduced oxygenation, but fetal reserve can be affected by several factors including gestational age, additional pregnancy complications, placental insufficiency, and prolonged labor. When these mechanisms fail, the fetus is at risk for neurologic effects or fetal death, even if the mother recovers completely.[39,41] Therefore, when signs of acute cardiac and/or respiratory distress arise, expedited delivery via cesarean delivery can be considered, particularly at term. A risk-benefit discussion of delivery at decreasing gestational ages should be undertaken in collaboration with maternal-fetal medicine specialists when the situation allows.

Diagnosis and Treatment of Anaphylaxis in Pregnancy

Diagnosis

Anaphylaxis is a clinical diagnosis, which includes a series of clinical factors, including exposure to a known allergen, cardiopulmonary compromise, and cutaneous symptoms.[42] Given the pathophysiological differences in pregnancy, there are important considerations when diagnosing anaphylaxis in this population. Blood pressure may be lower at baseline, or tolerated secondary to neuraxial anesthesia, delaying recognition of hypotension indicating severe anaphylaxis. Cutaneous symptoms may occur less frequently as a manifestation of anaphylaxis in the pregnant population.[9] Uterine contractions are reported as a symptom in anaphylaxis, in both pregnant and nonpregnant patients.[43] In pregnant patients, this may be misidentified as preterm labor, delaying the diagnosis of anaphylaxis.

Given that anaphylaxis is a clinical diagnosis, there is a wide differential to consider. Before labor and delivery, pregnant women have essentially the same differential diagnosis as the general population. In the labor and delivery period, there are unique considerations including hypotension related to epidural anesthesia, preeclampsia- or eclampsia-associated symptoms, amniotic fluid embolism, or placental abruption.[5,11] Amniotic fluid embolism has been referred to as an "anaphylactoid syndrome of pregnancy" because of its resemblance to anaphylaxis, with sudden cardiorespiratory collapse and DIC.[44] When amniotic fluid and fetal components enter the pregnant woman's bloodstream, physical obstruction, as well as intense cytokine response, contributes to symptoms.[44] The classic triad of amniotic fluid embolism, hypotension, hypoxia, and DIC, can mimic severe anaphylaxis.[45] Furthermore, the onset of amniotic fluid embolisms is often postpartum, particularly after cesarean delivery.[45] This timing is also when patients receive common anaphylaxis culprits such as anesthetic agents and/or antibiotics for surgical prophylaxis.

Anaphylaxis in pregnancy is a rare event; however, given the grave outcomes associated with delayed diagnosis, it is critical to recognize the condition promptly. Cesarean delivery is the most frequently reported event associated with anaphylaxis in the pregnant population, accounting for 34% (16 of 47) of cases in a recent systematic review.[11] Although nearly 30% of women undergoing vaginal delivery receive antibiotics, 100% of women undergoing cesarean delivery receive antibiotics for surgical site infection prophylaxis.[46] Having a high index of suspicion during these procedures is warranted. Cases are also frequently associated with antibiotic (21%) or anesthetic administration (23%), as well as latex exposure (20%).[11] If symptoms concerning for anaphylaxis emerge, considering recent exposures to common culprits in this population can facilitate diagnosis.

Prompt treatment is indicated once an anaphylaxis diagnosis is suspected; however, after stabilization of the pregnant woman and fetus, further evaluation by a board-certified allergist/immunologist is recommended. Obtaining a perievent serum tryptase level 30 minutes to 4 hours after the onset of symptoms can help confirm the diagnosis of anaphylaxis during subsequent evaluation.[47] Based on careful review of the exposures before onset of symptoms, the allergy/immunology physician can determine the testing indicated to identify a culprit and guide future avoidance. The current literature suggests this is not commonly completed, as one systematic review identified only 17% of included articles that described allergy testing to detect or confirm the anaphylactogenic agent.[5]

As noted previously, cesarean delivery accounts for many cases of pregnancy-associated anaphylaxis. Evaluation of these cases is similar to that of other intraoperative anaphylaxis cases. Although skin testing protocols for many intraoperative agents have not been well validated, testing for immediate hypersensitivity is recommended.[48] Over 90% of women who undergo cesarean delivery undergo repeat cesarean delivery in subsequent pregnancies[49,50]; this reinforces the importance of identifying the culprit agent to avoid reexposure in future pregnancies.

It is also important to consider systemic mast cell disorders in cases of anaphylaxis in pregnancy. Pregnancy and delivery can trigger mast cell degranulation, which can prompt anaphylactic events.[51,52] These patients may have a history of other episodes of anaphylaxis without clear trigger, or to common triggers for which patients with mast cell disorders are vulnerable, such as nonsteroidal anti-inflammatory drugs (NSAIDs) or hymenoptera venom.[53] Obtaining an acute serum tryptase level is the reference standard to evaluate mast cell activation.[53] Further evaluation of serum KITD816 V and bone marrow biopsy can be considered if indicated, based on clinical history and tryptase levels.[53]

A rare consideration includes exercise-induced anaphylaxis (EIA) during the labor period. There is a report of this published in 1985, in which a woman experienced symptoms consistent with anaphylaxis during the labor period of 2 separate pregnancies.[54] In a study following individuals with EIA for 19 years, 7 subjects with EIA, most of whom had reduced exercise to eliminate symptoms throughout pregnancy, nevertheless, had episodes during pregnancy. One subject reported pruritis and urticaria during labor.[55]

Treatment

Given the life-threatening nature of anaphylaxis to both the mother and fetus, prompt and aggressive treatment is warranted. Despite the unique physiology of pregnancy, there are no published guidelines outlining anaphylaxis management in pregnant women[9]; this is likely due to the rare nature of these events and lack of collective data to inform specific guidelines. General anaphylaxis guidelines address acute cardiopulmonary collapse with medication management including epinephrine, corticosteroids, antihistamine therapy, and fluid resuscitation. These recommendations extend to pregnant women. One descriptive study demonstrated this, with most pregnant women receiving epinephrine (93%), antihistamines (88%), corticosteroids (97%), and intravenous fluids (87%) in cases of anaphylaxis.[9]

The treatment of choice for anaphylaxis is epinephrine, which is critical to administer promptly.[1] In nonpregnancy anaphylaxis, delayed administration of epinephrine has been associated with greater risk for untoward outcomes.[26,56] In pregnant women, avoidance of epinephrine has been suggested. As a potent alpha- and beta-adrenergic agonist, epinephrine may induce uterine vasoconstriction, which could result in fetal bradycardia, acidosis, and hypoxia.[9,41] Some studies suggest ephedrine, a "mixed-acting" sympathomimetic, could accomplish the desired resuscitation in the pregnant women and cause less uterine vasoconstriction[41]; however, the peripheral vasoconstriction achieved by epinephrine contributes to improved hemodynamics seen with its administration. Despite the consideration of ephedrine for treatment in pregnant women, epinephrine is still the recommended first-line treatment in cases of anaphylaxis and should be administered promptly in suspected cases.[5]

In addition to epinephrine, to optimize blood flow to both the woman and fetus, the patient should be placed in the left lateral decubitus position, which reduces caval compression from the uterus.[11] This recommendation varies from that for Trendelenburg positioning in the general population. Aggressive fluid resuscitation is also critical.

If anaphylaxis occurs in labor, immediate delivery of the fetus should be considered after maternal stabilization, because this will protect the neonate as well as reduce compression of the vena cava in the pregnant woman.[5] Cesarean delivery is recommended in women experiencing severe anaphylaxis without adequate maternal resuscitation; this attempts to minimize neonatal hypoxia during anaphylactic events, which can lead to neonatal encephalopathy.[9]

Other treatments commonly used as secondary treatment of anaphylaxis include antihistamines and corticosteroids. These medications are generally not contraindicated in pregnancy. Antihistamines can reduce cutaneous symptoms associated with anaphylaxis, but its administration should not delay epinephrine use.[1] A large systematic review, including more than 200,000 subjects, found no evidence of teratogenicity associated with antihistamine use.[57] Given their longer history of use and larger quantity of safety data, first-generation antihistamines are generally preferred.[58] Several second-generation antihistamines carry a pregnancy category "B" (loratadine, cetirizine, levocetirizine). Loratadine is the most well-studied second-generation antihistamine, and the evidence suggests no increased risk of major malformations.[59] Glucocorticoids are also used as an adjunctive therapy in anaphylaxis.[1] The majority of data regarding corticosteroid use in pregnancy derives from its use in autoinflammatory conditions. Corticosteroids, particularly short courses, are generally well tolerated in pregnancy.[60]

Specific symptoms may warrant alternative treatment. As mentioned earlier, uterine contractions are a reported symptom of anaphylaxis in women. A recent systematic review suggests beta-2 agonists may be optimal to halt uterine contractions associated with anaphylaxis.[43] Multiple cases describe the use of nebulized or subcutaneous terbutaline in conjunction with epinephrine to successfully halt uterine contractions associated with anaphylaxis.[43] NSAIDs were also noted to reduce symptoms; however, given their potential role as a cofactor in anaphylaxis, their use in this setting requires caution. From an obstetric standpoint, NSAIDs are avoided in the third trimester due to the potential risk of closure of the fetal ductus arteriosus.[61]

In the event of cardiac arrest from anaphylaxis, high-quality cardiopulmonary resuscitation should be initiated immediately, in the same manner as in nonpregnant patients. Manual uterine displacement to the left should be performed to relieve obstruction of the great veins from the uterus. Early defibrillation with standard adult energies should be provided if the rhythm is shockable. All standard resuscitation drugs and doses, including epinephrine and amiodarone, should be used. Finally, preparations should be made immediately for cesarean delivery with initiation of delivery at 4 minutes and completion of delivery by 5 minutes if return of spontaneous circulation is not achieved. In addition to fetal benefits, delivery will facilitate more effective resuscitation of the mother via relief of aortocaval compression from the uterus.[62,63]

A high index of suspicion can avoid costly delays in diagnosis and treatment, allowing for adequate resuscitation of both the patient and fetus. In general, pregnant patients should promptly receive the same treatment as nonpregnant patients with anaphylaxis. Minor practice variations, such as patient positioning to account for hemodynamics associated with the gravid uterus, exist; however, these should not delay prompt administration of epinephrine and other life-saving measures.

Prevention

Recognition of potential triggers is key to prevention of anaphylaxis in pregnancy. Most commonly, anaphylaxis in pregnancy is associated with medication exposure. In cases of known prior medication reactions, prevention requires obtaining an accurate drug allergy history and careful avoidance of potential allergens. Ideally, history of reaction to an agent that may be required during the pregnancy would be evaluated before conception; however, there are many cases wherein this evaluation can be conducted safely in pregnant patients. For example, penicillin allergy evaluation, including skin testing and graded dose challenge, has been shown to be a safe and effective means to delabel "penicillin allergic" pregnant patients.[64,65] In general, skin testing carries a low risk of systemic reaction and it is reasonable to pursue in pregnant patients.[66] If hypersensitivity is confirmed, or comorbidities increase the risk of further allergy evaluation, desensitization can be performed when a medication to which IgE-mediated (anaphylactic) potential is confirmed or cannot be ruled out, and there is no equally efficacious alternative that can be used.[3]

CLINICS CARE POINTS

- Diagnosis of anaphylaxis in pregnant patients requires a high index of suspicion, because cutaneous symptoms are much less common in pregnant patients during anaphylaxis than in the general population.
- When positioning a pregnant patient during anaphylaxis, the patient should be placed in the lateral decubitus position to prevent uterine caval compression that can occur with the typically recommended Trendelenburg positioning.
- When pregnant women are diagnosed with anaphylaxis, referral for evaluation by a board-certified allergist/immunologist is warranted to identify the causative agent; this is particularly important for patients with anaphylaxis associated with cesarean delivery, because repeat cesarean delivery is common and reexposure can be avoided.

DISCLOSURE

M.M. Kuder, M. Hopkins, and R. Baird have nothing to disclose. D.M. Lang has carried out clinical research with, has received honoraria from, and/or has served as a consultant for ARS, AstraZeneca, Genentech, Novartis, and Sanofi-Regeneron.

REFERENCES

1. Shaker MS, Wallace DV, Golden DBK, et al. Anaphylaxis—a 2020 practice parameter update, systematic review, and Grading of Recommendations, Assessment, Development and Evaluation (GRADE) analysis. J Allergy Clin Immunol 2020;145(4). https://doi.org/10.1016/j.jaci.2020.01.017.
2. Wood RA, Camargo CA, Lieberman P, et al. Anaphylaxis in America: the prevalence and characteristics of anaphylaxis in the United States. J Allergy Clin Immunol 2014;133(2):461–7.
3. Wang J, Lieberman JA, Camargo CA, et al. Diverse perspectives on recognition and management of anaphylaxis. Ann Allergy Asthma Immunol 2021;127(1). https://doi.org/10.1016/j.anai.2021.01.019.
4. Motosue MS, Bellolio MF, Van Houten HK, et al. Risk factors for severe anaphylaxis in the United States. Ann Allergy Asthma Immunol 2017;119. https://doi.org/10.1016/j.anai.2017.07.014.
5. Carra S, Schatz M, Mertes PM, et al. Anaphylaxis and pregnancy: a systematic review and call for public health actions. J Allergy Clin Immunol Pract 2021; 9(12). https://doi.org/10.1016/j.jaip.2021.07.046.
6. Tacquard C, Chassard D, Malinovsky JM, et al. Anaphylaxis-related mortality in the obstetrical setting: analysis of the French National Confidential Enquiry into

Maternal Deaths from 2001 to 2012. Br J Anaesth 2019;123(1). https://doi.org/10.1016/j.bja.2018.12.009.

7. Gonzalez-Estrada A, Silvers SK, Klein A, et al. Epidemiology of anaphylaxis at a tertiary care center: A report of 730 cases. Ann Allergy Asthma Immunol 2017; 118(1):80–5.

8. Mulla ZD, Ebrahim MS, Gonzalez JL. Anaphylaxis in the obstetric patient: analysis of a statewide hospital discharge database. Ann Allergy Asthma Immunol 2010;104(1). https://doi.org/10.1016/j.anai.2009.11.005.

9. McCall SJ, Bunch KJ, Brocklehurst P, et al. The incidence, characteristics, management and outcomes of anaphylaxis in pregnancy: a population-based descriptive study. BJOG An Int J Obstet Gynaecol 2018;125(8). https://doi.org/10.1111/1471-0528.15041.

10. McCall SJ, Kurinczuk JJ, Knight M. Anaphylaxis in pregnancy in the united states: risk factors and temporal trends using national routinely collected data. J Allergy Clin Immunol Pract 2019;7. https://doi.org/10.1016/j.jaip.2019.04.047.

11. Simionescu AA, Danciu BM, Stanescu AMA. Severe anaphylaxis in pregnancy: a systematic review of clinical presentation to determine outcomes. J Pers Med 2021;11(11). https://doi.org/10.3390/jpm11111060.

12. Webb LM, Lieberman P. Anaphylaxis: A review of 601 cases. Ann Allergy Asthma Immunol 2006;97(1). https://doi.org/10.1016/S1081-1206(10)61367-1.

13. Lieberman P, Nicklas RA, Randolph C, et al. Anaphylaxis—a practice parameter update 2015. Ann Allergy Asthma Immunol 2015;115(5). https://doi.org/10.1016/j.anai.2015.07.019.

14. Berggren EK, Presley L, Amini SB, et al. Are the metabolic changes of pregnancy reversible in the first year postpartum? Diabetologia 2015;58(7). https://doi.org/10.1007/s00125-015-3604-x.

15. Zeeman GG, Cunningham FG, Pritchard JA. The magnitude of hemoconcentration with eclampsia. Hypertens Pregnancy 2009;28(2). https://doi.org/10.1080/10641950802556092.

16. Lindheimer MD, Davison JM, Katz AI. The kidney and hypertension in pregnancy: twenty exciting years. Semin Nephrol 2001;21(2). https://doi.org/10.1053/snep.2001.20937.

17. Øin P, Maltau JM, Noddeland H, et al. Oedema-preventing mechanisms in subcutaneous tissue of normal pregnant women. BJOG An Int J Obstet Gynaecol 1985;92(11). https://doi.org/10.1111/j.1471-0528.1985.tb03021.x.

18. Cong J, Yang X, Zhang N, et al. Quantitative analysis of left atrial volume and function during normotensive and preeclamptic pregnancy: a real-time three-dimensional echocardiography study. Int J Cardiovasc Imaging 2015;31(4). https://doi.org/10.1007/s10554-015-0628-8.

19. Mahendru AA, Everett TR, Wilkinson IB, et al. Maternal cardiovascular changes from pre-pregnancy to very early pregnancy. J Hypertens 2012;30(11). https://doi.org/10.1097/HJH.0b013e3283588189.

20. Cunningham F, Leveno K, Bloom S, et al. Maternal Physiology. In: Williams obstetrics. 25th edition. McGraw Hill; 2018.

21. Monga M, Mastrobattista JM. 7 - Maternal cardiovascular. Respir Ren Adaptation Pregnancy 2014;i.

22. Stewart RD, Nelson DB, Matulevicius SA, et al. Cardiac magnetic resonance imaging to assess the impact of maternal habitus on cardiac remodeling during pregnancy. Am J Obstet Gynecol 2016;214(5). https://doi.org/10.1016/j.ajog.2015.11.014.

23. Resnik JL, Hong C, Resnik R, et al. Evaluation of B-type natriuretic peptide (BNP) levels in normal and preeclamptic women. Am J Obstet Gynecol 2005;193(2). https://doi.org/10.1016/j.ajog.2004.12.006.

24. Bieniarz J, Branda LA, Maqueda E, et al. Aortocaval compression by the uterus in late pregnancy. III. Unreliability of the sphygmomanometric method in estimating uterine artery pressure. Am J Obstet Gynecol 1968;102(8). https://doi.org/10.1016/0002-9378(68)90400-6.

25. Kinsella SM, Lohmann G. Supine hypotensive syndrome. Obstet Gynecol 1994;83(5). https://doi.org/10.5005/jp/books/11286_10.

26. Pumphrey RSH. Fatal posture in anaphylactic shock [1]. J Allergy Clin Immunol 2003;112(2). https://doi.org/10.1067/mai.2003.1614.

27. Kenny LC, McCrae KR, Gary Cunningham F. Platelets, coagulation, and the liver. In: Chesley's hypertensive disorders in pregnancy. Fourth Edition; 2014. https://doi.org/10.1016/B978-0-12-407866-6.00017-1.

28. Sharief LT, Lawrie AS, Mackie IJ, et al. Changes in factor XIII level during pregnancy. Haemophilia 2014;20(2). https://doi.org/10.1111/hae.12345.

29. Hegewald MJ, Crapo RO. Respiratory Physiology in Pregnancy. Clin Chest Med 2011;32(1). https://doi.org/10.1016/j.ccm.2010.11.001.

30. Kolarzyk E, Szot WM, Lyszczarz J. Lung function and breathing regulation parameters during pregnancy. Arch Gynecol Obstet 2005;272(1). https://doi.org/10.1007/s00404-004-0691-1.

31. Heenan AP, Wolfe LA. Plasma osmolality and the strong ion difference predict respiratory adaptations in pregnant and nonpregnant women. Can J Physiol Pharmacol 2003;81(9). https://doi.org/10.1139/y03-072.

32. Bobrowski RA. Pulmonary physiology in pregnancy. Clin Obstet Gynecol 2010;53(2). https://doi.org/10.1097/GRF.0b013e3181e04776.

33. Jensen D, Wolfe LA, Slatkovska L, et al. Effects of human pregnancy on the ventilatory chemoreflex response to carbon dioxide. Am J Physiol - Regul Integr Comp Physiol 2005;288(5 57–5). https://doi.org/10.1152/ajpregu.00862.2004.

34. Izakson A, Cohen Y, Landau R. Physiologic Changes in the Airway and the Respiratory System Affecting Management in Pregnancy. In: Principles and practice of maternal critical care. 2020. https://doi.org/10.1007/978-3-030-43477-9_20.

35. Conrad KP, Stillman IE, Lindheimer MD. The kidney in normal pregnancy and preeclampsia. In: Chesley's hypertensive disorders in pregnancy. Fourth Edition; 2014. https://doi.org/10.1016/B978-0-12-407866-6.00016-X.

36. Lindheimer M, Grunfeld JP. Renal Disorders. In: Medical disorders during pregnancy. 3rd ed. Mosby; 2000.

37. Djurisic S, Hviid TVF. HLA class Ib molecules and immune cells in pregnancy and preeclampsia. Front Immunol 2014;5(DEC). https://doi.org/10.3389/fimmu.2014.00652.

38. Michimata T, Sakai M, Miyazaki S, et al. Decrease of T-helper 2 and T-cytotoxic 2 cells at implantation sites occurs in unexplained recurrent spontaneous abortion with normal chromosomal content. Hum Reprod 2003;18(7). https://doi.org/10.1093/humrep/deg280.

39. Simons FER, Schatz M. Anaphylaxis during pregnancy. J Allergy Clin Immunol 2012;130(3). https://doi.org/10.1016/j.jaci.2012.06.035.

40. Cousins L. Fetal oxygenation, assessment of fetal well-being, and obstetric management of the pregnant patient with asthma. J Allergy Clin Immunol 1999;103(2 SUPPL). https://doi.org/10.1016/s0091-6749(99)70260-5.

41. Chaudhuri K, Gonzales J, Jesurun CA, et al. Anaphylactic shock in pregnancy: A case study and review of the Literature. Int J Obstet Anesth 2008;17(4). https://doi.org/10.1016/j.ijoa.2008.05.002.
42. Sampson HA, Muñoz-Furlong A, Campbell RL, et al. Second symposium on the definition and management of anaphylaxis: Summary report - Second National Institute of Allergy and Infectious Disease/Food Allergy and Anaphylaxis Network symposium. J Allergy Clin Immunol 2006;117(2):391–7. https://doi.org/10.1016/j.jaci.2005.12.1303.
43. D'Astous-Gauthier K, Graham F, Paradis L, et al. Beta-2 Agonists May be Superior to Epinephrine to Relieve Severe Anaphylactic Uterine Contractions. J Allergy Clin Immunol Pract 2021;9(3):1232–41. https://doi.org/10.1016/J.JAIP.2020.10.047.
44. Haftel A, Chowdhury Y. Amniotic Fluid Embolism. In: StatPearls. Statpearls Publishing; 2022.
45. Stafford IA, Moaddab A, Dildy GA, et al. Amniotic fluid embolism syndrome: analysis of the Unites States International Registry. Am J Obstet Gynecol MFM 2020; 2. https://doi.org/10.1016/j.ajogmf.2019.100083.
46. Erratum: Practice Bulletin No. 199. Use of prophylactic antibiotics in labor and delivery. Obstet Gynecol 2018;132:e103–19. https://doi.org/10.1097/AOG.0000000000002833. Obstet Gynecol. 2019;134(4). doi: 10.1097/AOG.0000000000003499.
47. Chu J, Johnston TA, Geoghegan J. Maternal collapse in pregnancy and the puerperium: green-top guideline No. 56. BJOG An Int J Obstet Gynaecol 2020; 127(5):e14–52. https://doi.org/10.1111/1471-0528.15995.
48. Pitlick MM, Volcheck GW. Perioperative Anaphylaxis. Immunol Allergy Clin N Am 2022;42(1):145–59.
49. Mascarello KC, Matijasevich A, Barros AJD, et al. Repeat cesarean section in subsequent gestation of women from a birth cohort in Brazil. Reprod Health 2017;14(1):1–7.
50. Osterman M. Recent Trends in Vaginal Birth After Cesarean Delivery: United States, 2016–2018. 2020. https://www.cdc.gov/nchs/products/databriefs/db359.htm#Key_findings. [Accessed 22 February 2022].
51. Watson KD, Arendt KW, Watson WJ, et al. Systemic mastocytosis complicating pregnancy. Obstet Gynecol 2012;119(2 PART 2). https://doi.org/10.1097/AOG.0b013e318242d3c5.
52. Matito A, Álvarez-Twose I, Morgado JM, et al. Clinical impact of pregnancy in mastocytosis: A study of the Spanish network on mastocytosis (REMA) in 45 cases. Int Arch Allergy Immunol 2011;156(1). https://doi.org/10.1159/000321954.
53. Gülen T, Akin C. Anaphylaxis and Mast Cell Disorders. Immunol Allergy Clin N Am 2022;42(1):45–63.
54. Smith HS, Hare MJ, Hoggarth CE, et al. Delivery as a cause of exercise-induced anaphylactoid reaction: Case report. BJOG An Int J Obstet Gynaecol 1985; 92(11). https://doi.org/10.1111/j.1471-0528.1985.tb03038.x.
55. Shadick NA, Liang MH, Partridge AJ, et al. The natural history of exercise-induced anaphylaxis: Survey results from a 10-year follow-up study. J Allergy Clin Immunol 1999;104(1):123–7.
56. Chooniedass R, Temple B, Becker A. Epinephrine use for anaphylaxis: Too seldom, too late: Current practices and guidelines in health care. Ann Allergy Asthma Immunol 2017;119(2). https://doi.org/10.1016/j.anai.2017.06.004.
57. Seto A, Einarson T, Koren G. Pregnancy outcome following first trimester exposure to antihistamines: Meta-analysis. Am J Perinatol 1997;14(3):119–24.

58. Kar S, Krishnan A, Preetha K, et al. A review of antihistamines used during pregnancy. J Pharmacol Pharmacother 2012;3(2). https://doi.org/10.4103/0976-500X.95503.

59. Shawky RM, Seifeldin NS. The relation between antihistamine medication during early pregnancy & birth defects. Egypt J Med Hum Genet 2015;16(4):287–90.

60. Bandoli G, Palmsten K, Forbess Smith CJ, et al. A Review of Systemic Corticosteroid Use in Pregnancy and the Risk of Select Pregnancy and Birth Outcomes. Rheum Dis Clin North Am 2017;43(3). https://doi.org/10.1016/j.rdc.2017.04.013.

61. Simhan HN. Practice Bulletin No. 171: Management of Preterm Labor. Obstet Gynecol 2016;128(4). https://doi.org/10.1097/AOG.0000000000001711.

62. Peltolta L, Plaat F. Maternal Resuscitation. In: Einav S, Weiniger C, Landau R, editors. Principles and practice of maternal critical care. Cham, Switzerland: Springer; 2020. p. 373–82.

63. Jeejeebhoy FM, Zelop CM, Lipman S, et al. Cardiac arrest in pregnancy: a scientific statement from the American heart association. Circulation 2015;132(18). https://doi.org/10.1161/CIR.0000000000000300.

64. Kuder MM, Lennox MG, Li M, et al. Skin testing and oral amoxicillin challenge in the outpatient allergy and clinical immunology clinic in pregnant women with penicillin allergy. Ann Allergy Asthma Immunol 2020;125:646–51.

65. Patel V, Fadugba O, Ralston S, et al. Safety and Outcomes for Penicillin Skin Testing in Pregnancy. J Allergy Clin Immunol 2021;147(2). https://doi.org/10.1016/j.jaci.2020.12.528.

66. Valyasevi MA, Van Dellen RG. Frequency of systematic reactions to penicillin skin tests. Ann Allergy Asthma Immunol 2000;85(5):363–5.

Management of Allergic Skin Disorders in Pregnancy

Eleanor M. Pope, BA, Leah Laageide, MD, Lisa A. Beck, MD*

KEYWORDS

- Allergy • Pregnancy • Lactation • Atopic dermatitis • Chronic urticaria
- Contact dermatitis

KEY POINTS

- The most prevalent allergic skin disorders in pregnancy include atopic dermatitis, chronic urticaria, and allergic contact dermatitis.
- Disease activity of these skin disorders may vary in pregnancy.
- Treatments may include topical and systemic medications.
- To ensure maternal and infant health and to prevent secondary complications, it is vital to balance prescribing effective yet safe medication dosages and maintaining adequate disease control.

INTRODUCTION

The safe management of allergic skin disorders during pregnancy is essential to maternal and fetal health. In this review, we address gaps in knowledge on the course and best management of atopic dermatitis (AD), chronic urticaria (CU), and allergic contact dermatitis (ACD) in pregnancy. Each section describes disease activity in pregnancy and disease-specific topical and systemic treatments. **Tables 1–3** provide guidance for all relevant topical and systemic therapies during pregnancy, respectively. We briefly address concerns regarding breastfeeding (**Table 4**). Data are limited on the safety and efficacy of many commonly used treatments in human pregnancies and therefore, recommendations are largely based on observational studies. It is hoped that publications from Food and Drug Administration (FDA)-mandated post-marketing pregnancy registries for more recently approved therapies will provide greater clarity on best practices for pregnant patients with moderate to severe allergic skin diseases.

UR Medicine Dermatology, 40 Celebration Drive, Rochester, NY 14620
* Corresponding author.
E-mail address: Lisa_Beck@urmc.rochester.edu

Immunol Allergy Clin N Am 43 (2023) 117–132
https://doi.org/10.1016/j.iac.2022.05.012
0889-8561/23/© 2022 Elsevier Inc. All rights reserved.

immunology.theclinics.com

Table 1
Guidance for topical therapy during pregnancy

Therapy	Recommendations
Moisturizers	• First line • Patient's choice
Topical corticosteroids	• First line • Low-medium potency recommended (groups 4–6) • High potency (groups 2–3) as rescue therapy or on limited skin areas • Avoid fluticasone propionate • Consider UV therapy if use exceeds 200 g/mo
Topical calcineurin inhibitors	• Use on limited skin areas is permissible • Preferred use on face and areas prone to striae formation • Tacrolimus recommended (not much data on safety or efficacy of pimecrolimus)
Topical phosphodiesterase-4 inhibitors (crisaborole)	• Not recommended because of lack of experience/data
Topical antibiotics	• Escalate topical corticosteroids first
Topical JAK inhibitors (ruxolitinib)	• Not recommended because of lack of experience/data

Change to Risk Classification of Drugs in Pregnancy

In 2014, the FDA published the "Pregnancy and Lactation Labeling Rule" to replace the pregnancy letter categories (ie, A, B, C, D, and X) previously used to classify drug risk in pregnancy. This new "narrative" system went into effect June 30, 2015, changing the content and format of information presented in prescription drug labeling. The Pregnancy and Lactation Labeling Rule aims to assist health care providers and pregnant women in assessing risk/benefit and in making informed decisions

Table 2
Topical steroid potencies

Potency	Examples
Least potent (group 7)	• Hydrocortisone 1%, 2.5% cream, ointment, lotion
Low (group 6)	• Desonide 0.05% cream, lotion • Fluocinolone acetonide 0.01% cream • Triamcinolone 0.025% cream, lotion
Lower-mid (group 5)	• Fluocinolone acetonide 0.025% cream • Triamcinolone 0.1% lotion, 0.025% ointment
Medium (groups 4)	• Fluocinolone acetonide 0.025% ointment • Mometasone furoate 0.1% cream, lotion • Triamcinolone acetonide 0.1% cream, ointment
High (group 3)	• Betamethasone dipropionate 0.05% cream • Mometasone furoate 0.1% ointment
High (group 2)	• Betamethasone dipropionate 0.05% cream, ointment • Desoximetasone 0.25% cream, ointment • Fluocinonide 0.05% cream, ointment
Super high (group 1)	• Betamethasone dipropionate, augmented 0.05% ointment • Clobetasol propionate 0.05% cream, lotion, ointment • Fluocinonide 0.1% cream • Halobetasol propionate 0.05% cream, lotion, ointment

Table 3
Guidance for systemic therapy during pregnancy

Therapy	Recommendations
Systemic corticosteroids	• May be used as rescue therapy • Prioritize other therapies first (ie, escalate topical corticosteroids) • Prednisolone preferred • Recommend use only up to 0.5 mg/kg/d and avoid >20 mg/d • Use no more than 2–3 wk
Cyclosporine	• Reserve as rescue therapy for severe disease • Default first-line immunosuppressive for continuous treatment/long-term control • Can cause maternal hypertension and renal dysfunction
Azathioprine	• May be used under strict indications if no other therapy is possible • Avoid initiating after conception • Halve dose if already taking at time of conception
Methotrexate	• Absolutely contraindicated • Wait 1–6 mo after stopping treatment to conceive
Mycophenolate mofetil	• Absolutely contraindicated • Women should use nonhormonal contraception until 2–3 mo after stopping therapy
Oral antihistamines	• Not considered first choice or optimal therapy for AD in any patient population • Loratadine first choice • Cetirizine second choice (may also relieve pregnancy-associated nausea)
Dupilumab	• Not advised at this time because of lack of experience/data • Case reports show no adverse effects • Limited data have not identified a drug-associated risk
Systemic JAK inhibitors	• Avoid becoming pregnant during treatment and for at least 4 wk after last dose
Phototherapy	• UVB (broadband or narrow) or UVA1 recommended • Psoralen plus UVA not advised
Omalizumab	• May be used as rescue therapy • Registries show no increase in rate of birth defects or miscarriage

about taking a medication during pregnancy and lactation.[1] Although this amended regulation allows patients more accessible and consistent prescription drug information and thus greater autonomy in their care, this transition may also create a challenge for providers who are more familiar with the old "category" system. To facilitate counseling of relevant medications, we recommend consulting section 8 of the medication's FDA label, found online or in the prescription packaging (eg, https://www.opzelura.com/prescribing-information.pdf). Section 8 includes risk summaries and animal data for pregnancy (section 8.1) and lactation (section 8.2) and contact information for pregnancy exposure registries.

Food and Drug Administration–Approved Therapies and General Recommendations

For the treatment of AD in pregnancy, recommended therapies include moisturizers, topical steroids, topical tacrolimus, phototherapy, and systemic steroids or

Table 4
Guidance for therapies during breastfeeding

Therapy	Recommendations
Topical corticosteroids	• Safe to use • Apply immediately after feeding • Clean nipple before next feeding
Topical calcineurin inhibitors	• Safe to use • Apply immediately after feeding • Clean nipple before next feeding
Topical PDE-4 inhibitors (crisaborole)	• Not recommended
Topical JAK inhibitors (ruxolitinib)	• Not recommended
Phototherapy	• Safe to use
Systemic corticosteroids	• Safe to use as rescue therapy • Wait to breastfeed 4 h after ingestion
Oral antihistamines	• Safe to use • Nonsedating, second generation preferred • Use caution with first generation and monitor child for irritability/drowsiness
Cyclosporine	• May be used off-label under strict indications
Azathioprine	• Use debated • Wait to breastfeed for 4 h after ingesting or discard milk produced within 4 h after dose • Monitor child for signs of immunosuppression/periodically check child blood counts
Methotrexate	• Contraindicated
Mycophenolate mofetil	• Contraindicated
Dupilumab	• Not recommended currently because of lack of experience/data • Case reports show no adverse effects
Omalizumab	• Safe to use

cyclosporine as a last resort.[2] Guidelines are similar for the treatment of ACD in pregnancy, with topical steroids being first line and systemic steroids reserved for severe cases.[2,3] For CU in pregnancy, first-line treatment is nonsedating second-generation H_1 antihistamines; systemic steroids, cyclosporine, and omalizumab may be reserved for recalcitrant cases.[4–7]

ATOPIC DERMATITIS
Disease Activity in Pregnancy

AD is a chronic, relapsing inflammatory skin disease, affecting up to 10% of adults in industrialized countries[8] and the most common skin disease in pregnancy.[2,9] AD is characterized by type 2 immune deviation, skin barrier dysfunction, and pruritus,[10] and bacterial and viral skin infections, allergen sensitization, and collectively, a negative impact on quality of life measures.[2] During pregnancy, the immune system shifts toward a type 2 immune response.[2] The high levels of estrogen and progesterone enhance the activity of Th2 and T-regulatory cells, which collectively suppress Th1 and Th17 activity.[10] This shift is thought to reduce the immunologic response against the fetus, creating a favorable environment for acceptance of the allogenic fetus and reducing the risk of miscarriage.[2,10] The type 2 response has a humoral component with the induction of IgE and production of the inflammatory cytokines implicated in

AD, including interleukin (IL)-4, IL-5, and IL-13. Unfortunately, the immunologic state of pregnancy may lead to worsening of AD.[2] Furthermore, the physical and psychological stress of pregnancy may also exacerbate preexisting AD.[2] Importantly, there is little to no evidence to suggest AD directly affects fertility or rate of miscarriage and does not cause birth defects or preterm birth.[11]

The effect of pregnancy on AD disease activity is highly variable with some patients improving, worsening, or staying the same.[12] One report cited 25% of pregnant women see improvements in their AD, 50% deteriorate, and 10% flare in the postpartum period.[11] This is consistent with the estimate that 52% to 61% of cases worsen during pregnancy, most notably during the second and third trimesters.[10,13] However, a recent cross-sectional study reported only 17.7% of pregnant women experienced worsening of their AD, which led the authors to conclude "most will not experience worsening AD during pregnancy."[14]

A Danish birth registry identified an overrepresentation of premature rupture of membranes and staphylococcal neonatal septicemia in mothers with AD, but no associations with any other significant prenatal, obstetric, or birth outcomes.[15] Rather, it is the potential complications of undertreated, moderate to severe AD (ie, eczema herpeticum, secondary staphylococcus infections, neonatal septicemia) that poses maternal and fetal risk.[2,8] Physicians are quite risk-averse and offer restricted treatment options; consequently, pregnant women with AD are often inadequately managed and so experience recurrent flares and even infections.[2]

Disease Management and Treatment

Adequate management of AD during pregnancy is imperative to reduce maternal and fetal risk. However, treating pregnant or lactating women is a challenge, because there are no large, well-controlled clinical studies on the effects of AD treatments in this population.[8] Recommendations include advising patients with AD before conception, with the goal of minimizing baseline disease activity and avoiding irritants and relevant allergens.[11] The European Task Force on Atopic Dermatitis (ETFAD) recommends a safety-first approach for the treatment of future mothers and pregnant or lactating women. In order of preference, safe treatments include moisturizers, topical steroids, and topical tacrolimus; UV therapy or moderate sun exposure; and systemic treatments (ie, systemic steroids and cyclosporine A [CyA]) for severe cases.[2] Azathioprine (AZA) may only be used with strict indications, methotrexate (MTX) and mycophenolate mofetil (MMF) are absolutely contradicted, and there is still not clear data on the risk of dupilumab. The following section provides more detail on the management of AD during pregnancy, including topical, systemic, and emerging therapies. **Tables 1–3** provide a quick reference.

Topical treatments

Basic emollients with a high lipid content, tepid baths, and avoidance of basic soaps are key.[2] Topical corticosteroids (TCS) are first line in pregnant and nonpregnant women because of their minimal systemic side effects, although local side effects may be slightly greater in pregnancy especially when used in areas prone to striae formation. TCS may be used proactively or reactively. They have no association with preterm delivery, birth defects, fetal death, or low Apgar scores, although potent TCS may be associated with low birthweight.[2,16] Group 6 and 7 TCS are typically not potent enough to be beneficial in AD, groups 3 to 5 are often suitable, group 2 may be used in the short term, and group 1 should be avoided unless necessary for rescue therapy.[2] Importantly, fluticasone propionate is not metabolized by the placenta and should not be used.[2]

To date, there are no studies on the use of topical calcineurin inhibitors in pregnancy. Systemic absorption of topical tacrolimus is low, and available data suggest the risk of congenital defects is not increased.[2,17] Although topical pimecrolimus is absorbed even less,[18] its FDA label currently says not to use because of lack of experience. Topical tacrolimus is recommended because of a large amount of existing data and may be preferable to TCS especially for use on the face and areas prone to striae formation.[2]

There are no studies on the use of crisaborole in pregnancy. Its FDA label says it is contraindicated, and should not be used preconceptionally, in pregnancy, or during lactation because of lack of experience.[2]

Ruxolitinib is a topical potent, selective inhibitor of JAK1 and JAK2, recently FDA approved for short-term and noncontinuous use in mild to moderate AD in patients 12 years and older. There are no published studies on ruxolitinib in human pregnancies and observational data are insufficient at this time to make a formal recommendation; it is advised to avoid topical ruxolitinib in the pregnant and breastfeeding population.[19]

Topical antibiotics are used, although it is preferable to escalate the potency of a topical steroid rather than initiate topical antibiotics. Mupirocin is preferred because of its reduce allergenicity as compared with neomycin and bacitracin and its superior efficacy in treating methicillin-sensitive and methicillin-resistant *Staphylococcus aureus* infections.[20]

Phototherapy

There are no published studies on the safety and efficacy of phototherapy in pregnancy. Broad-spectrum and narrow-band UVB and UVA1 therapy are not thought to impose a risk to the fetus and are used liberally if topical therapy fails. UVB therapy does decrease folic acid levels and should be supplemented preconceptionally and in the first trimester.[21] Phototherapy may also exacerbate pregnancy-induced hyperpigmentation (ie, melasma); facial shielding may be advised depending on patient skin type. Lastly, psoralen plus UVA therapy is not a safe option because psoralen should not be used 3 months before conception, during pregnancy, or while breastfeeding.[2]

Systemic anti-inflammatories

Evidence for treatment of AD in pregnancy with systemic anti-inflammatories is observational and limited. Therapy should be initiated on an individual basis and in close collaboration with an experienced obstetrician. Although systemic corticosteroids (SCS) are used in nonpregnant patients in short courses for acute or severe flares, the risk/benefit ratio for their use is generally considered unfavorable. During pregnancy, SCS increase the risk of gestational diabetes, preeclampsia/eclampsia, premature rupture of membranes, and preterm delivery; repeated treatment courses may lead to decreased birthweight and gastroesophageal reflux disease.[2,16] Therefore, when possible, it is recommended to prioritize other therapies, such as escalating topical steroid therapy.[2] SCS are fortunately rarely needed in pregnant patients with AD; however, they are considered reasonably safe to use with proper monitoring of the mother and child. Additionally, in patients with concomitant asthma, the benefits of SCS in controlling asthmatic attacks clearly outweigh the risks during pregnancy.[12] The general recommendation is to limit their use and use only for the patient that has failed adequate administration of topical steroids and UV therapy. Preference is given for prednisolone (and not dexamethasone) at doses only up to 0.5 mg/kg/d for less than 2 to 3 weeks.[2]

CyA crosses the placenta but has no increased risk of congenital malformations or fetal death; it may have an increased risk of low birthweight.[2] Most of the data on CyA during pregnancy come from transplant recipients who generally receive higher doses than dermatologic patients.[16] CyA is considered a safe treatment alternative in cases recalcitrant to other therapies and is used off-label if there is a clear need for long-term control. CyA is considered the default immunosuppressive treatment of patients that need continuous treatment during pregnancy. Extra attention should be given to the patient's renal function and blood pressure.[2]

AZA has been used off-label in cases of severe and uncontrolled AD where phototherapy and other systemic therapies have failed. For example, it has been used in other systemic inflammatory diseases (eg, bowel disease, rheumatic disease, organ transplants) during pregnancy without consistent evidence of birth defects.[22] According to its FDA label, AZA is contraindicated during pregnancy. The ETFAD also recommends avoiding AZA during pregnancy but does stipulate that if a woman is already receiving AZA at the time of conception and there are no safer alternatives, treatment is continued, and the dosage should be reduced by 50%.[2]

MTX is well known to be associated with severe birth defects even at low doses and is therefore absolutely contraindicated during pregnancy. There is a discrepancy between waiting periods with some sources recommending stopping treatment 6 months before planned pregnancies and others recommending only 1 to 3 months; the risk/benefit of a shorter waiting period should be discussed on an individual basis.[2]

MMF is considered teratogenic and associated with specific embryonal malformations. MMF is absolutely contraindicated during pregnancy and should never be used in women who are planning pregnancy, pregnant, or breastfeeding. The FDA requires contraceptive counseling and use during and for 3 months after stopping therapy.[2]

Oral antihistamines

Oral antihistamines may be used if clinically indicated. Even in nonpregnant patients, they have limited efficacy in managing AD and have little effect on pruritus.[2] They are sometimes used for their sedative effects, but not considered first choice or an optimal therapy for AD in any patient population. In pregnancy, loratadine, a second-generation H_1 antihistamine, is preferred based on extensive experience.[23] Cetirizine may also be used and may relieve pregnancy-associated nausea and vomiting.[12] The sedating antihistamines may be used for strict indications with accompanying counseling on the long-term side effects (eg, motoric and cognitive function) and a risk/benefit discussion.[23]

Dupilumab

Dupilumab, a fully human IgG4 monoclonal antibody against the IL-4 receptor α that inhibits signaling of IL-4 and IL-13, is the first biologic treatment FDA approved for the treatment of moderate to severe AD[24] and becoming an increasingly popular option for severe or recalcitrant disease. As an IgG antibody, intrauterine exposure to dupilumab from midgestation on is likely to be quite high; it is also excreted in breast milk.[24] Although postmarketing data on dupilumab in pregnancy are limited,[9] there are a few case reports of pregnant patients with AD treated with dupilumab who achieved dramatic skin improvement and no adverse events for either mother or child.[13] In one report, the patient received a loading dose of 600 mg starting at 24 weeks of pregnancy followed by 300 mg every other week and had an uncomplicated delivery of a healthy male infant.[9] In another report, the patient was on 300 mg every other week at the time of conception and continued dupilumab until almost 25 weeks of gestation and had an uncomplicated delivery of a healthy female infant.[24] Furthermore, animal studies do not indicate direct or indirect harmful effects. The available data have not identified a drug-associated risk of major birth defects, miscarriage, or adverse maternal or fetal outcomes[24]; however, because of lack of experience and limited data, contraception is advised during therapy and dupilumab use during pregnancy is possible only if the potential benefits to the mother are higher than the potential risks to the fetus.[8] It is encouraged to enroll patients in the pregnancy registry study (https://clinicaltrials.gov/ct2/show/NCT03936335) to monitor outcomes, adverse or otherwise, in women exposed to dupilumab during pregnancy and lactation.[24]

JAK inhibitors
The data on the effects of any of the JAK inhibitors on human fertility and pregnancy are scant. Animal models suggest potential effects on fetal development and pregnancy outcomes. Therefore, it is strongly recommended to use effective birth control while taking an oral JAK inhibitor and to avoid becoming pregnant during therapy and for at least 4 weeks after the last dose.[8] It remains unclear whether these risks are lower with topical JAK inhibitors and moreover, how much the risk relates to the body surface area treated with the topical. Strict avoidance of topical JAK inhibitors in women planning pregnancies is also advisable.[19]

Emerging biologics
There are several new monoclonal antibodies that target IL-13, OX40, OX40 L, IL-5 receptor α, and IL-31 for treatment of AD. In fact, tralokinumab-ldrm, an inhibitor of IL-13, was FDA approved late December 2021 for the treatment of moderate to severe AD in adults 18 years or older.[25] There are no data on the effects of these new biologics on fertility, pregnancy, or breastfeeding and at this point, they should be avoided in pregnancy.[8]

In conclusion, there is limited evidence on the use of many AD treatments in human pregnancies and the impact of new medications on fertility is largely unknown. Importantly, the lack of adverse effects on animal fertility does not exclude a potential impact on humans. Patients with AD should consider planning a pregnancy when their disease is in remission or at least taking the minimum effective dose of medications with the best safety profiles, while ensuring adequate control to prevent secondary complications. Emollients and moisturizers should be used liberally. Low to mid potency TCS are first-line therapy.[8] Systemic therapies, including SCS and CyA, may be used on an individual basis with a careful assessment of potential risks and benefits with the patient's dermatologist and obstetrician.

CHRONIC URTICARIA
Disease Activity in Pregnancy

CU is characterized by greater than 6 weeks of recurrent pruritic wheals, angioedema, or both, and has a lifetime prevalence of approximately 20%.[26] It is further divided into chronic spontaneous urticaria (CSU) and chronic inducible urticaria (CIndU), the latter including nine subtypes.[4,5] Diagnosis is generally clinical and may be difficult because subtypes can coexist and the differential is broad, including mast cell activation syndrome, polymorphous light eruption, the urticarial form of bullous pemphigoid, drug reactions, cutaneous lupus erythematous, urticarial vasculitis, Schnitzler syndrome, Wells syndrome, and hereditary or acquired angioedema.[5,26,27]

Females have a higher prevalence of CU (3:1), greater disease activity, poorer prognosis, and decreased responsiveness to antihistamines or omalizumab.[28–34] The reasons for gender differences and the impact of pregnancy on disease severity remain unclear. Possible explanations include higher rates of autoimmunity in females and influences on sex hormones on menses, pregnancy, menopause, and hormonal therapies.[29] Despite an undefined pathogenic mechanism for CU, perivascular, Th2 cellular infiltrates are considered its predominant immunologic driver, whereas elevated plasma Th1/17 cytokines favor a role for type 1 and 3 immunity.[35–39] Central to CSU and CIndU pathogenesis is mast cell and basophil degranulation with the release of histamine, leukotrienes, prostaglandins, and other proinflammatory mediators.[5] In CSU, triggers of mast cell degranulation include idiopathic and/or circulating autoantibodies: IgE targeting self-antigens (type I autoimmunity) or IgG/IgM activating dermal mast cells and basophils (type IIb autoimmunity) targeting the α subunit of the high-affinity IgE receptor (FcϵR1) or cross-linking IgE present on the high-affinity IgE receptor.[26,40–42] Some patients with CU experience exacerbations from aspirin, nonsteroidal anti-inflammatory drugs, food, and/or stress.[26,43] In CIndU, mast cell degranulation stems from an indirect response to physical stimuli, such as cold, deep pressure, vibration, and/or sunlight.[4] Provocation tests are commonly used to diagnose CIndU, whereas CSU remains a clinical diagnosis that occasionally requires a skin biopsy to rule out differential diagnoses.[26]

As highlighted in the section on AD disease activity in pregnancy, regulatory T cells play a central role in the immune-tolerant state via a shift toward the Th2 axis, a deviation that may explain gestational exacerbations of Th2-driven diseases (eg, AD, allergic rhinitis, asthma) or improvement in Th1/Th17-driven diseases (eg, psoriasis, rheumatoid arthritis).[44,45] To date, limited data exist on incidence and disease pattern of urticaria and angioedema in pregnancy; accordingly, CU is not considered a "pregnancy-related dermatosis."[46]

Gestational changes in sex hormones, however, have shown effects on mast cell and basophil activity.[28,47,48] Progesterone inhibits mast cell secretion and basophil activation, whereas estrogen increases histamine release in rat mast cells and human basophils.[49] These observations may highlight why sex differences in CU prevalence are only observed between puberty and menopause.[29] High levels of synthetic estrogens via consumed substances or pollutants have also demonstrated rapid mast cell and histamine release; in fact, high levels of circulating mast cells have been shown to exacerbate pruritic urticarial papules and plaques of pregnancy.[46,50] Lastly, a few studies found lower levels of dehydroepiandrosterone, an androgenic immunomodulatory hormone, in patients with CU.[51,52]

Although the severity of CU may vary in response to hormonal exposures or pregnancy trimesters, no effect on fertility, labor, or delivery has been identified.[51,53] In the first international, multicenter study of CU in pregnancy (PREG-CU UCARE), about half of women (51.1%; n = 148/288) experienced skin improvement and a minority reported new or recurrent angioedema (17.4%; n = 50/288), irrespective of trimester. When stratified by trimester, skin exacerbations were most common in the first and third trimesters.[46] Because CU seems to be more commonly associated with cytokines reflective of type 2 immunity, questions remain regarding the hormonal influences on mast cells and basophils and their releasability.[46] Perhaps elevated levels of progesterone, estrogen, and cortisol are the key contributors to mast cell and basophil degranulation, and therefore CU activity. After birth, 37.4% (n = 265) of women reported worsening skin symptoms and/or angioedema from their pregestational baseline. When stratified by risk factors, exacerbations of CU during pregnancy were more commonly observed in women with no previous history of angioedema, or low CU disease activity, untreated disease, or the CIndU subtype before pregnancy.[28]

Disease Management and Treatment

With no cure or ability to predict the timing and likelihood of spontaneous remission, the goal of CU treatment is symptom control.[5] To help guide treatment decisions, validated patient-reported measures, such as urticaria and angioedema activity scores, are becoming customary in clinical practice. Avoidance of eliciting factors and searching for underlying factors is also important. For CIndU tolerance, induction may be a useful option.[54] Pharmacologically, the goal is reducing the downstream features of mast cell and/or basophil mediators (ie, histamine and leukotrienes) and free total IgE. To control symptoms, treatments should be used daily and not on an as-needed basis.[26,55]

Systemic treatments

First-line treatments are second-generation, nonsedating H_1 antihistamines with up-titration every 1 to 4 weeks until four-fold the manufacturer recommended dosage is reached.[4,56] Sedating, first-generation antihistamines are generally not recommended, but still used in particularly refractory cases.[57,58] For patients unresponsive to second-generation antihistamines, omalizumab may be added as treatment of either CSU or CIndU.[6,59] Initial dosing is 150 to 300 mg every 4 weeks with higher doses (5 mg/kg) or shorter intervals available off-label to patients with insufficient benefit with approved dosing.[6,60] Lastly, CyA (3.5–5 mg/kg/d) may be added to second-generation H_1 antihistamines if patients are not sufficiently controlled with these measures.[7,61] In cases of severe exacerbation, short courses of SCS (20–50 mg/d prednisone for maximum 10 days) may be added.[5,62]

There is a paucity of literature on CU management in pregnant or lactating women. However, treatment algorithms emphasize using the lowest effective medication dose.[4] In the context of the new, 2015 pregnancy and lactation labeling guidelines, the nonsedating, second-generation antihistamines remain first-line treatment in Europe and the United States. Use is safe during all trimesters, but discontinuation is encouraged 3 to 7 days before delivery to avoid potential side effects in infants from immature metabolism.[63,64] Preferred agents in pregnancy and breastfeeding include low-dose loratadine followed by cetirizine, largely because of safety profile and low concentrations in breastmilk.[56,65]

Leukotriene antagonists, including montelukast and zafirlukast (but not zileuton), may be added with no concern for neonatal structural abnormalities or perinatal problems.[12] More recently, the use of leukotriene antagonists in patients with CU with angioedema lesions has been shown to be beneficial.[66] If indicated, cyclosporine may be used but poses a risk for premature labor and gestational toxemia and can achieve high concentrations in breastmilk.[67]

Omalizumab

Little is known about the safety and efficacy of omalizumab during pregnancy and breastfeeding. There is reason to suspect that omalizumab may cross the placenta as an anti-IgE/IgE immune complex bound to the neonatal fetal receptor (FcRn), raising concerns that omalizumab could affect fetal immune development.[68] To date, the EXPECT Xolair Pregnancy Registry, the largest prospective observational study on perinatal and neonatal outcomes in women treated for asthma, has not found an increased risk of congenital abnormalities.[69] Less is known about the safety of omalizumab during pregnancy in CSU patients, with only about 13 cases reported in the literature. All cases, however, resulted in normal pregnancies with no gestational or fetal complications.[5] **Tables 1–3** provide a quick reference.

ALLERGIC CONTACT DERMATITIS
Disease Activity in Pregnancy

ACD, a type IV–mediated delayed hypersensitivity reaction, is caused by cutaneous exposure to an exogenous substance that elicits an inflammatory response.[70] It may present as an acute, subacute, or chronic dermatitis, and is characterized by pruritus and typically sharply delineated lesions consisting of erythema, induration, vesicles, and/or desquamation.[3] Although this is a common inflammatory skin disorder in the general population and more common in females, there are no data on the prevalence of ACD during pregnancy.[12] A history of AD may also be a contributing factor.[3]

Disease Management and Treatment

The mainstay of treatment of ACD is avoidance of the allergen.[3] Thus, identification of the causative allergy is necessary for resolution of ongoing ACD[71] and the gold standard for diagnosis is patch testing. It is advised that patch testing should be deferred until after pregnancy[71] and women who are breastfeeding should also not be patch tested.[12] However, there is no clear evidence of adverse effects on pregnancy outcomes or evidence to suggest the immunologic changes of pregnancy would alter the accuracy of patch testing.[71] **Tables 1–3** provide a quick reference.

Topical and systemic treatments

The same treatment guidelines for AD in pregnancy apply to ACD in pregnancy because the recommended therapies overlap. Midpotency TCS are recommended as first-line treatment of exacerbations in nonpregnant patients[3] and are also safe to use in pregnant patients for severe ACD. In the pregnant population it is recommended to use only up to 0.5 mg/kg/d for 2 to 3 weeks and to avoid greater than 20 mg/d if possible.[2] Antihistamines have generally not been shown to be helpful in treating the pruritus associated with ACD and are therefore not recommended in pregnant patients with ACD.[12]

CONCERNS REGARDING BREASTFEEDING

In general, few to no studies have examined the safety of various dermatologic treatments on breastfeeding and recommendations are based on observational studies. TCS and topical calcineurin inhibitors are safe to use, with the caveat they should ideally be applied immediately after breastfeeding and the nipple should be cleaned before the next feeding.[2] SCS are safe to use as rescue therapy, but breastfeeding should be delayed 4 hours after ingestion.[2] For CyA and AZA, their use is highly debated and may only be used under extreme circumstances.[2] Both MTX and MMF are contraindicated during breastfeeding.[2] Finally, biologics including dupilumab and omalizumab are not recommended at this time because of a lack of safety data, although case reports have shown no adverse effects.[24,69] **Table 4** provides a quick reference.

SUMMARY

This review has covered the management of AD, CU, and ACD during pregnancy and while breastfeeding. We demonstrated the complex interplay of the hormonal and immunologic effects of pregnancy on allergic skin disorders. We focused on disease course, safety and efficacy of topical and systemic treatments, and postpartum considerations to best advise patients with gestational planning. The Hippocratic oath to "do no harm" must be balanced with the need to achieve adequate management of these disorders, because poorly controlled allergic skin disease also affects the health of mother and child.

CLINICS CARE POINTS

- Consider planning a pregnancy when the allergic skin disorder is under good control or during remission.
- Prescribe the minimum effective dose of medications with the best safety profiles.
- Ensure adequate control to prevent secondary complications.
- Dermatologists and allergists need to work closely with obstetricians when more aggressive systemic treatments are necessary.

DISCLOSURE

Atopic Dermatitis Research Network (ADRN) 3 grant U01AI152011.

CONFLICTS OF INTEREST

L.A. Beck is a consultant for AbbVie, Allakos, Astra-Zeneca, AlBio, Sanofi/Genzyme, DermTech, Sanofi-Aventis, and Stealth biotherapeutics; and an investigator for Abb-Vie, Astra-Zeneca, Kiniska, LEO Pharma, Pfizer, Regeneron, and Sanofi. L. Laageide is an investigator for AbbVie, AstraZeneca, Kiniska, Sanofi, Pfizer, Regeneron, and DermTech. E. Pope is an investigator for DermTech.

REFERENCES

1. Research CfDEa. PLLR labeling final rule. U.S. food and drug administration. Available at: https://www.fda.gov/drugs/labeling-information-drug-products/pregnancy-and-lactation-labeling-drugs-final-rule. Accessed October 1, 2021.
2. Vestergaard C, Wollenberg A, Barbarot S, et al. European task force on atopic dermatitis position paper: treatment of parental atopic dermatitis during preconception, pregnancy and lactation period. J Eur Acad Dermatol Venereol 2019; 33(9):1644–59.
3. Nassau S, Fonacier L. Allergic contact dermatitis. Med Clin North Am 2020; 104(1):61–76.
4. Zuberbier T, Aberer W, Asero R, et al. The EAACI/GA^{2}LEN/EDF/WAO guideline for the definition, classification, diagnosis and management of urticaria. Allergy 2018;73(7):1393–414.
5. Saini S, Shams M, Bernstein JA, et al. Urticaria and angioedema across the ages. J Allergy Clin Immunol Pract 2020;8(6):1866–74.
6. Saini S, Rosen KE, Hsieh HJ, et al. A randomized, placebo-controlled, dose-ranging study of single-dose omalizumab in patients with H1-antihistamine-refractory chronic idiopathic urticaria. J Allergy Clin Immunol 2011;128(3): 567–73.e1.
7. Grattan CE, O'Donnell BF, Francis DM, et al. Randomized double-blind study of cyclosporin in chronic 'idiopathic' urticaria. Br J Dermatol 2000;143(2):365–72.
8. Napolitano M, Ruggiero A, Fontanella G, et al. New emergent therapies for atopic dermatitis: a review of safety profile with respect to female fertility, pregnancy, and breastfeeding. Dermatol Ther 2021;34(1):e14475.
9. Mian M, Dunlap R, Simpson E. Dupilumab for the treatment of severe atopic dermatitis in a pregnant patient: a case report. JAAD Case Rep 2020;6(10): 1051–2.

10. Kanda N, Hoashi T, Saeki H. The roles of sex hormones in the course of atopic dermatitis. Int J Mol Sci 2019;20(19). https://doi.org/10.3390/ijms20194660.
11. Weatherhead S, Robson SC, Reynolds NJ. Eczema in pregnancy. BMJ 2007; 335(7611):152–4.
12. Gonzalez-Estrada A, Geraci SA. Allergy medications during pregnancy. Am J Med Sci 2016;352(3):326–31.
13. Tuttle KLF J, Beck LA. Novel systemic treatments in atopic dermatitis: are there sex differences? Int J Women's Dermatol 2021;7(5):606–14.
14. Rakita U, Kaundinya T, Silverberg JI. Lack of association between atopic dermatitis severity and worsening during pregnancy: a cross-sectional study. J Am Acad Dermatol 2021. https://doi.org/10.1016/j.jaad.2021.09.066.
15. Hamann CR, Egeberg A, Wollenberg A, et al. Pregnancy complications, treatment characteristics and birth outcomes in women with atopic dermatitis in Denmark. J Eur Acad Dermatol Venereol 2019;33(3):577–87.
16. Murase JE, Heller MM, Butler DC. Safety of dermatologic medications in pregnancy and lactation: Part I. Pregnancy. J Am Acad Dermatol 2014;70(3): 401.e1-14, quiz 415.
17. Reitamo S, Wollenberg A, Schöpf E, et al. Safety and efficacy of 1 year of tacrolimus ointment monotherapy in adults with atopic dermatitis. The European tacrolimus ointment study group. Arch Dermatol 2000;136(8):999–1006.
18. Draelos Z, Nayak A, Pariser D, et al. Pharmacokinetics of topical calcineurin inhibitors in adult atopic dermatitis: a randomized, investigator-blind comparison. J Am Acad Dermatol 2005;53(4):602–9.
19. Cartron AM, Nguyen TH, Roh YS, et al. Janus kinase inhibitors for atopic dermatitis: a promising treatment modality. Clin Exp Dermatol 2021;46(5):820–4.
20. Dadashi M, Hajikhani B, Darban-Sarokhalil D, et al. Mupirocin resistance in *Staphylococcus aureus*: a systematic review and meta-analysis. J Glob Antimicrob Resist 2020;20:238–47.
21. El-Saie LT, Rabie AR, Kamel MI, et al. Effect of narrowband ultraviolet B phototherapy on serum folic acid levels in patients with psoriasis. Lasers Med Sci 2011; 26(4):481–5.
22. Akbari M, Shah S, Velayos FS, et al. Systematic review and meta-analysis on the effects of thiopurines on birth outcomes from female and male patients with inflammatory bowel disease. Inflamm Bowel Dis 2013;19(1):15–22.
23. Simons FE, Simons KJ. Histamine and H1-antihistamines: celebrating a century of progress. J Allergy Clin Immunol 2011;128(6):1139–50, e4.
24. Lobo Y, Lee RC, Spelman L. Atopic dermatitis treated safely with dupilumab during pregnancy: a case report and review of the literature. Case Rep Dermatol 2021;13(2):248–56.
25. Wollenberg A, Blauvelt A, Guttman-Yassky E, et al. Tralokinumab for moderate-to-severe atopic dermatitis: results from two 52-week, randomized, double-blind, multicentre, placebo-controlled phase III trials (ECZTRA 1 and ECZTRA 2). Br J Dermatol 2021;184(3):437–49.
26. Zuberbier T, Abdul Latiff AH, Abuzakouk M, et al. The International EAACI/GA^2-LEN/EuroGuiDerm/APAAACI guideline for the definition, classification, diagnosis, and management of urticaria. Allergy 2021. https://doi.org/10.1111/all.15090.
27. Kolkhir P, Borzova E, Grattan C, et al. Autoimmune comorbidity in chronic spontaneous urticaria: a systematic review. Autoimmun Rev 2017;16(12):1196–208.
28. Kocatürk E, Al-Ahmad M, Krause K, et al. Effects of pregnancy on chronic urticaria: results of the PREG-CU UCARE study. Allergy 2021;76(10):3133–44.

29. Fricke J, Ávila G, Keller T, et al. Prevalence of chronic urticaria in children and adults across the globe: systematic review with meta-analysis. Allergy 2020; 75(2):423–32.
30. Zhong H, Song Z, Chen W, et al. Chronic urticaria in Chinese population: a hospital-based multicenter epidemiological study. Allergy 2014;69(3):359–64.
31. Maurer M, Ortonne JP, Zuberbier T. Chronic urticaria: an internet survey of health behaviours, symptom patterns and treatment needs in European adult patients. Br J Dermatol 2009;160(3):633–41.
32. Gregoriou S, Rigopoulos D, Katsambas A, et al. Etiologic aspects and prognostic factors of patients with chronic urticaria: nonrandomized, prospective, descriptive study. J Cutan Med Surg 2009;13(4):198–203.
33. Sánchez Borges M, Tassinari S, Flores A. [Epidemiologic features in patients with antihistamine-resistant chronic urticaria]. Rev Alerg Mex 2015;62(4):279–86. Características epidemiológicas en pacientes con urticaria crónica espontánea resistente al tratamiento con antihistamínicos.
34. Straesser MD, Oliver E, Palacios T, et al. Serum IgE as an immunological marker to predict response to omalizumab treatment in symptomatic chronic urticaria. J Allergy Clin Immunol Pract 2018;6(4):1386–8.e1.
35. Pierdominici M, Maselli A, Colasanti T, et al. Estrogen receptor profiles in human peripheral blood lymphocytes. Immunol Lett 2010;132(1–2):79–85.
36. Kay AB, Clark P, Maurer M, et al. Elevations in T-helper-2-initiating cytokines (interleukin-33, interleukin-25 and thymic stromal lymphopoietin) in lesional skin from chronic spontaneous ('idiopathic') urticaria. Br J Dermatol 2015;172(5): 1294–302.
37. Kay AB, Ying S, Ardelean E, et al. Calcitonin gene-related peptide and vascular endothelial growth factor are expressed in lesional but not uninvolved skin in chronic spontaneous urticaria. Clin Exp Allergy 2014;44(8):1053–60.
38. Giménez-Arnau AM, DeMontojoye L, Asero R, et al. The pathogenesis of chronic spontaneous urticaria: the role of infiltrating cells. J Allergy Clin Immunol Pract 2021;9(6):2195–208.
39. Krasselt M, Baerwald C. Sex, symptom severity, and quality of life in rheumatology. Clin Rev Allergy Immunol 2019;56(3):346–61.
40. Maurer M, Eyerich K, Eyerich S, et al. Urticaria: Collegium Internationale Allergologicum (CIA) update 2020. Int Arch Allergy Immunol 2020;181(5):321–33.
41. Asero R, Marzano AV, Ferrucci S, et al. Co-occurrence of IgE and IgG autoantibodies in patients with chronic spontaneous urticaria. Clin Exp Immunol 2020; 200(3):242–9.
42. Ying S, Kikuchi Y, Meng Q, et al. TH1/TH2 cytokines and inflammatory cells in skin biopsy specimens from patients with chronic idiopathic urticaria: comparison with the allergen-induced late-phase cutaneous reaction. J Allergy Clin Immunol 2002;109(4):694–700.
43. Shakouri A, Compalati E, Lang DM, et al. Effectiveness of *Helicobacter pylori* eradication in chronic urticaria: evidence-based analysis using the grading of recommendations assessment, development, and evaluation system. Curr Opin Allergy Clin Immunol 2010;10(4):362–9.
44. Robertson SA, Care AS, Moldenhauer LM. Regulatory T cells in embryo implantation and the immune response to pregnancy. J Clin Invest 2018;128(10): 4224–35.
45. Murase JE, Chan KK, Garite TJ, et al. Hormonal effect on psoriasis in pregnancy and post partum. Arch Dermatol 2005;141(5):601–6.

46. Woidacki K, Zenclussen AC, Siebenhaar F. Mast cell-mediated and associated disorders in pregnancy: a risky game with an uncertain outcome? Front Immunol 2014;5:231.
47. Cocchiara R, Albeggiani G, Di Trapani G, et al. Modulation of rat peritoneal mast cell and human basophil histamine release by estrogens. Int Arch Allergy Appl Immunol 1990;93(2–3):192–7.
48. Woidacki K, Popovic M, Metz M, et al. Mast cells rescue implantation defects caused by c-kit deficiency. Cell Death Dis 2013;4(1):e462.
49. Zaitsu M, Narita S, Lambert KC, et al. Estradiol activates mast cells via a non-genomic estrogen receptor-alpha and calcium influx. Mol Immunol 2007;44(8): 1977–85.
50. Narita S, Goldblum RM, Watson CS, et al. Environmental estrogens induce mast cell degranulation and enhance IgE-mediated release of allergic mediators. Environ Health Perspect 2007;115(1):48–52.
51. Kasperska-Zajac A, Brzoza Z, Rogala B. Lower serum concentration of dehydroepiandrosterone sulphate in patients suffering from chronic idiopathic urticaria. Allergy 2006;61(12):1489–90.
52. Choi IS, Cui Y, Koh YA, et al. Effects of dehydroepiandrosterone on Th2 cytokine production in peripheral blood mononuclear cells from asthmatics. Korean J Intern Med 2008;23(4):176–81.
53. Lawlor F. Urticaria and angioedema in pregnancy and lactation. Immunol Allergy Clin N Am 2014;34(1):149–56.
54. Beissert S, Ständer H, Schwarz T. UVA rush hardening for the treatment of solar urticaria. J Am Acad Dermatol 2000;42(6):1030–2.
55. Kowalski ML, Woessner K, Sanak M. Approaches to the diagnosis and management of patients with a history of nonsteroidal anti-inflammatory drug-related urticaria and angioedema. J Allergy Clin Immunol 2015;136(2):245–51.
56. Powell RJ, Leech SC, Till S, et al. BSACI guideline for the management of chronic urticaria and angioedema. Clin Exp Allergy 2015;45(3):547–65.
57. Bousquet J, Khaltaev N, Cruz AA, et al. Allergic rhinitis and its impact on asthma (ARIA) 2008 update (in collaboration with the World Health Organization, GA(2) LEN and AllerGen). Allergy 2008;63(Suppl 86):8–160.
58. Viegas LP, Ferreira MB, Kaplan AP. The maddening itch: an approach to chronic urticaria. J Investig Allergol Clin Immunol 2014;24(1):1–5.
59. Maurer M, Altrichter S, Bieber T, et al. Efficacy and safety of omalizumab in patients with chronic urticaria who exhibit IgE against thyroperoxidase. J Allergy Clin Immunol 2011;128(1):202–9, e5.
60. Metz M, Vadasz Z, Kocatürk E, et al. Omalizumab updosing in chronic spontaneous urticaria: an overview of real-world evidence. Clin Rev Allergy Immunol 2020;59(1):38–45.
61. Vena GA, Cassano N, Colombo D, et al. Cyclosporine in chronic idiopathic urticaria: a double-blind, randomized, placebo-controlled trial. J Am Acad Dermatol 2006;55(4):705–9.
62. Zuberbier T, Ifflander J, Semmler C, et al. Acute urticaria: clinical aspects and therapeutic responsiveness. Acta Derm Venereol 1996;76(4):295–7.
63. Zuberbier T. A summary of the new International EAACI/GA2LEN/EDF/WAO guidelines in urticaria. World Allergy Organ J 2012;5(Suppl 1):S1–5.
64. Zuberbier T. Pharmacological rationale for the treatment of chronic urticaria with second-generation non-sedating antihistamines at higher-than-standard doses. J Eur Acad Dermatol Venereol 2012;26(1):9–18.

65. Powell RJ, Du Toit GL, Siddique N, et al. BSACI guidelines for the management of chronic urticaria and angio-oedema. Clin Exp Allergy 2007;37(5):631–50.

66. Akenroye AT, McEwan C, Saini SS. Montelukast reduces symptom severity and frequency in patients with angioedema-predominant chronic spontaneous urticaria. J Allergy Clin Immunol Pract 2018;6(4):1403–5.

67. Kaplan A, Ledford D, Ashby M, et al. Omalizumab in patients with symptomatic chronic idiopathic/spontaneous urticaria despite standard combination therapy. J Allergy Clin Immunol 2013;132(1):101–9.

68. Bundhoo A, Paveglio S, Rafti E, et al. Evidence that FcRn mediates the transplacental passage of maternal IgE in the form of IgG anti-IgE/IgE immune complexes. Clin Exp Allergy 2015;45(6):1085–98.

69. Namazy JA, Blais L, Andrews EB, et al. Pregnancy outcomes in the omalizumab pregnancy registry and a disease-matched comparator cohort. J Allergy Clin Immunol 2020;145(2):528–36.e1.

70. Fonacier L, Bernstein DI, Pacheco K, et al. Contact dermatitis: a practice parameter-update 2015. J Allergy Clin Immunol Pract 2015;3(3 Suppl):S1–39.

71. Mowad CM, Anderson B, Scheinman P, et al. Allergic contact dermatitis: patient diagnosis and evaluation. J Am Acad Dermatol 2016;74(6):1029–40.

Primary Antibody Immunodeficiency and the Pregnant Patient

Shouling Zhang, MD, Charlotte Cunningham-Rundles, MD, PhD*

KEYWORDS

- Primary immunodeficiency (PI) • Immunoglobulin replacement therapy (IGRT) • IVIG
- SCIG • Pregnancy

KEY POINTS

- Primary immune defects of antibody production do not preclude a normal pregnancy.
- Routine immunizations recommended in pregnancy (i.e., inactivated flu vaccine, Tdap) are also recommended in pregnant women with PI. Antimicrobials may be used with some exceptions.
- Immunoglobulin replacement therapy (IGRT) is safe in pregnancy and should be continued in patients with primary antibody immunodeficiency.
- In primary immunodeficiency, dosing adjustments in IGRT are needed to account for maternal placental transfer of IgG, fetal gestational age, and changing body habitus in the pregnant patient.

INTRODUCTION

Primary immunodeficiencies (PI), also known as inborn errors of immunity, represent a growing number of now more than 450 genetic mutations that increase susceptibility to infections, autoimmunity, autoinflammatory disorders, allergy, malignancy, and/or immune dysregulation.[1,2] Primary immune defects are currently divided into 10 main categories (**Table 1**).[1] Examples of these defects are included. Immune defects are caused by mutations in genes that result in loss of expression, loss of function, or gain of function of the encoded protein. Heterozygous mutations may lead to either autosomal dominant defects, loss of function by haploinsufficiency, or negative dominance. Homozygous or biallelic mutations, and X-linked recessive mutations, usually lead to loss of function of the gene. However, with earlier diagnosis and better prognosis, patients are more likely to live longer and lead more normal lives. For women

Division of Allergy and Immunology, Icahn School of Medicine at Mount Sinai, New York, NY, USA
* Corresponding author. The Icahn School of Medicine at Mount Sinai, 1425 Madison Avenue, New York, NY 10029.
E-mail address: Charlotte.Cunningham-Rundles@mssm.edu

Immunol Allergy Clin N Am 43 (2023) 133–144
https://doi.org/10.1016/j.iac.2022.07.009   **immunology.theclinics.com**

Table 1
Types of primary immunodeficiencies

Type	Examples
1. Immunodeficiencies affecting cellular and humoral immunity	Severe combined immune deficiency
2. Combined immunodeficiencies with associated/syndromic features	Wiskott Aldrich, Hyper immunoglobulin (Ig) E, etc.
3. Predominantly antibody deficiencies	IgA deficiency, common variable immune deficiency, IgG-subclass defects
4. Diseases of immune dysregulation	Autoimmune lymphoproliferative disease CARD11, etc.
5. Congenital defects of phagocyte number or function	Chronic granulomatous disease, neutropenia, etc.
6. Defects in intrinsic and innate immunity	STAT1, Warts hypogammaglobulinemia myelokathexis, etc.
7. Autoinflammatory disorders	Adenosine deaminase type 2, Familial Mediterranean Fever, etc.
8. Complement deficiencies	Complement C2, properdin
9. Bone marrow failure syndromes	Fanconi, dyskeratosis congenita
10. Phenocopies of inborn errors of immunity	Thymoma/anti-cytokine antibodies

Data from Tangye SG, Al-Herz W, Bousfiha A, et al. Human Inborn Errors of Immunity: 2019 Update on the Classification from the International Union of Immunological Societies Expert Committee [published correction appears in J Clin Immunol. 2020 Feb 22;:]. *J Clin Immunol.* 2020;40(1):24-64.

with immune defects, this is likely to include the desire to have children, leading to questions about the safety of ongoing treatments and the management of existing or newly arising medical conditions. The largest majority of patients with primary immune defects are those with defects of antibody production, in particular, immunoglobulin (Ig)G defects, common variable immune deficiency (CVID), and all subjects with loss of antibody production. Because of the relative prevalence of these conditions, questions about the medical management of pregnancy commonly arise. These questions usually concern the safe use of new or prophylactic antibiotics, the application of immunizations that are commonly prescribed, and the use of immunoglobulin replacement therapy (IGRT). Here we outline the use of these in patients with primary immune defects that impair antibody production.

USES OF IMMUNIZATIONS AND ANTIBIOTICS IN THE IMMUNE-DEFICIENT PATIENT

For the immune-deficient patient, routine immunization practices are modified. In general, pregnant women receive 2 vaccines during pregnancy: (1) the inactivated flu vaccine (the injection and not the live nasal flu vaccine) and (2) the Tdap (tetanus, diphtheria, and pertussis) vaccine.[3] Although the inactivated flu vaccine is advised for all patients before the start of flu season each year, the Tdap vaccine is not required if a patient is receiving immune globulin therapy, as these antibodies are contained in these solutions.[4,5] In addition, for patients with little or no antibody production, these vaccines would not elicit an antibody response. However, the reason for flu vaccine in subjects with little or no antibody production, is that the vaccine can elicit specific and robust T cell responses to flu.[6] According to the Centers for Disease Control and Prevention and the American College of Obstetricians and Gynecologists, the COVID-19 vaccination is also recommended for people who are pregnant, breastfeeding, trying to get pregnant, or might become pregnant in the future.[7,8] Pregnant individuals with PI may also receive the COVID-19 vaccine booster shot.[7,8] Recent studies demonstrate the safety of the vaccine, and a lowered risk of COVID-19 infection among vaccinated individuals.[9–11] Antibody production has also been observed among pregnant and lactating women.[12] Although data on patients with PI are still limited, variable antibody responses to this vaccine have also been observed. Other vaccines, as for all pregnant patients, are never given in pregnancy: human papillomavirus (HPV) vaccine; measles, mumps, and rubella (MMR) vaccine; live influenza vaccine (nasal flu vaccine); varicella (chicken pox) vaccine; yellow fever; typhoid fever; and Japanese encephalitis.[3]

Patients with primary immune defects often require intermittent or continuous prophylactic use of antibiotics. However, the general rules for the use of antibiotics, applied to all women during pregnancy, are followed. In immune deficiency, the commonly prescribed antibiotics are the penicillins and derivatives, cephalosporins, and macrolides (i.e., erythromycin, azithromycin), which are considered safe.[4,13] Sulfamethoxazole and trimethoprim, tetracyclines, and fluoroquinolones are generally not used in pregnancy and should be avoided.[13] There is uncertainty regarding the use of antifungal agents. Topical antifungals that have limited absorption and amphotericin B are preferred, but more studies are needed regarding safe use in pregnancy.[14]

IMMUNOGLOBULIN REPLACEMENT THERAPY

The main treatment for primary humoral immunodeficiencies is IGRT. As this treatment is generally lifelong, and should not be interrupted, questions about this therapy in the course of pregnancy commonly arise.

Immunoglobulin replacement was first used in PI in 1952 for the treatment of congenital agammaglobulinemia.[15] Over time, these products have become the standard of care for all patients with lack of antibody production. Originally this was given by intramuscular (IM) injections, but these were painful, and did not supply sufficient amounts of immune globulin. For these reasons, there are currently no IM products approved for use in PI.[16] Intravenous (IV) formulations, which safely supply large amounts of IgG, were developed in the 1980s. Following this, subcutaneous (SC) products, which can be given in the home, have been developed. At this time, there are a number of IGRT products approved for IV or SC use that have varying compositions (**Table 2**).[16,17] Available concentrations of various IV and SC products, salt and sugar content, IgA content, and maximum recommended infusion rates are outlined. Additional clinical considerations are also listed (see **Table 2**).

Aside from immune deficiency, a number of other indications for immunoglobulin replacement have been identified, and some may have application in the pregnant patient. A major use has been in autoimmunity, first starting in 1981, when an IV formulation was first used for acute immune thrombocytopenic purpura (ITP) in children.[18] Shortly after, intravenous immunoglobulin (IVIG) was found to be beneficial in both children and adults with chronic ITP.[19] IGRT has been approved by the US Food and Drug Administration for PI, ITP, B-cell chronic lymphocytic leukemia, chronic inflammatory demyelinated polyneuropathy, Kawasaki disease, multifocal motor neuropathy, human immunodeficiency virus infection, and bone marrow transplantation.[16,20] In PI, the main goal of IGRT, either IV or SC, is to prevent infections through antibody replacement.[5] Aside from the preceding indications, within obstetrics, IVIG also may be used in early-onset hemolytic disease of the fetus and newborn, neonatal alloimmune thrombocytopenia, gestational alloimmune liver disease, refractory or severe cases of antiphospholipid syndrome (APS), including life-

Table 2
Immunoglobulin replacement therapy products in intravenous (IV) and subcutaneous (SC) forms for primary immunodeficiency

Product	Route	Available Concentrations, %	Maximum Recommended Infusion Rate	Sugar Content	Sodium Content	Osmolarity/ Osmolality	IgA Content	Other Considerations
1. Asceniv	IV	10	4.8 mL/kg/h	No added sugars	0.100–0.140 M sodium chloride	370–510 mOsm/kg	≤ 200 µg/mL	—
2. Bivigam	IV	10	3.6 mL/kg/h	No added sugars	0.100–0.140 M sodium chloride	370–510 mOsm/kg	≤ 200 µg/mL	—
3. Carimune	IV	3, 6, 9, 12	3% 0.10 mL/kg/min 6% 0.050 mL/kg/min 9% 0.033 mL/kg/min 12% 0.025 mL/kg/min	1.67 g sucrose per g of protein	<20 mg sodium chloride per g of protein	192–1074 mOsm/kg	720 µg/mL	—
4. Flebogamma DIF	IV	5, 10	5% 6.0 mL/kg/h 10% 4.8 mL/kg/h	None	Trace amounts	240–370 mOsm/kg	5% and 10% Average: < 3 µg/mL	—
5. Gammagard Liquid	IV, SC	10	IV 5 mL/kg/h SC ≥40 kg body weight (BW): 30 mL/site at 20–30 mL/h site. <40 kg BW: 20 mL/site at 15–20 mL/h/site	No added sugars	No added sodium	240–300 mOsm/kg	37 µg/mL	—
6. Gammagard S/D	IV	5, 10	5% 4 mL/kg/h 10% 8 mL/kg/h	5% 20 mg/mL glucose 10% 40 mg/mL glucose	5% 8.5 mg/mL sodium chloride10% 17 mg mL sodium chloride	5% 636 mOsm/kg 10% 1250 mOsm/L	5% ≤ 1 µg/mL ≤ 2.2 µg/mL 10%N/A	Only product for anti-IgA antibodies and history of hypersensitivity (minimal IgA content)

Product	Route	Concentration (%)	Infusion rate	Stabilizer	Sodium	Osmolality	IgA content	Comments
7. Gammaked	IV, SC	10	*IV* 4.8 mL/kg/h *SC* 20 mL/h	None	Trace amounts	258 mOsm/kg	46 µg/mL	—
8. Gammaplex	IV	5, 10	4.8 mL/kg/h	5% 5% D-sorbitol (polyol) 10% None	5% 30–50 mmol/L 10% < 30 mM	5% 460–500 mOsm/L 10% Typically, 280 mOsmol/kg	5% Average: <4 µg/mL 10% Specification value: < 20 µg/mL	—
9. Gammunex-C	IV, SC	10	*IV* 4.8 mL/kg/h *SC* 20 mL/h/site	None	Trace amounts	258 mOsm/kg	Average: 46 µg/mL	—
10. Octagam	IV	5, 10	5% <4.2 mL/kg/h 10% <7.2 mL/kg/h	5% 100 mg/mL maltose 10% 90 mg/mL maltose	≤30 mmol/L	310–380 mOsm/kg	5% <100 µg/mL 10% Average of 106 µg/mL	May yield falsely elevated blood glucose
11. Panzyga	IV	10	For new patients: 4.8 mL/kg/h For experienced patients: up to 7.2 or 8.4 mL/kg/h	None	Trace amounts	240–310 mOsmol/kg	Average: 100 µ/mL	—
12. Privigen	IV	10	4.8 mL/kg/h	None	Trace amounts	Isotonic (320 mOsmol/kg)	≤ 25 µg/mL	—
13. Cutaquig	SC	16.5	Up to 100 mL/h/all sites combined First 6 infusions ≤ 20 mL/h/site (30 mL/h/all sites combined) Subsequent infusions:	79 mg/mL Maltose	≤30 mmol/L	310–380 mOsm/kg	≤0.6 mg/mL	—

(continued on next page)

Table 2
(continued)

Product	Route	Available Concentrations, %	Maximum Recommended Infusion Rate	Sugar Content	Sodium Content	Osmolarity/ Osmolality	IgA Content	Other Considerations
			25 mL/h/site (Up to 100 mL/h/all sites combined) Subsequent infusions may gradually increase to 50 mL, then to 80 mL; if well tolerated, use a max of 100 mL/h/all sites combined					
14. Cuvitru	SC	20	First 2 infusions: 10–20 mL/h/site Subsequent infusions: ≤60 mL/h/site	No added sugars	No added sodium	280–292 mOsm/kg	80 µg/mL	—
15. Hizentra	SC	20	Up to 25 mL/h/injection site (50 mL/h for all sites combined)	None	Trace amounts (≤10 mmol/L)	380 mOsmol/kg	Average: ≤50 µg/mL	—
16. Hyqvia	SC	10	< 40 kg BW: maximum 160 mL/site > 40 kg BW: maximum 300 mL/site	No added sugars	8.5 mg/mL sodium chloride in recombinant human hyaluronidase, no added sodium in IG 10%	240–300 mOsm/kg	Average: 37 µg/mL	—
17. Xembify	SC	20	25 mL/h/site	None	Trace amounts	280–404 mOsm/kg	≤0.07 mg/mL	—

Data from Immune Deficiency Foundation (IDF): Characteristics of Immunoglobulin Products Used to Treat Primary Immunodeficiencies (PI). Available at: https://primaryimmune.org/immunoglobulin-products.

threatening catastrophic APS, as well as in acute or chronic ITP.[21] This therapy is not recommended for recurrent pregnancy loss.[21,22] Other instances of off-label use of IGRT in pregnancy that could arise in a patient with an immune defect have been reported, including fetal-neonatal alloimmune thrombocytopenia and severe fetal-neonatal alloimmune hemolysis due to anti-erythrocyte antibodies.[22]

EARLY USE OF IMMUNOGLOBULIN REPLACEMENT THERAPY IN PREGNANCY IN PATIENTS WITH PRIMARY IMMUNODEFICIENCY

With the introduction of IVIG, several early case series and cohort studies examined the use of this therapy in pregnancy among patients with PI. Early reports by Sorensen and colleagues[23] (1984) described 2 pregnant patients with CVID who tolerated IVIG in the third trimester and had subsequent, uneventful, term deliveries of healthy newborns. One patient was on subcutaneous immunoglobulin (SCIG) before IVIG, and the second patient was on IM replacement before switching to IVIG. In both pregnancies, maternal serum IgG levels declined as fetal gestational age increased. This was ascribed to an increase in maternal IgG distribution space, as there is an expansion in plasma volume.[23] In this case, with transition to a higher doses of IVIG, maternal IgG levels rose steadily, thus illustrating the need for higher doses of IGRT in the later stages of pregnancy.[23] With the subsequent introduction of SCIG, this therapy was also tried in pregnant patients with PI. An early case study from 1982 of a pregnant woman with CVID and splenectomy, revealed that a slow, SCIG infusion of 20 mL/day was better tolerated in this case than IM replacement, and that normal serum IgG levels could be maintained on this rate with no significant infections during pregnancy.[24] A subsequent case series by Gardulf and colleagues[25] found that rapid, SCIG infusion was also well tolerated in 11 pregnancies among 9 women with PI. Weekly infusions were self-administered at 100 mg/kg per week throughout the pregnancy, and there were no adverse systemic reactions.[25] All 11 newborns were healthy and term.[25] Although most had CVID, 2 women had IgG-subclass deficiencies, and one had combined IgA and IgG2 deficiency, exemplifying how SCIG was safe in other instances of PI.[25] More recently introduced, the use of facilitated SCIG using recombinant human hyaluronidase, given every 3 to 4 weeks, was examined, and was also reported as successful in a case study of CVID during pregnancy in a patient with difficult venous access who refused IVIG.[26] Overall, most studies of IGRT during pregnancy in PI are from case studies or case series demonstrating a variety of options in IVIG and SCIG dosing, infusion rate, and frequency. In summary, IGRT has been considered safe and effective in pregnancy for those with PI, when dosed appropriately, as discussed in the following.[5,20,21,23–26]

DOSING OF IMMUNOGLOBULIN REPLACEMENT THERAPY

For woman with immune deficiency, the main goal of IGRT is to prevent infections. Clinical history and trough serum IgG levels guide dosing. In CVID, the most common PI, infection prevention is usually accomplished with doses of 400 to 600 mg/kg body weight per month.[5] However, individual differences in target trough levels for serum IgG vary according to baseline serum IgG levels, metabolism, and comorbidities involving lung disease or previous history of autoimmunity.[27] In pregnancy, however, additional considerations are needed for proper dosing. This is illustrated in a case series of 4 pregnant patients with CVID in Japan that examined the relationship between dosing of IGRT and pregnancy using different strategies of dose adjustment.[28] In all 4 cases, pre-pregnancy IVIG regimens in women with CVID were not able to maintain maternal IgG levels throughout pregnancy, which was attributed to a change in IgG distribution from maternal weight gain and blood volume expansion.[28] The investigators also identified that IVIG efficiency significantly decreased as gestational age increased.[28] From this case series, flexible adjustments in the dose and frequency of IVIG was recommended with a goal of maintaining stable serum IgG trough levels.[28] Aside from blood volume expansion, another major consideration is that IgG in maternal serum will be transported via the placenta to the infant, facilitated and regulated by the neonatal Fc receptor.[29,30] The amount of IgG transported from mother to infant gradually increases as the pregnancy progresses.[31] The transport involves mostly the IgG isotype 1, whereas IgA, IgM, or IgE are not passed to the infant.[31,32] For an immune-deficient mother, this may lead to lower than desirable levels of serum IgG, especially in the last trimester, because of placental transfer of maternal IgG, further contributing to the need to increase doses of IGRT.[3,31–33] Changes in total body weight during pregnancy will occur and IGRT should be increased to maintain maternal serum levels of IgG.[23,28] Similarly, adjustments in IGRT dosing also should be considered postpartum with weight loss. Weight-based modifications in infusion rate are also important to consider in both pre- and post-pregnancy (see **Table 2**).

Both IVIG and SCIG can be given in pregnancy, and patients may also switch between treatment routes. This is likely, however, to require new insurance authorization approvals for the alteration of products and routes of administration. Practical considerations for SCIG include baseline body habitus, subcutaneous tissue availability, patient comfort and convenience, and ease of SCIG use.[34] Because SCIG is typically administered into SC tissues of the abdomen, thighs, or upper arms using short needles of a tiny gauge, patients who typically self-inject into the abdomen may need guidance in injecting other body areas as pregnancy progresses. A woman may also prefer to switch to the IVIG route sooner, because of concerns about introducing a needle into the expanding abdomen. We recommend discussing different options for administering IGRT with patients throughout pregnancy to personalize care.

Another dosing consideration is frequency of IGRT. As patients approach delivery, timing of IGRT before delivery also may require coordination of care depending on patient preferences. It may be useful to schedule an IVIG infusion before a patient's anticipated delivery date to maximize the duration not requiring IGRT postpartum, but individual patient preferences should be considered.[23] IGRT dosing regimens before, during, and after pregnancy are important to consider in PI, and may be flexible according to patient preferences.

SAFETY CONSIDERATIONS

Although IVIG and SCIG are considered safe for use in pregnancy,[20–26,28] a few additional safety considerations include awareness of the contraindications of IGRT. These contraindications include hypersensitivity to immune globulins or any formula component.[35] The presence of anti-IgA antibodies with a history of hypersensitivity to IGRT is a contraindication for IV use, except in the case of Gammagard S/D, which contains very low amounts of this immune globulin.[35] However, as an alternative, subjects with anti-IgA antibodies have also been safely treated with SCIGs.[36,37] Additional contraindications for specific products include hyperprolinemia (Hizentra, Privigen), corn hypersensitivity (Octagam 5%), hereditary intolerance to fructose (Gammaplex 5%), possible sucrose or fructose intolerance in infants/neonates (Gammaplex 5%), and hypersensitivity to hyaluronidase, human albumin, or any component of the hyaluronidase formulation (HyQvia).[35]

Hematologic factors are also important to consider in pregnancy among those with PI. Several autoimmune manifestations occur in PI, such as ITP and autoimmune hemolytic anemia, and may be part of the clinical history of the patient, or may develop later.[38] A case study of a pregnant patient with CVID with previous ITP noted a significant drop in platelet count to 16,000 right before delivery that necessitated an urgent platelet transfusion.[39] Knowledge of baseline platelet count among patients with PI with risk of hematologic complications may be useful to guide management. Larger, immunomodulatory doses of immune globulin can be used in these cases, as for other patients with these autoimmune conditions. For all immunoglobulin products (IV, SC), it is important to note that there is a risk of thrombosis that has led to a black box warning on all products.[40] These conditions include thromboembolic events, such as myocardial infarction, stroke, deep vein thrombosis, and pulmonary embolism. These adverse events are quite rare, and are much more likely to occur in patients with autoimmune or neurologic disease receiving larger doses of IVIG, but have been reported in patients with PI.[41]

Risk factors for this include large doses of immune globulin, advanced age, prolonged immobilization, hypercoagulable conditions, diabetes mellitus, dehydration, history of venous or arterial thrombosis, use of estrogens, indwelling central vascular catheters, hyperviscosity and hypertension, and cardiovascular risk factors according to the US FDA.[40] For providers, careful consideration of these risk factors, and close monitoring for any signs or symptoms of thrombosis during or after infusion, are recommended.[40]

FUTURE DIRECTIONS

There are several areas that could benefit from additional studies of IGRT in pregnancy among those with PI. More research on IVIG dosing in pregnancy across different PI conditions is recommended. Although most case series and cohort studies have focused on CVID, additional studies evaluating specifics of IGRT dosing in other immune defects are also needed. Multicenter trials evaluating off-label obstetric uses of IVIG are also recommended, as some of these conditions may coexist with PI.[22] Larger studies of pregnancy in PI are needed to evaluate effectiveness of different IGRT regimens. Patient-centered studies examining patient preferences for different routes of IGRT and reasons for specific preferences are also encouraged.

SUMMARY

Pregnancy in PI involves careful consideration of IGRT dosing. Fortunately, immunoglobulin replacement, both IV and SC, is generally considered safe in pregnancy. Patient preferences should be considered when tailoring an effective and feasible treatment plan for patients with PI. Patient convenience is an important consideration, as is flexibility in treatment route. Future studies examining IGRT dosing across PI conditions, as well as patient preferences, are encouraged. Together, these can improve our understanding of IGRT management in pregnancy for individuals with PI.

CLINICS CARE POINTS

- When taking care of pregnant women with PI, encourage routine immunizations that are recommended in pregnancy (i.e., inactivated flu vaccine, Tdap, COVID vaccine).
- When prescribing antimicrobials for pregnant women with PI, follow general guidelines for antimicrobial use in pregnancy.
- When prescribing IGRT for pregnant women with PI, consider dosing adjustments for maternal placental transfer of IgG, fetal gestational age, and changing body habitus.

> Consideration of individual patient preferences throughout pregnancy is also encouraged.

DISCLOSURE

S. Zhang: None. C. Cunningham-Rundles, MD, PhD: None relevant to this article.

REFERENCES

1. Tangye SG, Al-Herz W, Bousfiha A, et al. Human inborn errors of immunity: 2019 update on the classification from the International Union of Immunological Societies Expert Committee. J Clin Immunol 2020;40(1):24–64.
2. Bousfiha A, Jeddane L, Picard C, et al. Human inborn errors of immunity: 2019 update of the IUIS Phenotypical Classification. J Clin Immunol 2020;40(1):66–81.
3. Dancis J, Lind J, Oratz M, et al. Placental transfer of proteins in human gestation. Am J Obstet Gynecol 1961;82:167–71.
4. Bonilla FA, Khan DA, Ballas ZK, et al. Practice parameter for the diagnosis and management of primary immunodeficiency. J Allergy Clin Immunol 2015;136(5): 1186–205, e1181-1178.
5. Orange JS, Hossny EM, Weiler CR, et al. Use of intravenous immunoglobulin in human disease: a review of evidence by members of the Primary Immunodeficiency Committee of the American Academy of Allergy, Asthma and Immunology. J Allergy Clin Immunol 2006;117(4 Suppl):S525–53.
6. Friedmann D, Goldacker S, Peter HH, et al. Preserved cellular immunity upon influenza vaccination in most patients with common variable immunodeficiency. J Allergy Clin Immunol Pract 2020;8(7):2332–2340 e2335.
7. CDC. Centers for Disease Control and Prevention: COVID-19 Vaccines While Pregnant or Breastfeeding. 2021. Available at: https://www.cdc.gov/coronavirus/2019-ncov/vaccines/recommendations/pregnancy.html. Accessed 21 Dec, 2021.
8. ACOG. American College of Obstetricians and Gynecologists (ACOG): COVID-19 Vaccination Considerations for Obstetric–Gynecologic Care. 2021. Available at: https://www.acog.org/clinical/clinical-guidance/practice-advisory/articles/2020/12/covid-19-vaccination-considerations-for-obstetric-gynecologic-care. Accessed Dec 21, 2021.
9. Shimabukuro TT, Kim SY, Myers TR, et al. Preliminary findings of mRNA Covid-19 vaccine safety in pregnant persons. N Engl J Med 2021;384(24):2273–82.
10. Goldshtein I, Nevo D, Steinberg DM, et al. Association between BNT162b2 vaccination and incidence of SARS-CoV-2 infection in pregnant women. JAMA 2021; 326(8):728–35.
11. Dagan N, Barda N, Biron-Shental T, et al. Effectiveness of the BNT162b2 mRNA COVID-19 vaccine in pregnancy. Nat Med 2021;27(10):1693–5.
12. Gray KJ, Bordt EA, Atyeo C, et al. Coronavirus disease 2019 vaccine response in pregnant and lactating women: a cohort study. Am J Obstet Gynecol 2021; 225(3):303.e301–17.
13. Bookstaver PB, Bland CM, Griffin B, et al. A review of antibiotic use in pregnancy. Pharmacotherapy 2015;35(11):1052–62.
14. Pilmis B, Jullien V, Sobel J, et al. Antifungal drugs during pregnancy: an updated review. J Antimicrob Chemother 2015;70(1):14–22.
15. Bruton OC. Agammaglobulinemia. Pediatrics 1952;9(6):722–8.

16. US Food and Drug Administration. Immune Globulins. Available at: https://www.fda.gov/vaccines-blood-biologics/approved-blood-products/immune-globulins. Accessed Sep 28, 2021.

17. Foundation ID. Characteristics of immunoglobulin products used to treat primary immunodeficiencies (PI). In: Foundation ID, ed. Available at: https://primaryimmune.org/immunoglobulin-products2020:18.

18. Imbach P, Barandun S, d'Apuzzo V, et al. High-dose intravenous gammaglobulin for idiopathic thrombocytopenic purpura in childhood. Lancet (London, England) 1981;1(8232):1228–31.

19. Bussel JB, Kimberly RP, Inman RD, et al. Intravenous gammaglobulin treatment of chronic idiopathic thrombocytopenic purpura. Blood 1983;62(2):480–6.

20. Perez EE, Orange JS, Bonilla F, et al. Update on the use of immunoglobulin in human disease: a review of evidence. J Allergy Clin Immunol 2017;139(3s):S1–46.

21. D'Mello RJ, Hsu CD, Chaiworapongsa P, et al. Update on the use of intravenous immunoglobulin in pregnancy. NeoReviews 2021;22(1):e7–24.

22. Branch DW, Porter TF, Paidas MJ, et al. Obstetric uses of intravenous immunoglobulin: successes, failures, and promises. J Allergy Clin Immunol 2001;108(4 Suppl):S133–8.

23. Sorensen RU, Tomford JW, Gyves MT, et al. Use of intravenous immune globulin in pregnant women with common variable hypogammaglobulinemia. Am J Med 1984;76(3a):73–7.

24. Berger M, Cupps TR, Fauci AS. High-dose immunoglobulin replacement therapy by slow subcutaneous infusion during pregnancy. JAMA 1982;247(20):2824–5.

25. Gardulf A, Andersson E, Lindqvist M, et al. Rapid subcutaneous IgG replacement therapy at home for pregnant immunodeficient women. J Clin Immunol 2001;21(2):150–4.

26. Więsik-Szewczyk E, Jahnz-Różyk K. A case report of pregnancy in a patient with common variable immunodeficiency emphasizing the need for personalized immunoglobulin replacement. Medicine 2018;97(44):e12804.

27. Cunningham-Rundles C. How I treat common variable immune deficiency. Blood 2010;116(1):7–15.

28. Egawa M, Kanegane H, Imai K, et al. Intravenous immunoglobulin (IVIG) efficiency in women with common variable immunodeficiency (CVID) decreases significantly during pregnancy. J Maternal-Fetal Neonatal Med 2019;32(18):3092–6.

29. Simister NE, Mostov KE. An Fc receptor structurally related to MHC class I antigens. Nature 1989;337(6203):184–7.

30. Firan M, Bawdon R, Radu C, et al. The MHC class I-related receptor, FcRn, plays an essential role in the maternofetal transfer of gamma-globulin in humans. Int Immunol 2001;13(8):993–1002.

31. Malek A, Sager R, Kuhn P, et al. Evolution of maternofetal transport of immunoglobulins during human pregnancy. Am J Reprod Immunol 1996;36(5):248–55. New York, NY : 1989.

32. Palmeira P, Quinello C, Silveira-Lessa AL, et al. IgG placental transfer in healthy and pathological pregnancies. Clin Develop Immunol 2012;2012:985646.

33. Costa-Carvalho BT, Vieria HM, Dimantas RB, et al. Transfer of IgG subclasses across placenta in term and preterm newborns. Braz J Med Biol Res 1996;29(2):201–4.

34. Skoda-Smith S, Torgerson TR, Ochs HD. Subcutaneous immunoglobulin replacement therapy in the treatment of patients with primary immunodeficiency disease. Ther Clin Risk Manag 2010;6:1–10.

35. Immune globulin (Intravenous, subcutaneous, and intramuscular). Drug information; 2021. https://www.uptodate.com/contents/immune-globulin-intravenous-subcutaneous-and-intramuscular-drug-information. [Accessed 10 January 2021]. Accessed.
36. Bonilla FA. Intravenous immunoglobulin: adverse reactions and management. J Allergy Clin Immunol 2008;122(6):1238–9.
37. Quinti I, Soresina A, Agostini C, et al. Prospective study on CVID patients with adverse reactions to intravenous or subcutaneous IgG administration. J Clin Immunol 2008;28(3):263–7.
38. Cunningham-Rundles C. Hematologic complications of primary immune deficiencies. Blood Rev 2002;16(1):61–4.
39. Sheikhbahaei S, Sherkat R, Camacho-Ordonez N, et al. Pregnancy, child bearing and prevention of giving birth to the affected children in patients with primary immunodeficiency disease; a case-series. BMC Pregnancy Childbirth 2018; 18(1):299.
40. FDA. Safety & Availability (Biologics) > FDA Safety Communication: New boxed warning for thrombosis related to human immune globulin products. 2013. 2021. Available at: http://wayback.archive-it.org/7993/20170112095644/http://www.fda.gov/BiologicsBloodVaccines/SafetyAvailability/ucm375096.htm. Accessed Dec 15, 2021.
41. Brown HC, Ballas ZK. Acute thromboembolic events associated with intravenous immunoglobulin infusion in antibody-deficient patients. J Allergy Clin Immunol 2003;112(4):797–9.

Hereditary Angioedema During Pregnancy
Considerations in Management

Marc A. Riedl, MD, MS

KEYWORDS

- Hereditary angioedema • Pregnancy • Women • Management • Treatment
- Estrogen • C1INH deficiency

KEY POINTS

- Pregnancy has a highly variable and unpredictable effect on hereditary angioedema (HAE) symptoms and can result in worsening, improvement, or no change in the HAE clinical course.
- Prepregnancy education and counseling is an important component of HAE management to familiarize patients and families with the genetics of HAE and potential changes in symptoms and treatment plans during pregnancy.
- Evidence-based guidelines recommend plasma-derived C1INH for acute and preventative treatment during pregnancy based on available safety data for HAE medications during pregnancy and lactation.
- Collaborative care by obstetrics and the HAE specialist is important around the time of delivery to ensure acute and short-term prophylactic HAE treatment plans are in place as appropriate thereby minimizing the risk of HAE symptoms during and following childbirth.

INTRODUCTION

Hereditary angioedema (HAE) is a rare autosomal-dominant genetic disorder causing recurrent episodes of severe, debilitating, and life-threatening angioedema.[1] HAE affects females and males in equal numbers, although females may suffer more frequent and severe angioedema episodes in part because of symptom exacerbating effects of estrogen.[2] Pregnancy presents a unique and complex time for women affected by HAE because physiologic and hormonal changes can influence HAE symptoms and the safety of treatment plans must be carefully considered. Following a brief summary of HAE for context, this review focuses on the clinical management of HAE during pregnancy.

Division of Rheumatology, Allergy & Immunology, Department of Medicine, University of California - San Diego, 8899 University Center Lane, Suite 230, La Jolla, CA 92122, USA
E-mail address: mriedl@ucsd.edu

Immunol Allergy Clin N Am 43 (2023) 145–157
https://doi.org/10.1016/j.iac.2022.05.011
immunology.theclinics.com
0889-8561/23/© 2022 Elsevier Inc. All rights reserved.

BACKGROUND

HAE is categorized into subtypes based on underlying pathophysiology.[3] HAE is most commonly caused by C1 esterase inhibitor deficiency (HAE-C1INH) because of mutations in SERPING1. HAE-C1INH can further be divided into HAE-C1INH type 1, with low quantitative and functional C1INH levels, and HAE-C1INH type 2, with normal quantitative but low functional C1INH levels. A third subtype of HAE is HAE with normal C1INH (HAE-nl-C1INH).[4] Laboratory studies of C1INH level and function are normal in this condition, although the clinical phenotype is extremely similar to HAE-C1INH.[5] HAE-nl-C1INH is further subcategorized into identified associated mutations in factor XII (FXII), plasminogen (PLG), angiopoetin-1 (AGPT1), kininogen-1 (KNG1), myoferlin (MYO), and heparan sulfate 3-O-sulfotransferase 6 (HS3ST6).[6] A subset of individuals affected by HAE-nl-C1INH have no currently identified associated mutations and are classified as HAE-unknown (U).

The hallmark symptoms of HAE are recurrent episodes of localized swelling predominantly affecting the skin, gastrointestinal tract, and airway.[2] Episodic and transient vascular leak within the subcutaneous (SC) and submucosal tissues causes angioedema symptoms that are often unpredictable and severe. Untreated angioedema episodes caused by HAE follow a typical pattern of gradually increasing in severity for approximately 24 hours, followed by persistent symptoms for 1 to 2 days and then gradual resolution over 1 to 2 days, such that the usual duration of symptoms is 3 to 5 days per episode.[7,8] The frequency of angioedema episodes in HAE is highly variable between affected individuals, but also may vary widely over a single individual's lifetime. Attack frequency can range from weekly to less than once a year. Cutaneous angioedema is the most common manifestation of HAE and frequently affects the face, extremities, and urogenital region.[2] Gastrointestinal angioedema is also common in HAE and frequently causes severe debilitating abdominal pain most often caused by small intestinal obstruction from submucosal swelling.[2] HAE abdominal attacks are often associated with nausea, vomiting, or diarrhea and the severe pain is frequently mistaken for an acute abdominal event leading to unnecessary surgery or other invasive procedures.[9] Airway angioedema caused by HAE is less common than cutaneous or gastrointestinal involvement; however, at least 50% of affected patients experience airway angioedema.[2] If not recognized and effectively treated, death by asphyxiation from HAE airway angioedema is a real risk.[10] In the absence of effective HAE therapy, mortality rates associated with airway episodes may exceed 30%.[11]

Angioedema caused by HAE-C1INH is caused by dysregulation of the contact (kallikrein-bradykinin) system.[12] C1INH deficiency leads to decreased inhibition of factor XIIa and plasma kallikrein, which in turn causes increased production of bradykinin because of excessive cleavage of high-molecular-weight kininogen. Bradykinin acts through the B2-receptor on endothelial cells to increase vascular permeability ultimately leading to vascular leak in SC and submucosal tissues manifesting clinically as protracted and often severe episodes of angioedema. The pathophysiology of swelling caused by HAE-nl-C1INH is less clearly established, at least for some forms of the condition.[13] Mutations associated with HAE-FXII have been shown to result in increased FXII activation.[14] Mutations associated with HAE-PLG, HAE-KNG1, and HAE-HS3ST6 are hypothesized to contribute to dysregulation of the contact system through various specific mechanisms.[15–17] In contrast, mutations associated with HAE-AGPT1 and HAE-MYO have putative effects on overall vascular permeability such that contact system activation may be a contributing factor, but not the sole cause of angioedema in families affected by these rare subtypes.[18,19]

Based on this understanding of contact system dysregulation as the underlying cause of recurrent angioedema in HAE-C1INH, numerous targeted therapeutics have been developed and are available for the clinical management of HAE.[20] These medications have been studied for two primary indications or strategies to manage HAE: acute treatment of angioedema symptoms when they occur, or long-term preventative treatment to reduce the frequency and severity of angioedema episodes.[21,22] For acute treatment of HAE symptoms, four medications are Food and Drug Administration (FDA)–approved with variable regulatory approval in other countries: plasma-derived (pd) C1INH, recombinant human (rh) C1INH, icatibant, and ecallantide. The C1INH concentrates, administered intravenously (IV) for acute treatment of HAE, address the underlying C1INH deficiency, thus reducing bradykinin production.[23,24] Icatibant, given SC, is a B2-receptor antagonist, blocking the vascular effects of bradykinin.[25] Ecallantide, given SC, is a plasma-kallikrein inhibitor, thus reducing kallikrein activity and subsequent formation of bradykinin.[26]

Other medications have been shown effective in significantly reducing the frequency of HAE symptoms when dosed regularly for long-term preventative treatment. These include pd-C1INH concentrates administered IV or SC every 3 to 4 days, a monoclonal antibody inhibiting plasma kallikrein (lanadelumab) administered SC every 2 or 4 weeks, and an oral kallikrein inhibitor (berotralstat) administered daily.[27–30] Additionally, oral attenuated androgens, such as danazol, are also effective for long-term preventative treatment in HAE.[31] However, androgens are currently used less often in clinical practice because of the increased risk of adverse effects and toxicities compared with modern targeted therapies, particularly with long-term use.[32] Antifibrinolytic medications, such as tranexamic acid, have inferior efficacy compared with other medications for long-term prophylaxis (LTP) in HAE-C1INH.[33] In contrast, study data suggest tranexamic acid may be useful in preventing angioedema symptoms caused by HAE-nl-C1INH.[34]

An additional strategy used in the management of HAE is short-term prophylactic treatment, with medication administered just before medical procedures or other anticipated trauma/events with a high risk of triggering HAE symptoms.[35] Clinical data support the benefit of C1INH concentrates administered IV within a few hours before procedures or oral androgens given daily for several days before procedures for short-term prophylaxis.[36,37] However, these medications are not FDA–labeled for this indication.

Having summarized HAE symptoms, pathophysiology, and treatment options, the remainder of the review focuses on important considerations in HAE management during pregnancy. For planning and discussion in the clinical setting, a useful approach is to consider three phases of HAE management during this important life event: (1) prepregnancy, (2) pregnancy, and (3) delivery/postdelivery (**Box 1**).

PREPREGNANCY

Although pregnancy may be planned or unplanned, it is helpful to discuss the topic with every woman of childbearing age who is diagnosed with HAE. Ideally, this allows the patient and family to anticipate any HAE-associated issues and consider treatment options and plans ahead of time. Before pregnancy, counseling potential parents on the genetic nature of HAE and the autosomal inheritance pattern is important so that families understand the risk of children inheriting the condition. For HAE-C1INH, the risk is 50% for each individual offspring when one parent is affected by HAE-C1INH.[38] For HAE-nl-C1INH, the inheritance pattern also seems to be autosomal-dominant, although strong estrogen effects on symptom expression lead

---

Box 1
Hereditary angioedema management considerations surrounding pregnancy

Prepregnancy
- Genetic counseling for patient/family on HAE inheritance pattern (autosomal-dominant with variable expression)
- Review with patient/family variable course of HAE symptoms during pregnancy: possible increase, decrease, or no change in symptoms
- Review HAE medication safety data for pregnancy and evidence-based guideline recommendations for pd-C1INH use
- Adjust prescribed medications before pregnancy when planned and possible
- For assisted reproductive procedures (ie, ovulation induction), discuss risk of worsening HAE symptoms with exogenous estrogen administration; adjust management plan to include pd-C1INH long-term prophylaxis if needed

Pregnancy
- Review medication safety data and management plan
- Ensure reliable access to HAE medication and clear administration plan including back-up medical facility if home or self-administration is unsuccessful
- Ensure regular communication between patient and HAE clinical care team to review symptom changes during pregnancy
- Adjust HAE treatment plan as needed; consider pd-C1INH long-term prophylactic treatment for women who will benefit based on individualized care plan and shared-decision making
- Recommend short-term prophylactic treatment (pd-C1INH IV) for diagnostic procedures, such as amniocentesis or chorionic villous sampling
- Monitor weight periodically and adjust dosing of weight-based HAE medication

Delivery and Postdelivery
- Communicate with obstetrics team regarding management plan surrounding childbirth
- Ensure access to acute HAE medication (pd-C1INH IV, at least 2 doses) for use as needed during delivery period
- Uncomplicated labor and normal spontaneous vaginal delivery rarely triggers HAE symptoms; if forceps, vacuum assistance required, administration of pd-C1INH IV recommended
- For surgical delivery: short-term prophylaxis with pd-C1INH IV recommended and use of regional anesthesia recommended when possible
- Monitor for HAE symptoms postpartum because of potential increased risk of attacks; ensure access to effective acute HAE medication
- During breastfeeding, pd-C1INH recommended for HAE treatment based on current safety data
- Discuss importance of testing child for HAE

---

to males rarely being symptomatic.[39] Genetic counseling in HAE is not intended to discourage childbearing because the development of new therapies has substantially reduced the historical morbidity and burden of disease associated with HAE. In addition, disease expression is highly variable and the severity of a parent's HAE does not predict the child's clinical course.[40] However, it is important for prospective parents to understand the probability of children having the condition and the important role of testing for HAE in early childhood.

A second important issue in the prepregnancy period is discussion of medications used to manage HAE based on available safety data in pregnancy. This is presented in greater detail in the section on pregnancy. However, for women attempting to become pregnant, it is prudent to adjust their HAE management plan to include medications currently recommended by evidence-based guidelines for optimal safety (ie, pd-C1INH concentrates).[41–43] Because pregnancy may not be confirmed until weeks after implantation, the most cautious approach includes avoidance of medications with unknown safety in pregnancy during the first trimester. In addition, the long half-life of monoclonal antibodies, such as lanadelumab, means that discontinuation of the medication at the time pregnancy is confirmed may still result in fetal drug exposure given evidence that IgG1 monoclonal antibodies cross the placenta, albeit at low levels early in pregnancy.[44] Because the safety of lanadelumab in pregnancy is currently unknown, it is reasonable and advisable to ideally discontinue this medication greater than or equal to 3 months (>5 half-lives) before conception.

Assisted reproductive technology to address infertility issues also raises important questions for women with HAE. Specifically, the ovulation induction procedures may involve increased risk of angioedema attacks because the estrogens administered frequently exacerbate HAE symptoms.[45] Although the diagnosis of HAE does not preclude these fertility efforts, women and families should understand the risks of worsening HAE symptoms with any exogenous estrogen therapy (eg, ovulation induction, contraception, hormone replacement). Frequently, HAE management plans must be adjusted because of increased frequency and severity of HAE symptoms during ovulation induction; specifically LTP with pd-C1INH should be considered (discussed later) .

PREGNANCY

Once pregnancy is confirmed, the HAE management plan should again be reviewed in detail with the patient. This is to ensure that: (1) HAE-specific medications used during pregnancy maximize safety based on available data, (2) the patient and family know how to effectively manage HAE symptoms, and (3) the patient is aware that HAE symptoms may change during pregnancy necessitating reevaluation and adjustment of the HAE management plan.

Based on currently available safety data, recent evidence-based guidelines for the management of HAE recommend pd-C1INH concentrates as preferred medication for acute treatment and prophylaxis (long-term or short-term) during pregnancy.[41–43] Current pregnancy safety data for HAE medications are summarized next.

Acute Treatments

Plasma-derived C1INH (Berinert)
Because pd-C1INH concentrates have been used to treat HAE for more than 40 years, considerable historical data on use during pregnancy exist. A recent systematic literature review reported published data on 1562 doses of pd-C1INH in 136 pregnancies, showing a favorable safety profile and supporting the current evidence-based guideline recommendations as the preferred medication for HAE treatment during pregnancy.[46] International registry data on pd-C1INH use in pregnancy has yielded similarly reassuring results.[47]

Recombinant human C1INH (Ruconest)
rh-C1INH is produced from the isolated gene for human C1INH, resulting in an amino acid sequence identical to that of endogenous human C1INH.[48] Protein glycosylation differences result in a shorter plasma half-life compared with plasma-derived products. Published cases series on rh-C1INH use in pregnancy include 242 doses in 17 women with no pregnancy-related adverse events and full-term healthy babies delivered for all women.[49,50] Based on these data, rh-C1INH is a reasonable consideration for treatment during pregnancy, particularly if pd-C1INH is not readily available.

Icatibant (Firazyr, generic products)
Data on the use of icatibant in pregnancy are limited to case series with a small number of attacks treated: experience with 20 doses in nine women has been published,

although one report does not specify the number of doses administered in a single patient while pregnant.[50–53] Of 11 pregnancy outcomes reported, one preterm delivery occurred but no other adverse pregnancy-related events. However, the dataset remains too small to reach conclusions on safety. Animal studies have shown evidence of adverse events including premature birth, abortion, fetal death, and preimplantation loss, although no evidence of teratogenicity.[54] Further work and data are needed to evaluate the safety of icatibant in pregnancy.

Ecallantide (Kalbitor)
No human data are available on the safety of ecallantide use in pregnancy. Animal studies have shown some evidence of developmental toxicity.[55]

Prophylactic Treatments

Plasma-derived C1INH (Cinryze, Haegarda)
Based on the data outlined previously, evidence-based guidelines recommend pd-C1INH concentrates given IV or SC every 3 to 4 days for LTP treatment of HAE during pregnancy.[41–43]

Lanadelumab (Takhzyro)
No human data on the safety of lanadelumab in pregnancy are available. IgG1 monoclonal antibodies, such as lanadelumab, are transported across the placenta particularly during the third trimester of pregnancy.[44] Animal studies have not shown any evidence of harm to the developing fetus.[56]

Berotralstat (Orladeyo)
No human data on the safety of berotralstat in pregnancy are available. Animal studies have been reassuring.[57]

Androgens (Danazol, others)
Attenuated androgens are contraindicated during pregnancy because they cross the placenta and may affect fetal development, particularly with regard to virilization of the fetus.[58,59]

Antifibrinolytics (tranexamic acid)
Antifibrinolytics cross the placenta but no specific pregnancy-related adverse events have been reported.[60] Animal studies of tranexamic acid have shown no evidence of teratogenicity.[61] Given the inferior preventative efficacy of tranexamic acid in HAE-C1INH, use should only be considered when C1INH concentrates are unavailable.

Based on the previously mentioned data and evidence-based guidelines, HAE management plans during pregnancy are generally centered on the use of pd-C1INH concentrates for on-demand treatment of attacks, with consideration of LTP with pd-C1INH for patients who benefit from this added to the acute treatment plan.[41–43] This approach maximizes the safety profile of the HAE medication used during pregnancy, although logistically, requires that the patient is reliably able to administer C1INH therapy IV for acute treatment of symptoms. Many patients are able to self-administer IV C1INH or receive treatment with the assistance of family or friends, although adequate training of the patient and/or caregiver is required.[62,63] Patients should have a backup plan for health care professional assistance with medication dosing through home-health, outpatient clinic, urgent care, or hospital services if needed.

In addition to the acute treatment plan, LTP with pd-C1INH is an important consideration for patients who experience frequent, severe, or disruptive symptoms. SC pd-C1INH for LTP is usually preferred over IV because of the easier route of administration and improved efficacy demonstrated in controlled studies.[27,28] As pregnancy progresses, SC administration sites on the abdomen may become more challenging and infusion sites using the upper thighs, upper arms, or other regions with adequate SC tissue is considered. pd-C1INH IV should also be administered for short-term prophylaxis before any invasive procedure required during pregnancy, such as amniocentesis or chorionic villous sampling. Most C1INH treatments are weight-based (pd-C1INH IV 20 U/kg for acute treatment, rh-C1INH IV 50 U/kg up to 4200 U for acute treatment, pd-C1INH SC 60 U/kg for LTP), so monitoring weight and adjusting doses appropriately during pregnancy is important for optimal efficacy.

HAE symptoms often change during pregnancy, likely attributable to hormonal, physiologic, and anatomic changes. Regular communication and follow-up between the patient and the HAE specialist is necessary to ensure optimal care. Women and families should be counseled that HAE symptoms may worsen during pregnancy, with one study showing increased attack rates in 83% of women while pregnant.[64] The largest study of HAE and pregnancy demonstrated significant clinical variability with 38% of women experiencing increased symptoms, 30% decreased symptoms, and 32% with no change in symptoms during pregnancy.[65] Additional data from this study suggest that women with menses as a historical trigger for HAE symptoms are more likely to have worsening of HAE during pregnancy.[65] Carrying a fetus affected by the familial HAE mutation is associated with a higher frequency of third-trimester attacks.[66] However, the clinical course is unpredictable and may be different for the same woman from one pregnancy to the next.[67] Management plans may require adjustments based on clinical course, with special consideration given to pd-C1INH prophylaxis in patients with increased or poorly controlled symptoms. Abdominal HAE symptoms are most frequently reported during pregnancy, potentially because of fetal movement and uterine stretching.[66] A clinical challenge not unique to pregnancy, but important to highlight, is differentiating HAE abdominal attacks from other causes of abdominal pain. If abdominal pain from a suspected HAE attack during pregnancy does not clearly respond to effective HAE medication, patients should have immediate evaluation for other pregnancy-related issues or complications as the underlying cause.

Although pregnancy often affects HAE symptom frequency and severity, data on the effects of HAE on pregnancy outcomes have largely been reassuring. Most studies indicate that women with HAE do not experience increased rates of spontaneous abortion, premature births, cesarean delivery, or other pregnancy complications compared with the general population.[65,66] One study observed a higher rate of spontaneous abortion or premature labor in women with HAE compared with non-HAE relatives.[68]

DELIVERY AND POSTDELIVERY

As pregnancy progresses and delivery approaches, communication between the patient, HAE specialist, and obstetrics team is important to ensure proper planning. Labor and normal spontaneous vaginal delivery seem to rarely trigger HAE symptoms with angioedema episodes occurring during 6% to 8% of these events.[66] If normal spontaneous vaginal delivery is planned, it is reasonable to proceed without specific prophylactic treatment, although at least two doses of effective acute medication (ie, C1INH concentrate) should be readily available for administration if any angioedema symptoms occur.[67] In addition, if procedural intervention or instrumentation (ie, forceps) becomes necessary during the course of delivery, IV pd-C1INH treatment should be given because of the likelihood of this increased trauma causing angioedema.[67] Likewise, if surgical delivery is planned or becomes necessary, IV pd-C1INH concentrate should be administered for short-term prophylactic treatment, ideally at least 1 hour before the procedure or as soon as the need for an emergent surgical procedure is confirmed.[41–43] Regional anesthesia is preferred for surgery when possible because of a risk of laryngeal edema with intubation for general anesthesia. Providing a written management plan outlining these measures and contact information for the HAE specialist is useful for the obstetrics team to ensure coordination of care.

Clinical monitoring is important following delivery, because of an increased risk of HAE symptoms in the first few days postpartum.[66] Vulvar angioedema may occur more frequently following delivery.[69] The patient should have reliable access to acute HAE medication that is used as needed for HAE attacks at the hospital or at home during this higher-risk period. Some women may wish to switch to SQ non-C1INH acute treatments postdelivery if these have been successfully used and tolerated before pregnancy, although breastfeeding plans should be carefully considered in this decision.

Breastfeeding may also be associated with an increased frequency in HAE attacks.[66] Safety data for HAE medications during breastfeeding are limited. Based on historical safety data for pd-C1INH concentrate use over many years, current evidence-based HAE management guidelines recommend C1INH concentrates as the preferred treatment of acute and prophylactic therapy during breastfeeding.[41–43] Androgens and antifibrinolytics are secreted in breast milk.[61,70] Androgens are contraindicated during breastfeeding given numerous potential adverse effects; tranexamic acid has been found to be generally safe during breastfeeding.[71] Animal studies have demonstrated icatibant, lanadelumab, and berotralstat are excreted in breast milk; the clinical importance of this for human breastfeeding is unknown.[54,56,57] It is not known whether ecallantide is excreted in human milk.[55]

Children born to a parent with confirmed HAE should be tested for the condition. Recommended complement system testing for HAE-C1INH (C4, C1INH level, C1INH function) may be done at any time after birth, although some levels, particularly C4, may be difficult to interpret before 12 months of age because of ongoing development of the complement system in the first months of life.[72] Recent data suggest C1INH testing, in particular C1INH function, are accurate and reliable in the first few months of life.[73] Genetic testing with sequencing of SERPING1 or other known familial mutations associated with HAE-nl-C1INH can be done any time after birth. Because it is unusual for HAE symptoms to occur before 2 years of age, completion of C1INH testing following the first birthday may be reasonable to ensure reliable results. However, monitoring infants for clinical symptoms is essential because this may warrant earlier testing.

MANAGEMENT OF HEREDITARY ANGIOEDEMA WITH NORMAL C1INH

The management of HAE-nl-C1INH during and surrounding pregnancy largely mirrors the recommendations for HAE-C1INH, because medication safety for mother and fetus is of paramount importance and HAE symptoms may be dangerous and detrimental to the pregnancy. However, data on the efficacy of these management approaches are predominantly derived from studies of HAE-C1INH and efficacy in HAE-nl-C1INH is less certain. Because symptoms and risks for HAE conditions are similar, and the pathophysiology of HAE-nl-C1INH is largely believed to involve contact system dysregulation, it is reasonable to carefully use these strategies and treatments, recognizing that future research efforts are needed to determine any differences in the pregnancy course and management of HAE-nl-C1INH.

SUMMARY

The clinical course of HAE is highly variable and unpredictable during pregnancy. Optimal management requires patient and family education, careful attention to medications administered, consistent monitoring, and collaboration between the obstetrics team and HAE specialists. Current treatment guidelines recommend pd-C1INH therapy for acute and prophylactic treatment during pregnancy, with adjustment of the treatment plan often necessary because of the variable effect of pregnancy on HAE. Delivery, postpartum care, and breastfeeding require additional planning and monitoring. Fortunately, HAE-related complications seem rare; safely and effectively treating or preventing symptoms, anticipating HAE triggers, and avoiding iatrogenic complications during pregnancy is paramount.

CLINICS CARE POINTS

- Prepregnancy discussions with women and families affected by HAE are beneficial in providing education/information on genetics of HAE, possible changes in HAE symptoms during pregnancy, and adjusting medication use for optimal safety.
- The clinical course of HAE during pregnancy is highly variable and unpredictable, although at least one-third of women experience worsening HAE symptoms with pregnancy.
- Based on available safety data, evidence-based guidelines recommend pd-C1INH for HAE acute treatment, and when indicated, for prophylactic treatment during pregnancy and lactation.
- Immediate access to IV pd-C1INH for acute treatment may be sufficient for uncomplicated labor and spontaneous vaginal delivery, which rarely trigger HAE symptoms; if instrumentation (ie, forceps) or surgical delivery is required, dosing of IV pd-C1INH for short-term prophylaxis is recommended.

DISCLOSURE

M.A. Riedl has received research grants from BioCryst, CSL Behring, Ionis, Kalvista, Pharvaris, and Takeda; consultancy fees from Astria, BioCryst, Biomarin, CSL Behring, Cycle Pharma, Fresenius-Kabi, Ipsen, Kalvista, Ono Pharma, Pfizer, Pharming, Pharvaris, RegenexBio, and Takeda; and fees for speaker presentations from CSL Behring, Grifols, Pharming, and Takeda. All grants provided to the institution and all fee payments regulated and processed through the institutional compensation plan.

REFERENCES

1. Busse PJ, Christiansen SC. Hereditary angioedema. N Engl J Med 2020;382(12): 1136–48.
2. Bork K, Meng G, Staubach P, et al. Hereditary angioedema: new findings concerning symptoms, affected organs, and course. Am J Med 2006;119:267–74.
3. Proper SP, Lavery WJ, Bernstein JA. Definition and classification of hereditary angioedema. Allergy Asthma Proc 2020;41(Suppl 1):S03–7.
4. Riedl MA. Hereditary angioedema with normal C1-INH (HAE type III). J Allergy Clin Immunol Pract 2013;1(5):427–32.
5. Magerl M, Germenis AE, Maas C, et al. Hereditary angioedema with normal C1 inhibitor: update on evaluation and treatment. Immunol Allergy Clin N Am 2017; 37(3):571–84.
6. Veronez CL, Csuka D, Sheikh FR, et al. The expanding spectrum of mutations in hereditary angioedema. J Allergy Clin Immunol Pract 2021;9(6):2229–34.

7. Bork K, Staubach P, Hardt J. Treatment of skin swellings with C1-inhibitor concentrate in patients with hereditary angioedema. Allergy 2008;63(6):751–7.

8. Bork K, Meng G, Staubach P, et al. Treatment with C1 inhibitor concentrate in abdominal pain attacks of patients with hereditary angioedema. Transfusion 2005;45(11):1774–84.

9. Hahn J, Hoess A, Friedrich DT, et al. Unnecessary abdominal interventions in patients with hereditary angioedema. J Dtsch Dermatol Ges 2018;16(12):1443–9.

10. Bork K, Hardt J, Witzke G. Fatal laryngeal attacks and mortality in hereditary angioedema due to C1-INH deficiency. J Allergy Clin Immunol 2012;130(3):692–7.

11. Minafra FG, Gonçalves TR, Alves TM, et al. The mortality from hereditary angioedema worldwide: a review of the real-world data literature. Clin Rev Allergy Immunol 2021;62(1):232–9.

12. Kaplan AP, Joseph K. Pathogenesis of hereditary angioedema: the role of the bradykinin-forming cascade. Immunol Allergy Clin N Am 2017;37(3):513–25.

13. Sharma J, Jindal AK, Banday AZ, et al. Pathophysiology of hereditary angioedema (HAE) beyond the SERPING1 gene. Clin Rev Allergy Immunol 2021;60(3):305–15.

14. de Maat S, Björkqvist J, Suffritti C, et al. Plasmin is a natural trigger for bradykinin production in patients with hereditary angioedema with factor XII mutations. J Allergy Clin Immunol 2016;138(5):1414–23.

15. Bork K, Wulff K, Steinmüller-Magin L, et al. Hereditary angioedema with a mutation in the plasminogen gene. Allergy 2018;73(2):442–50.

16. Bork K, Wulff K, Rossmann H, et al. Hereditary angioedema cosegregating with a novel kininogen 1 gene mutation changing the N-terminal cleavage site of bradykinin. Allergy 2019;74(12):2479–81.

17. Bork K, Wulff K, Möhl BS, et al. Novel hereditary angioedema linked with a heparan sulfate 3-O-sulfotransferase 6 gene mutation. J Allergy Clin Immunol 2021;148(4):1041–8.

18. Bafunno V, Firinu D, D'Apolito M, et al. Mutation of the angiopoietin-1 gene (ANGPT1) associates with a new type of hereditary angioedema. J Allergy Clin Immunol 2018;141(3):1009–17.

19. Ariano A, D'Apolito M, Bova M, et al. A myoferlin gain-of-function variant associates with a new type of hereditary angioedema. Allergy 2020;75(11):2989–92.

20. Caballero T. Treatment of hereditary angioedema. J Investig Allergol Clin Immunol 2021;31(1):1–16.

21. Christiansen SC, Zuraw BL. Hereditary angioedema: on-demand treatment of angioedema attacks. Allergy Asthma Proc 2020;41(Suppl 1):S26–9.

22. Li HH. Hereditary angioedema: long-term prophylactic treatment. Allergy Asthma Proc 2020;41(Suppl 1):S35–7.

23. Craig TJ, Levy RJ, Wasserman RL, et al. Efficacy of human C1 esterase inhibitor concentrate compared with placebo in acute hereditary angioedema attacks. J Allergy Clin Immunol 2009;124(4):801–8.

24. Zuraw B, Cicardi M, Levy RJ, et al. Recombinant human C1-inhibitor for the treatment of acute angioedema attacks in patients with hereditary angioedema. J Allergy Clin Immunol 2010;126(4):821–7.

25. Cicardi M, Banerji A, Bracho F, et al. Icatibant, a new bradykinin-receptor antagonist, in hereditary angioedema. N Engl J Med 2010;363(6):532–41.

26. Levy RJ, Lumry WR, McNeil DL, et al. EDEMA4: a phase 3, double-blind study of subcutaneous ecallantide treatment for acute attacks of hereditary angioedema. Ann Allergy Asthma Immunol 2010;104(6):523–9.

27. Zuraw BL, Busse PJ, White M, et al. Nanofiltered C1 inhibitor concentrate for treatment of hereditary angioedema. N Engl J Med 2010;363(6):513–22.
28. Longhurst H, Cicardi M, Craig T, et al. Prevention of hereditary angioedema attacks with a subcutaneous C1 inhibitor. N Engl J Med 2017;376(12):1131–40.
29. Banerji A, Riedl MA, Bernstein JA, et al. Effect of lanadelumab compared with placebo on prevention of hereditary angioedema attacks: a randomized clinical trial. JAMA 2018;320(20):2108–21.
30. Zuraw B, Lumry WR, Johnston DT, et al. Oral once-daily berotralstat for the prevention of hereditary angioedema attacks: a randomized, double-blind, placebo-controlled phase 3 trial. J Allergy Clin Immunol 2021;148(1):164–72.
31. Gelfand JA, Sherins RJ, Alling DW, et al. Treatment of hereditary angioedema with danazol. Reversal of clinical and biochemical abnormalities. N Engl J Med 1976; 295(26):1444–8.
32. Riedl MA. Critical appraisal of androgen use in hereditary angioedema: a systematic review. Ann Allergy Asthma Immunol 2015;114(4):281–8.
33. Wintenberger C, Boccon-Gibod I, Launay D, et al. Tranexamic acid as maintenance treatment for non-histaminergic angioedema: analysis of efficacy and safety in 37 patients. Clin Exp Immunol 2014;178(1):112–7.
34. Vitrat-Hincky V, Gompel A, Dumestre-Perard C, et al. Type III hereditary angio-oedema: clinical and biological features in a French cohort. Allergy 2010; 65(10):1331–6.
35. Craig T. Triggers and short-term prophylaxis in patients with hereditary angioedema. Allergy Asthma Proc 2020;41(Suppl 1):S30–4.
36. Zanichelli A, Ghezzi M, Santicchia I, et al. Short-term prophylaxis in patients with angioedema due to C1-inhibitor deficiency undergoing dental procedures: an observational study. PLoS One 2020;15(3):e0230128.
37. Farkas H, Zotter Z, Csuka D, et al. Short-term prophylaxis in hereditary angioedema due to deficiency of the C1-inhibitor: a long-term survey. Allergy 2012; 67(12):1586–93.
38. Germenis AE, Margaglione M, Pesquero JB, et al. International consensus on the use of genetics in the management of hereditary angioedema. J Allergy Clin Immunol Pract 2020;8(3):901–11.
39. Bork K, Wulff K, Witzke G, et al. Hereditary angioedema with normal C1-INH with versus without specific F12 gene mutations. Allergy 2015;70(8):1004–12.
40. Agostoni A, Ayg.ren-Pursun E, Binkley KE, et al. Hereditary and acquired angioedema: problems and progress: proceedings of the third C1 esterase inhibitor deficiency workshop and beyond. J Allergy Clin Immunol 2004;114(3):S51–131.
41. Busse PJ, Christiansen SC, Riedl MA, et al. US HAEA Medical Advisory Board 2020 guidelines for the management of hereditary angioedema. J Allergy Clin Immunol Pract 2021;9(1):132–50.
42. Maurer M, Magerl M, Betschel S, et al. The International WAO/EAACI guideline for the management of hereditary angioedema: the 2021 revision and update. Allergy 2022.
43. Betschel S, Badiou J, Binkley K, et al. The International/Canadian Hereditary Angioedema Guideline. Allergy Asthma Clin Immunol 2019;15:72.
44. Pentsuk N, van der Laan JW. An interspecies comparison of placental antibody transfer: new insights into developmental toxicity testing of monoclonal antibodies. Birth Defects Res B Dev Reprod Toxicol 2009;86(4):328–44.
45. Gompel A, Fain O, Boccon-Gibod I, et al. Exogenous hormones and hereditary angioedema. Int Immunopharmacol 2020;78:106080.

46. Brooks JP, Radojicic C, Riedl MA, et al. Experience with intravenous plasma-derived C1-inhibitor in pregnant women with hereditary angioedema: a systematic literature review. J Allergy Clin Immunol Pract 2020;8(6):1875–80.
47. Fox J, Vegh AB, Martinez-Saguer I, et al. Safety of a C1-inhibitor concentrate in pregnant women with hereditary angioedema. Allergy Asthma Proc 2017;38(3):216–21.
48. van Veen HA, Koiter J, Vogelezang CJ, et al. Characterization of recombinant human C1 inhibitor secreted in milk of transgenic rabbits. J Biotechnol 2012;162(2–3):319–26.
49. Moldovan D, Bernstein JA, Hakl R, et al. Safety of recombinant human C1 esterase inhibitor for hereditary angioedema attacks during pregnancy. J Allergy Clin Immunol Pract 2019;7(8):2938–40.
50. Hakl R, Kuklínek P, Krčmová I, et al. Treatment of hereditary angioedema attacks with icatibant and recombinant C1 inhibitor during pregnancy. J Clin Immunol 2018;38(7):810–5.
51. Farkas H, Kőhalmi KV, Veszeli N, et al. First report of icatibant treatment in a pregnant patient with hereditary angioedema. J Obstet Gynaecol Res 2016;42(8):1026–8.
52. Kaminsky LW, Kelbel T, Ansary F, et al. Multiple doses of icatibant used during pregnancy. Allergy Rhinol (Providence) 2017;8(3):178–81.
53. Zanichelli A, Mansi M, Periti G. Icatibant exposure during pregnancy in a patient with hereditary angioedema. J Investig Allergol Clin Immunol 2015;25(6):447–9.
54. Icatibant [package insert]. Available at: https://www.accessdata.fda.gov/drugsatfda_docs/label/2011/022150s000lbl.pdf. Accessed January 22, 2022.
55. Ecallantide [package insert]. Available at: https://www.accessdata.fda.gov/drugsatfda_docs/label/2014/125277s071lbl.pdf. Accessed January 22, 2022.
56. Lanadelumab [package insert]. Available at: https://www.accessdata.fda.gov/drugsatfda_docs/label/2018/761090s000lbl.pdf. Accessed January 22, 2022.
57. Berotralstat [package insert]. Available at: https://www.accessdata.fda.gov/drugsatfda_docs/label/2020/214094s000lbl.pdf. Accessed January 22, 2022.
58. Schwartz R. Ambiguous genitalia in a term female infant due to exposure to danazol in utero. Am J Dis Child 1982;136(5):474.
59. Reschini E, Giustina G, D'Alberton A, et al. Female pseudohermaphroditism due to maternal androgen administration: 25-year follow-up. Lancet 1985;1:1226.
60. Dunn CJ, Goa KL. Tranexamic acid: a review of its use in surgery and other indications. Drugs 1999;57:1005–32.
61. Tranexamic acid [package insert]. Available at: https://www.accessdata.fda.gov/drugsatfda_docs/label/2013/022430s004lbl.pdf. Accessed January 22, 2022.
62. Zanichelli A, Azin GM, Cristina F, et al. Safety, effectiveness, and impact on quality of life of self-administration with plasma-derived nanofiltered C1 inhibitor (Berinert®) in patients with hereditary angioedema: the SABHA study. Orphanet J Rare Dis 2018;13(1):51.
63. Riedl MA, Bygum A, Lumry W, et al. Safety and usage of C1-inhibitor in hereditary angioedema: Berinert Registry Data. J Allergy Clin Immunol Pract 2016;4(5):963–71.
64. Martinez-Saguer I, Rusicke E, Aygören-Pürsün E, et al. Characterization of acute hereditary angioedema attacks during pregnancy and breast-feeding and their treatment with C1 inhibitor concentrate. Am J Obstet Gynecol 2010;203(2):131.
65. Bouillet L, Longhurst H, Boccon-Gibod I, et al. Disease expression in women with hereditary angioedema. Am J Obstet Gynecol 2008;199(5):484.

66. Czaller I, Visy B, Csuka D, et al. The natural history of hereditary angioedema and the impact of treatment with human C1-inhibitor concentrate during pregnancy: a long-term survey. Eur J Obstet Gynecol Reprod Biol 2010;152(1):44–9.
67. Caballero T, Farkas H, Bouillet L, et al. International consensus and practical guidelines on the gynecologic and obstetric management of female patients with hereditary angioedema caused by C1 inhibitor deficiency. J Allergy Clin Immunol 2012;129:308–20.
68. Nielsen EW, Gran JT, Straume B, et al. Hereditary angioedema: new clinical observations and autoimmune screening, complement and kallikrein-kinin analyses. J Intern Med 1996;239:119–30.
69. Caballero T, Canabal J, Rivero-Paparoni D, et al. Management of hereditary angioedema in pregnant women: a review. Int J Womens Health 2014;6:839–48.
70. Danazol [package insert]. Available at: https://www.accessdata.fda.gov/drugsatfda_docs/label/2011/017557s033s039s040s041s042lbl.pdf. Accessed January 22, 2022.
71. Drugs and lactation Database (LactMed) [Internet]. Bethesda (MD): National Library of Medicine (US); 2021. 2006–. Tranexamic Acid.
72. Farkas H, Martinez-Saguer I, Bork K, et al. International consensus on the diagnosis and management of pediatric patients with hereditary angioedema with C1 inhibitor deficiency. Allergy 2017;72:300–13.
73. Pedrosa M, Phillips-Angles E, López-Lera A, et al. Complement study versus CINH gene testing for the diagnosis of type I hereditary angioedema in children. J Clin Immunol 2016;36(1):16–8.

Mastocytosis in Pregnancy

Nonie Arora, MD, MBA[a], Cem Akin, MD, PhD[b], Anna Kovalszki, MD[b],*

KEYWORDS

- Mastocytosis • Pregnancy • Mast cell disorder • Medication safety

KEY POINTS

- Well-managed mastocytosis is not a contraindication to pursuing pregnancy.
- Twenty percent to one-third of patients experience worsening of mastocytosis symptoms during pregnancy.
- Management of mastocytosis in pregnancy generally involves avoiding mast cell activation triggers, and continuation of antimediator treatments.
- Care ought to be taken when selecting medications during the labor and delivery process. The patient's obstetrician and anesthesiologist should be made aware of the diagnosis of mastocytosis.

INTRODUCTION

Mastocytosis is a rare clonal neoplastic disorder resulting from unregulated proliferation and activation of mast cells in tissues such as skin and the bone marrow. Mast cells are the major effector cells of allergic reactions along with basophils.[1] The population estimate of mastocytosis is 1 in 10,000 individuals, although it is likely underdiagnosed.[2] Mastocytosis has a significant impact on quality of life and has been associated with a high degree of morbidity.[3] There are 2 main categories of mastocytosis, that affecting only the skin (cutaneous) and that affecting noncutaneous tissues, most commonly bone marrow, with or without skin involvement (systemic).[1] Cutaneous mastocytosis usually presents in infancy and therefore is not pertinent to the discussion of mastocytosis in pregnancy. Cutaneous mastocytosis is manifested by typical lesions of urticaria pigmentosa and less commonly mastocytomas or diffuse cutaneous mastocytosis. Symptoms of cutaneous mastocytosis include pruritus, flushing, dermatographism, and rarely anaphylaxis in affected individuals.[1] Most cases of childhood-onset mastocytosis resolve before adulthood.[4] Those that begin in adulthood, while still potentially affecting the skin, are usually deemed systemic and do not typically resolve.

[a] Department of Internal Medicine, Michigan Medicine, 3116 Taubman Center, SPC 53681500 E. Medical Center Drive, Ann Arbor, MI 48109-5368, USA; [b] Allergy and Immunology Division, University of Michigan, 24 Frank Lloyd Wright Drive, Suite H-2100, Ann Arbor, MI 48106, USA
* Corresponding author.
E-mail address: vidadi@med.umich.edu

Immunol Allergy Clin N Am 43 (2023) 159–168
https://doi.org/10.1016/j.iac.2022.07.003   immunology.theclinics.com

Systemic mastocytosis (SM) involves extracutaneous organs such as the bone marrow, liver, spleen, lymph nodes, and gastrointestinal tract (and often still involves the skin).[5] SM is divided into nonadvanced variants (indolent SM [ISM] and smoldering SM) and advanced variants (SM with an associated hematologic neoplasm, aggressive SM, and mast cell leukemia). ISM makes up most of the patients with SM.[6] Patients with ISM have a comparable life expectancy to the age-matched general population and have low risk of progressing to advanced SM. Most patients with ISM suffer from episodic and chronic mast cell mediator release symptoms such as flushing, pruritus, tachycardia, hypotension, abdominal pain, and anaphylaxis. Systemic smoldering mastocytosis is a rare subtype characterized by high-degree mast cell burden ($\geq$30% mastocytosis in bone marrow biopsies and/or tryptase $\geq$200 ng/ mL), but there is no evidence of an associated hematologic disorder or end-organ dysfunction that characterizes aggressive SM.[6] In advanced SM, patients may present with a non-mast cell myeloid hematological disorder (termed associated hematological neoplasm or AHN) such as a myeloproliferative disorder or myelodysplastic syndrome (SM-AHN) or evidence of end-organ dysfunction caused by extensive mastocytosis infiltration (cytopenias, malabsorption, portal hypertension, pathologic fractures).[5] Anaphylactic episodes occur in 30% to 40% of patients with SM.[7] Uterine contractions associated with anaphylaxis as well as hypotension and the risk of placental hypoperfusion are potential risks in a pregnant patient. Gastrointestinal symptoms are also common in patients with mastocytosis, affecting about 30% of patients. These symptoms include bloating, abdominal pain, nausea, and diarrhea. In severe cases, this can lead to malabsorption and weight loss.[8] Mast cell leukemia is a rare variant characterized by greater than 10% mastocytosis in peripheral circulation or greater than 20% atypical mastocytosis in bone marrow aspirates. Patients with advanced SM have poor prognosis and shortened life expectancy and are generally considered candidates for mast cell cytoreduction.[9] Mast cell sarcoma is an extremely rare variant with poor prognosis that is characterized by a solid invasive mastocytosis tumor.[10] Because most mast cell cytoreductive options used in advanced mastocytosis are contraindicated in pregnancy, this review mostly focuses on indolent systemic mast cell disease complicating pregnancy.

Mast cell mediator release can be provoked by several physical and psychological stressors, infections, and medications (eg, nonsteroidal antiinflammatory drugs [NSAIDs], opioids, anesthetics).[11] Pregnancy is marked by significant physical and psychological stressors that can trigger and worsen symptoms of mastocytosis in about one-third of patients.[12] On the other hand, up to one-third of pregnant patients can experience improvement in symptoms during pregnancy, similar to other autoimmune diseases such as systemic lupus erythematosus and also allergic diseases such as asthma.[13]

Given constraints on research in pregnant women, and the rarity of mastocytosis, limited research has been done on the impact and treatment of mastocytosis on pregnancy. There are conflicting results on the physiologic and pathogenic effects of mast cells in pregnancy. Mediators of mast cells, in physiologic concentrations, in particular histamine, are essential to pregnancy and delivery, including implantation of the blastocyst, development of the placenta, and myometrial contractions.[11] In addition, mast cells produce a variety of inflammatory mediators and are thought to have a role in cervical ripening.[14] On the other hand, mast cells have also been implicated in recurrent pregnancy losses. They have been found throughout the endometrial layers in women with recurrent miscarriages and are thought to produce proinflammatory mediators.[15,16] Because elevated histamine levels can lead to uterine contractions, there are concerns that patients with mastocytosis may be at risk of preterm labor. Whether this is true clinically is not clear based on the current literature. One case review series suggested higher miscarriage rates in those with mastocytosis (25%–30% vs 8%–20% in the general population, n = 45),[13] whereas another case review series suggested that mastocytosis did not significantly change pregnancy or fetal outcomes (21% miscarriage rate, n = 23) as compared with the general population.[17] Additional research is required, especially given the small case numbers of these cohort studies.

DIAGNOSIS OF MASTOCYTOSIS

SM is diagnosed according to the World Health Organization criteria. The major criterion for diagnosis is multifocal clusters of neoplastic mast cells (>15 cells per cluster) in the bone marrow. The minor diagnostic criteria include elevated baseline serum tryptase of greater than 20 ng/mL, morphologic aberrations of mastocytosis such as spindle shapes and hypogranulation, abnormal mastocytosis CD25 expression, and the presence of KIT D816V mutation.[18] The 1 major plus 1 minor or 3 minor criteria must be fulfilled for the diagnosis of SM. The diagnostic tissue of choice is a bone marrow biopsy and aspirate.[18]

The total baseline serum tryptase should be measured in all patients. For patients experiencing suspected anaphylaxis, the basal tryptase level increases during the event but should mostly return to baseline after 4 to 6 hours. A formula of 20% above baseline + 2 ng/mL has been validated as a marker of anaphylaxis in cases in which the clinical presentation may be atypical.[1]

KIT D816V mutation is a somatic gain-of-function mutation present in greater than 90% of patients with SM in bone marrow aspirates. This mutation occurs in a hematopoietic mast cell progenitor and results in expansion of the mast cell clone carrying the mutation. KIT is a transmembrane receptor with intrinsic tyrosine kinase activity and under physiologic circumstances, binds stem cell factor to initiate tyrosine autophosphorylation of the receptor. KIT/SCF interaction is the most important event in proliferation and differentiation of mast cells. KIT D816V mutation affects the tyrosine kinase domain of the molecule at exon 17 and results in ligand-independent autophosphorylation.[4] KIT D816V mutation should be analyzed by a highly sensitive method such as allele-specific polymerase chain reaction (PCR) or digital droplet PCR with the capacity to detect less than 0.1% of mutated allele burden. Because KIT D816V is a somatic mutation, it is not transmitted to the child. Research is ongoing on state-of-the-art biomarkers that can be used to identify other predictors of anaphylaxis in obstetric patients.[19,20]

THERAPEUTIC OPTIONS FOR MASTOCYTOSIS IN PREGNANCY

The major principle in the management of pregnant patient with mastocytosis is to use the lowest dose of medication to prevent symptoms both for the benefit of the patient and with the belief that mast cell mediator release has greater potential for fetal harm than potential medication effect so long as high-risk medications to the fetus and lactating mother are avoided when feasible. Management generally involves avoiding flare triggers and antimediator drugs such as antihistamines, corticosteroids, and epinephrine, if needed.

Treatment of all types of mastocytosis involves therapy targeting the mediators of mast cells (**Table 1**).[11] Mast cells release several bioactive mediators, including histamine, prostaglandins, and leukotrienes that can be targeted by antimediator drugs. In advanced SM, cytoreductive therapy may also be required.[21] In addition, there are several investigational therapies currently evaluated in clinical trials for treatment of SM including monoclonal antibodies and small molecule tyrosine kinase

Table 1
Mastocytosis treatments and pregnancy risk

Group	Medication	Pregnancy Implications	Lactation Guidance
First-generation H1 antihistamines	Brompheniramine	Increased risk of birth defects. Avoid.	Use with caution
	Chlorpheniramine	No increased risk of birth defects	Excreted in breast milk, use with caution
	Dimenhydrinate	Crosses placenta, no increased risk of fetal abnormalities	Excreted in breast milk, use with caution
	Diphenhydramine	Crosses placenta, generally considered safe to use as needed	Excreted in breast milk, breast-feeding contraindicated
	Doxylamine	Historical association with neural tube defects, oral clefts, hypoplastic left heart	Breast-feeding contraindicated
	Hydroxyzine	Crosses placenta, not recommended in early pregnancy or before or during labor	Breast-feeding not recommended
	Meclizine	No increased risk of birth defects	Unknown if excreted into breast milk
Second-generation H1 antihistamines	Cetirizine	No increased risk of birth defects	Excreted in breast milk
	Levocetirizine	No increased risk of birth defects	Unknown if excreted into breast milk, not recommended
	Loratadine	No increased risk of birth defects, prior historical association with hypospadias	Small amounts excreted into breast milk
	Fexofenadine	Limited information available, alternatives generally used	Excreted in breast milk
	Desloratadine	Adverse events in animal studies	Excreted in breast milk
H2 antihistamines	Cimetidine	Crosses placenta, no increased risk of birth defects	Excreted in breast milk, breast-feeding not recommended
	Famotidine	Crosses placenta, no increased risk of birth defects	Excreted in breast milk, use with caution
Mast cell stabilizers	Cromolyn	Safe in pregnancy	No data on excretion into breast milk, use with caution
	Ketotifen	Adverse events in animal studies	Breast-feeding not recommended
Anti-IgE antibody	Omalizumab	No increased risk of birth defects (limited patient numbers)	Likely excreted in breast milk, not recommended

(continued on next page)

Table 1 (continued)			
Group	**Medication**	**Pregnancy Implications**	**Lactation Guidance**
Oral glucocorticoids	Hydrocortisone, prednisone, dexamethasone	Possible increased risk of oral clefts with use in first trimester	Excreted in breast milk, wait 4 h after dose
Leukotriene antagonist	Montelukast/ zafirlukast	No increased risk of birth defects	Unknown if excreted into breast milk, use with caution
	Zileuton	Potentially increased risk of birth defects, not recommended	Insufficient data. Avoidance recommended
Cytoreductive therapies	Cladribine	Teratogenic effects and fetal mortality observed	Not recommended
	KIT targeting tyrosine kinase inhibitors	Pregnancy not recommended (in mother or father)	Not recommended
	Interferon alpha-2b	No clear association, can be used in severe cases, contraindicated in combination therapy with ribavirin	Excreted in breast milk

Adapted from Lei D, Akin C, Kovalszki A. Management of Mastocytosis in Pregnancy: A Review. J Allergy Clin Immunol Pract. 2017;5(5):1217-1223.

inhibitors.[21,22] Currently available cytoreductive therapies can be associated with adverse events that are unacceptable to many patients, and there is a need for more targeted therapies with improved adverse event profiles.[21] These therapies are not studied in pregnant women and thus are not recommended at this time given fetal risk.

The Food and Drug Administration (FDA) has changed the labeling of medications for pregnancy to give priority to postmarketing surveillance data.[23] In addition, the ABCDX system for putative safety of drugs for use among pregnant women has been removed and replaced with a new labeling system, the FDA Pregnancy and Lactation Labeling Rule.[24] This rule requires labels to include narrative text to describe risk information, clinical considerations, and background data for the drug. The new rules cover 3 categories: (1) pregnancy, including labor and birth, (2) lactation, and (3) women and men of reproductive potential.[24] Thus, in this work, the authors present narrative information regarding pregnancy safety of medications instead of referring to the prior category risk system.

Antimediator Therapies

Antihistamines

Patients with mastocytosis have excessive amounts of basal histamine, which is increased during mast cell activation episodes.[25] Histamine release from mast cells leads to potential pulmonary, gastrointestinal, and cutaneous symptoms. Thus, first-generation and second-generation antihistamines are a mainstay in the treatment of mastocytosis, including in pregnancy. These drugs (which are mostly over-the-counter in most countries) can control the symptoms of pruritus, hives, and flushing and ameliorate gastrointestinal symptoms. High doses (about 2–4x those for allergic rhinitis) may be required in patients whose symptoms are refractory to standard dosing. The literature suggests that second-generation long-acting antihistamines are safe in pregnancy and do not lead to birth defects.[26] In pregnancy, loratadine and cetirizine are favored H1 blockers, as they have not been associated with risk and are less sedating. Fexofenadine is less studied in pregnancy and thus preferentially avoided.

First-generation antihistamines are sometimes used as needed to supplement second-generation antihistamines, especially to counteract the symptoms of a mastocytosis activation episode. Diphenhydramine is commonly used for this purpose and, although sedating, has not been associated with fetal harm and is considered safe to use. In contrast, hydroxyzine, another common first-generation H1 antihistamine, should be avoided especially in first trimester and shortly before or during labor, as its use has been associated with birth defects and increased seizure risk in newborns.

H2 blockers famotidine, and cimetidine are thought to be safe in pregnancy, with no associations to birth defects in postmarketing surveillance data.[26]

Mast cell stabilizers

Oral cromolyn sodium is commonly used as a mast cell stabilizer, although it can cause gastrointestinal side effects such as bloating, abdominal cramping, and diarrhea in some patients. In this way, it is different from antihistamines, which reduce the action of histamines after they have already been released from mast cells.[27] Although risk has not definitively been ruled out, it is generally considered acceptable for use in pregnancy. It is not known if is excreted in breast milk.[27] Ketotifen, another mast cell stabilizer/antihistamine, has been associated with some adverse events shown in animal studies and is not recommended.[12]

Leukotriene Antagonists

Patients with mastocytosis overproduce cysteinyl leukotrienes such as LTC4. Montelukast and zafirlukast, leukotriene receptor-blocking drugs, improve cutaneous and pulmonary symptoms in mastocytosis.[28] No adverse events have been observed in animal studies. In a study of montelukast use during pregnancy on infant outcomes in women with asthma, montelukast did not seem to increase the baseline rate of major malformations.[29] In contrast, zileuton, a 5-LO inhibitor blocking cysLT production should not be used in pregnancy, as animal studies indicated potential harm to fetus at high doses.[30]

Antiimmunoglobulin E (Omalizumab)

Omalizumab has been shown to prevent anaphylaxis and reduce gastrointestinal and cutaneous symptoms in patients with mastocytosis.[21] In the Observational Study of the Use and Safety of Xolair (omalizumab) during Pregnancy (EXPECT), 250 women were exposed to omalizumab during pregnancy. There was no evidence of an increased risk of major congenital abnormalities when compared with a disease-matched external comparison cohort.[31]

Glucocorticoids

Although the use of inhaled steroids is considered to be safe in pregnancy, there is conflicting and insufficient data about the use of systemic steroids. Some studies suggest increased risk of cleft lip especially in the first trimester.[32] Thus, care must be taken when prescribing them for mastocytosis, carefully weighing risks and benefits. Most patients with mastocytosis do not require persistent or long-term systemic steroid use. Occasional use for significant flares may be required, undertaken with concomitant discussion about risks with patient and overseeing obstetrician.

Cytoreductive Agents

Almost all cytoreductive agents, with the exception of interferon-α, are associated with potential fetal harm in pregnancy.

Cladribine, a nucleoside analogue, has shown transient improvement in advanced mastocytosis. Animal studies show teratogenic effects and fetal mortality, and it should be avoided entirely in pregnancy.[33]

KIT targeting tyrosine kinase inhibitors midostaurin, avapritinib, and imatinib show significant promise in treating advanced forms of SM, and avapritinib is also in clinical trials on ISM. These agents are not safe for use in pregnancy or lactation or to be used by partners of pregnant women due to increased risk of spontaneous abortion, teratogenicity, skeletal defects, pyloric stenosis, and hypospadias.[34,35]

Interferon Alpha-2b

Interferon alpha-2b was the earliest cytoreductive agent that was reported to reduce mast cell mediator release and mast cell infiltration, although the onset of action is delayed and remission rates with this agent remain low. It is associated with significant side effects including flulike symptoms and mood changes, limiting its current use as a first-line agent in SM. Mechanism of action of interferon-α in mastocytosis is not fully understood. It has not been clearly associated with maternal or fetal complications or malformations.[8] There was an association with intrauterine growth restriction, but causality could not be established due to a small sample size.

LABOR AND DELIVERY

The management of anesthesia during the labor and delivery period focuses on preventing anaphylaxis and being prepared to treat mast cell degranulation should it occur. Mast cell degranulation can occur perioperatively due to emotional stress, physical stress, allergen exposure, or drugs that promote the release of histamine (such as morphine). The risk of a potential reactions can be minimized by promoting a calm environment, normothermia, avoiding exposures to medications that have previously triggered the onset of flare, and avoidance of medications that are known to release histamine or other mediators if the patient's tolerance from prior pregnancies or surgeries is not known. Although evidence is currently lacking, some experts do recommend pretreatment with steroids, antihistamines, and potentially oral cromolyn sodium.[36] One case report suggests that nonpharmaceutical interventions (provider education, an advance meeting with the birthing team, involvement of a doula) can reduce anxiety and potentially improve pregnancy outcomes.[37]

Even with the most thorough birth plan, mast cell degranulation can occur spontaneously. Home births should be avoided, and medical personnel should have immediate access to epinephrine, adequate intravenous access, and a team to assist with resuscitation if shock develops.[36,38]

Certain medications such as codeine, morphine, certain muscle relaxants such as mivacurium or atracurium, and some antibiotics (including vancomycin) are associated with increased risk of mast cell mediator release, and it is generally recommended to use alternative agents if the patient's tolerance is not known. Fentanyl, benzodiazepines, and local anesthetics have been generally well tolerated. Of the muscle relaxants, succinylcholine and cisatracurium seem to have the least mastocytosis mediator release effect.[39] NSAIDs should be avoided as a precaution if the patient's tolerance is not known.

DISCUSSION OF PREGNANCY OUTCOMES

Only cohort and case studies are available regarding pregnancy outcomes in patients with mastocytosis. As discussed, the literature supports mixed outcomes on mast cell activation symptoms with approximately 20% to 33% of pregnant women with mastocytosis experience worsening during pregnancy.[13,17,40] Of note, symptoms generally worsened in the first or third trimester, when Th1-mediated proinflammatory conditions are more common. Irregular medication intake and reduction in medication dose may also contribute to the worsening of mastocytosis symptoms.[17]

In one study of 23 pregnancies, 4 of the patients developed worsening severity of their mastocytosis.[17] In a second study of 45 women, 5 women developed mastocytosis mediator–related symptoms during delivery (pruritus, erythema, flushing) and none developed anaphylaxis. Premedication was given before 17 of the 45 deliveries.[13] One case study describes women with SM who had a delivery complicated by anaphylactic shock despite pretreatment with dexamethasone and diphenhydramine.[36]

SUMMARY

Pregnant patients with mastocytosis should be ideally managed with a team of providers including obstetricians, allergists, and hematologists depending on the subtype of mastocytosis. Consultation with a high-risk obstetric specialist is recommended in those with a history of anaphylaxis and in patients with advanced mastocytosis. Treatment generally focuses on management of symptoms with antimediator therapy (H1 & H2 antihistamines, leukotriene antagonist, glucocorticoids, and epinephrine, if required).

CLINICS CARE POINTS

- Well-managed mastocytosis is not a contraindication to pursuing pregnancy.
- Twenty percent to one-third of patients experience worsening of mastocytosis symptoms during pregnancy, whereas other patients report stable or even improved symptoms.
- Management of mastocytosis in pregnancy generally involves avoiding mast cell activation triggers and prophylactic and/or therapeutic antihistamines, limited courses of corticosteroids, and epinephrine, as needed.
- Care ought to be taken when selecting medications during the labor and delivery process.

DISCLOSURE

N. Arora: no disclosures. C. Akin: consultancy agreements with Blueprint Medicines, Cogent, and Novartis, Research support from Blueprint Medicines and Cogent. A. Kovalszki: no disclosures.

REFERENCES

1. Theoharides TC, Valent P, Akin C. Mast Cells, Mastocytosis, and Related Disorders. N Engl J Med 2015;373(2):163–72. https://doi.org/10.1056/NEJMra 1409760.
2. Cohen SS, Skovbo S, Vestergaard H, et al. Epidemiology of systemic mastocytosis in Denmark. Br J Haematol 2014;166(4):521–8.
3. Pulfer S, Ziehfreund S, Gebhard J, et al. Health-Related Quality of Life and Influencing Factors in Adults with Nonadvanced Mastocytosis—A Cross-Sectional Study and Qualitative Approach. J Allergy Clin Immunol In Pract 2021;9(8): 3166–75.e2.
4. Carter MC, Metcalfe DD, Komarow HD. Mastocytosis. Immunol Allergy Clin 2014; 34(1):181–96.
5. Akin C, Metcalfe DD. Systemic mastocytosis. Annu Rev Med 2004;55:419–32.
6. Valent P, Akin C, Hartmann K, et al. Updated Diagnostic Criteria and Classification of Mast Cell Disorders: A Consensus Proposal. Hemasphere 2021;5(11): e646.
7. Siebenhaar F, Akin C, Bindslev-Jensen C, et al. Treatment strategies in mastocytosis. Immunol Allergy Clin 2014;34(2):433–47.
8. Nanagas VC, Kovalszki A. Gastrointestinal Manifestations of Hypereosinophilic Syndromes and Mast Cell Disorders: a Comprehensive Review. Clin Rev Allergy Immunol 2019;57(2):194–212.
9. Georgin-Lavialle S, Lhermitte L, Dubreuil P, et al. Mast cell leukemia. Blood 2013; 121(8):1285–95.
10. Weiler CR, Butterfield J. Mast cell sarcoma: clinical management. Immunol Allergy Clin North Am 2014;34(2):423–32.
11. Lei D, Kovalszki A. Mastocytosis in Pregnancy. Mastocytosis 2020;187–205.
12. Lei D, Akin C, Kovalszki A. Management of Mastocytosis in Pregnancy: A Review. J Allergy Clin Immunol Pract 2017;5(5):1217–23.
13. Matito A, Alvarez-Twose I, Morgado JM, et al. Clinical impact of pregnancy in mastocytosis: a study of the Spanish Network on Mastocytosis (REMA) in 45 cases. Int Arch Allergy Immunol 2011;156(1):104–11.
14. Norström A, Radulovic NV, Bullarbo M, et al. Mast cell involvement in human cervical ripening. Eur J Obstet Gynecol Reprod Biol 2019;238:157–63.
15. Elieh Ali Komi D, Shafaghat F, Haidl G. Significance of mast cells in spermatogenesis, implantation, pregnancy, and abortion: cross talk and molecular mechanisms. Am J Reprod Immunol 2020;83(5):e13228.
16. Derbala Y, Elazzamy H, Bilal M, et al. Mast cell–induced immunopathology in recurrent pregnancy losses. Am J Reprod Immunol 2019;82(1):e13128.
17. Ciach K, Niedoszytko M, Abacjew-Chmylko A, et al. Pregnancy and Delivery in Patients with Mastocytosis Treated at the Polish Center of the European Competence Network on Mastocytosis (ECNM). PLoS One 2016;11(1):e0146924.
18. Pardanani A. Systemic mastocytosis in adults: 2019 update on diagnosis, risk stratification and management. Am J Hematol 2019;94(3):363–77.
19. Simionescu AA, Stanescu AMA, Popescu FD. State-of-the-Art on Biomarkers for Anaphylaxis in Obstetrics. Life (Basel) 2021;11(9). https://doi.org/10.3390/ life11090870.
20. Valent P, Akin C, Metcalfe DD. Mastocytosis: 2016 updated WHO classification and novel emerging treatment concepts. Blood 2017;129(11):1420–7.
21. Giannetti MP. Treatment of systemic mastocytosis: Novel and emerging therapies. Ann Allergy Asthma Immunol 2021;127(4):412–9.

22. Bose P, Verstovsek S. Avapritinib for Systemic Mastocytosis. Expert Rev Hematol 2021;14(8):687–96.
23. Greene MF. FDA drug labeling for pregnancy and lactation drug safety monitoring systems. Semin Perinatol 2015;39(7):520–3.
24. Brucker MC, King TL. The 2015 US Food and Drug Administration Pregnancy and Lactation Labeling Rule. J Midwifery Womens Health 2017;62(3):308–16.
25. Butterfield J, Weiler CR. The utility of measuring urinary metabolites of mast cell mediators in systemic mastocytosis and mast cell activation syndrome. J Allergy Clin Immunol In Pract 2020;8(8):2533–41.
26. Gilboa SM, Ailes EC, Rai RP, et al. Antihistamines and birth defects: a systematic review of the literature. Expert Opin Drug Saf 2014;13(12):1667–98.
27. Minutello K, Gupta V. Cromolyn sodium. Treasure Island (FL): StatPearls Publishing; 2021.
28. Tolar J, Tope WD, Neglia JP. Leukotriene-receptor inhibition for the treatment of systemic mastocytosis. N Engl J Med 2004;350(7):735–6.
29. Sarkar M, Koren G, Kalra S, et al. Montelukast use during pregnancy: a multicentre, prospective, comparative study of infant outcomes. Eur J Clin Pharmacol 2009;65(12):1259–64.
30. Bonham CA, Patterson KC, Strek ME. Asthma Outcomes and Management During Pregnancy. Chest 2018;153(2):515–27.
31. Namazy JA, Blais L, Andrews EB, et al. Pregnancy outcomes in the omalizumab pregnancy registry and a disease-matched comparator cohort. J Allergy Clin Immunol 2020;145(2):528–36.e1.
32. Källén B. Maternal use of anti-asthmatic drugs and infant congenital malformations. maternal drug use and infant congenital malformations. Springer International Publishing; 2019. p. 353–65.
33. Cardet JC, Akin C, Lee MJ. Mastocytosis: update on pharmacotherapy and future directions. Expert Opin Pharmacother 2013;14(15):2033–45.
34. Hartmann K, Gotlib J, Akin C, et al. Midostaurin improves quality of life and mediator-related symptoms in advanced systemic mastocytosis. J Allergy Clin Immunol 2020;146(2):356–66. e4.
35. Castells M, Akin C. Finding the right KIT inhibitor for advanced systemic mastocytosis. Nat Med 2021;27(12):2081–2.
36. Watson KD, Arendt KW, Watson WJ, et al. Systemic mastocytosis complicating pregnancy. Obstet Gynecol 2012;119:486–9.
37. Kehoe SL, Bathgate SL, Macri CJ. Use of a Doula for Labor Coaching in a Patient With Indolent Systemic Mastocytosis in Pregnancy. Obstet Gynecol 2006;107(2 Part 2):514–6.
38. Madendag IC, Madendag Y, Tarhan I, et al. Mastocytosis in Pregnancy. Taiwanese J Obstet Gynecol 2010;49(2):192–6.
39. Hermans MAW, Arends NJT, Gerth van Wijk R, et al. Management around invasive procedures in mastocytosis: An update. Ann Allergy Asthma Immunol 2017;119(4):304–9.
40. Worobec AS, Akin C, Scott LM, et al. Mastocytosis complicating pregnancy. Obstet Gynecol 2000;95(3):391–5.

Use of Asthma Medication During Gestation and Risk of Specific Congenital Anomalies

Ruth P. Cusack, MBBch[a], Christiane E. Whetstone, BSc[b],
Gail M. Gauvreau, PhD, Professor[c],*

KEYWORDS

- Asthma medication • Congenital anomaly • Pregnancy

KEY POINTS

- Inhaled corticosteroids and long-acting β-agonists are safe in pregnancy.
- Low priority should be placed on stepping down treatment until after delivery in a well-controlled patient.
- Good education before and during pregnancy is important to ensure compliance to asthma medication.
- More data on the use of biological therapies for asthma in pregnancy is needed.

INTRODUCTION

Asthma is one of the most common medical conditions to affect pregnancy with a prevalence of between 5% and 13% of pregnancies,[1–3] with prevalence increasing in recent years in the United States.[4,5] Poorly controlled maternal asthma during pregnancy is common, affecting up to 28% of pregnancies,[1] and can affect maternal health (preeclampsia) and neonatal outcomes (congenital anomalies, preterm delivery, increased perinatal mortality, low birth weight).[5,6] These complications can potentially be reduced with appropriate management of asthma and its exacerbations during pregnancy.[7,8]

The treatment of asthma during pregnancy follows the same principles as asthma management in the general adult population with asthma medications divided into rescue therapy and maintenance therapy.[9,10] Using a stepwise approach to asthma therapy ensures the lowest amount of medication necessary is used to control the

[a] Department of Medicine, McMaster University, HSC 3U31 F, 1200 Main Street West, Hamilton, Ontario L8N 3Z5, Canada; [b] Department of Medicine, McMaster University, HSC 3U20, 1200 Main Street West, Hamilton, Ontario L8N 3Z5, Canada; [c] Department of Medicine, McMaster University, HSC 3U31E, 1200 Main Street W, Hamilton, Ontario L8N 3Z5, Canada
* Corresponding author.
E-mail address: gauvreau@mcmaster.ca

Immunol Allergy Clin N Am 43 (2023) 169–185
https://doi.org/10.1016/j.iac.2022.07.007
0889-8561/23/© 2022 Elsevier Inc. All rights reserved.

patient's symptoms, with increasing number and dosage of medications with increasing asthma severity. However, one of the biggest challenges in managing asthma during pregnancy is medication adherence, and despite clear guidelines, many women remain concerned about a potential negative effect of treatment on their unborn child. A cross-sectional study by Al Ghobain and colleagues[11] investigated the views of pregnant women with asthma and found that 46.8% of pregnant asthmatic women had stopped (or expressed a desire to stop) their asthma medications during pregnancy, and 48% believed asthma medications would harm them and their babies. Powell and colleagues[12] previously found pregnant women with asthma overestimated the teratogenic risk of asthma medications with 42% perceiving a teratogenic risk with oral corticosteroids (OCSs), 12% a risk with inhaled corticosteroids (ICSs), and 5% a risk with short-acting β-agonists (SABAs). Despite women's concerns regarding the risk of asthma medications during pregnancy, the benefit of asthma education cannot be underestimated with only 40% of women more likely to continue their asthma medication during pregnancy if their obstetrician alone recommended it.[13] There is also evidence of suboptimal management of asthma within primary care. An Australian anonymous mail survey of 174 general practitioners found 25.8% of respondents would stop or decrease patients' ICS dose during pregnancy, even if asthma was well controlled on current therapy, and 12.1% of respondents indicated they did not know how to manage a deterioration of asthma during pregnancy.[14]

The overall risk of congenital abnormalities with maternal asthma is slightly increased; however, there is a lack of consensus concerning the effects of asthma medications versus the disease itself on the development of congenital anomalies because confounding factors can contribute to some of these associations.[15–17] Maternal asthma exacerbations during the first trimester of pregnancy significantly increase the risk of congenital abnormalities (adjusted odds ratio [AOR] = 1.48; 95% confidence interval [CI], 1.04–2.09), because this is a critical period of embryogenesis when congenital anomalies happen.[18] Treatments that maintain asthma control during pregnancy are favorable to optimize both maternal and fetal health, and the risk of poor asthma control greatly outweighs the risk of treatment side effects, particularly with regard to congenital anomalies.

Congenital Anomalies: Definition, Detection, and Risk Factors

Congenital anomalies may be detected prenatally, at birth, or later in infancy such as hearing or visual anomalies. In recent decades there have been major improvements in congenital anomalies diagnosis because prenatal ultrasonography has become a standard part of prenatal care, with prenatal diagnosis of structural malformations of most organ systems detectable during pregnancy.[19]

Different congenital anomalies and patterns are due to a teratogenic insult at particular gestational stages (**Fig. 1**). After the egg is fertilized and before implantation, the result of a teratogenic insult is an all or nothing effect. The first 8 weeks of pregnancy, often before the first identification of pregnancy, is termed blastogenesis (weeks 0–4) and organogenesis (weeks 4–8), when the embryo develops into tissues and organs. Insults during blastogenesis can result in severe, often lethal anomalies that involve several organ systems. Insults during organogenesis tend to involve single organ structures; for example, weeks 3 to 5 are critical for central nervous system development, and weeks 7 to 9 for urogenital development. During the fetal period (after 8 weeks gestation), harmful influences may affect fetal growth and function (eg, hearing loss, cognitive impairment, lung immaturity). Therefore, timing of exposure of a particular event or insult, duration and frequency of exposure, can result in very different outcomes.

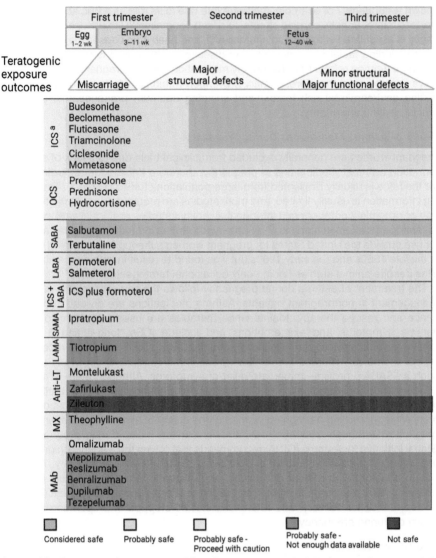

Fig. 1. Risk of teratogenic outcomes with asthma treatment. LAMA, long-acting muscarinic agonist; LT, leukotriene; mAb, monoclonal antibody; MX, methylxanthine; SAMA, short-acting muscarinic antagonist. [a]High-dose ICS (>1000 μg/d beclomethasone equivalent) in the first trimester could be associated with a small increased risk of congenital anomaly.

The risk factors for developing anomalies can be classified as modifiable (environmental, smoking, obesity, diabetes, medications, folic acid deficiency) and nonmodifiable (genetic), although in most cases the cause remains unknown. A genetic predisposition to specific teratogens has been studied extensively. Maternal and fetal genetic variants have been associated with an embryo's susceptibility to develop fetal alcohol syndrome.[20] Cigarette smoke exposure is a risk factor for the development of orofacial clefts and gastroschisis in the fetus; however, the risk is increased even further if the fetus carries specific, rare genotypes.[21,22] Specific medications are known teratogens. For example, methotrexate due to its role as a folic acid antagonist leads to microcephaly, cardiac effects, and limb anomalies[23]; lithium use in early pregnancy is associated with cardiac anomalies[24]; and phenytoin causes major malformations including facial clefts and cardiac disease.[25] Although it is preferable that all pregnant women refrain from taking any medications during pregnancy, this is not always possible, and therefore, primary prevention within the whole population by controlling environmental risk factors and ensuring optimum preconceptual care is a crucial health care priority.

Safety of Asthma Medications During Pregnancy

Pregnant women are generally excluded from clinical trials due to a lack of safety information on most medications in pregnancy; therefore knowledge regarding safety for the fetus is usually presented from large population studies (**Table 1**). Thus, existing information is usually limited, and more studies are required due to lack of information or potential confounders. Unfortunately animal studies are not always predictive of teratogenic effect in humans,[26] as observed with thalidomide, which was approved for use outside the United States for pregnant women suffering from morning sickness in the late 1950s and the early 1960s but was found to result in limb congenital anomalies despite animal studies finding only occasional teratogenic events.[27]

The treatment of asthma during pregnancy follows the same principles as asthma management in nonpregnant patients. Asthma medications are divided into maintenance and rescue therapy. Maintenance therapies are used long term to prevent asthma symptoms and exacerbations and include ICSs, long-acting β-agonists (LABA), antileukotrienes, anticholinergic agents, theophylline, and more recently biological therapies, whereas rescue therapies, primarily rapid-onset bronchodilators such as SABAs, provide immediate relief of symptoms. Although there is a general concern about any medication use in pregnancy, an important role for a clinician is to stress the importance of maintaining good control of asthma and medication adherence while reassuring a pregnant woman of the safety of asthma medications during pregnancy. Although treatment adjustments can be made during pregnancy, the Global Initiative for Asthma (GINA) recommends that "given the evidence in pregnancy and infancy for adverse outcomes from exacerbations during pregnancy, including due to a lack of ICS or poor adherence, and evidence for safety of usual doses of ICS and LABA, a low priority should be placed on stepping down treatment (however guided) until after delivery, and ICS should not be stopped in preparation for pregnancy or during pregnancy."[9]

Inhaled Corticosteroids

ICSs have been the cornerstone of asthma therapy for more than 40 years and are recommended as a first-line therapy for asthma in both adolescents and adults, recently replacing SABAs as the first-line therapy for mild asthma.[9] However, ICS adherence during pregnancy is poor with 39% of pregnant women reporting nonadherence[28] despite studies showing that ICS does not increase risk of congenital anomalies associated with its use,[29] ICS reduces asthma exacerbations in pregnancy,[30] and cessation of ICS increases the risk of developing exacerbations, which are a risk factor for congenital anomalies rather than asthma itself (AOR = 1.21; 95% CI, 1.05–1.39).[31]

Concerns raised about a potential association of congenital anomalies and moderate- to high-dose ICSs have been examined. A previous literature review[32] summarizing the risk of congenital malformations with the use of ICSs in pregnancy found that in 15 separate studies[29,33–46] comparing women with asthma using any ICS versus women with asthma not using ICS the adjusted relative risk ranged from 0.4 to 1.1.

Table 1
Summary data for asthma medications and risk of congenital anomalies

Drug Category	Preferred Drugs	Human Data	Considerations
Inhaled corticosteroids	Budesonide (more published data) Beclomethasone (reassuring data)	At low and moderate doses no increased risk of congenital anomalies. One study showed at >1000 μg/d beclomethasone equivalent in the first trimester there was a small increased risk of congenital anomaly[47]	If well controlled on an ICS before pregnancy this may be continued because changing drug may threaten asthma control
Inhaled SABAs	Salbutamol/albuterol (more published data)	Recommended as safe in pregnancy. Large population studies have found no association between β-agonists and congenital anomalies[51]	Goal is to minimize SABA use using ICSs to ensure adequate control
Inhaled LABAs	Salmeterol Formoterol Indacaterol Vilanterol	Similar safety profile to SABAs. Animal studies for once-daily LABAs are reassuring; however, no human data are available	LABA monotherapy should not be used. These agents are not first choice in pregnancy unless a once-daily fixed combination regime is required to ensure adherence
Combination therapy	Low-dose ICS-formoterol can be used as maintenance and reliever therapy	The use of ICS-LABA combination did not result in a significant increased risk of congenital anomalies compared with high-dose ICS alone during the first trimester[56]	Limited studies, however, probably safe in pregnancy with no increased congenital anomaly risk
Oral corticosteroids	Prednisone (more published data)	Conflicting data; however, recent studies suggest no increased risk of congenital anomalies[58,59]	Major benefit outweighs the risk in severe asthma

(continued on next page)

Table 1
(continued)

Drug Category	Preferred Drugs	Human Data	Considerations
Antileukotrienes	Montelukast (more published data)	A cohort study of 180 montelukast-exposed pregnancies found montelukast did not increase the risk of major congenital anomalies[63]	Zileuton not recommended in pregnancy due to fetal abnormalities in animal studies.[61] Montelukast probably safe as an add-on therapy in uncontrolled asthma
Anticholinergics	Ipratropium	Nebulized ipratropium recommended for acute, severe asthma not responding to β-agonists alone	No published data for tiotropium in pregnancy
Theophylline	N/A	No increased risk of congenital anomalies compared with inhaled beclomethasone; however, increased risk of discontinuation due to side effects[38]	No evidence of teratogenic effects. Blood levels should be monitored
Monoclonal antibody therapies	Omalizumab	No increased risk of congenital anomalies with omalizumab[69]	Probably safe in pregnancy; however, larger studies are needed
	Mepolizumab	No published human data	Pregnancy registry ongoing
	Reslizumab	No published human data	Pregnancy registry ongoing
	Benralizumab	No published human data	Pregnancy registry ongoing
	Dupilumab	A review of 23 pregnancies in study patients found no increased risk of congenital anomalies; however, low numbers of pregnancies, therefore more data needed[78]	EMA states dupilumab should only be used during pregnancy if the potential benefits outweigh the risks.[81] Pregnancy registry ongoing
	Tezepelumab	No published human data	No pregnancy registry

Abbreviations: EMA, European Medicines Agency; LABA, long-acting β-agonist; N/A, not applicable.

Bakhireva and colleagues[35] were the only investigators to report a significantly increased risk of congenital anomalies associated with ICS use when they compared 438 pregnant women using ICSs during pregnancy with nonasthmatic control pregnant women (4.1% vs 0.3% presence of major anomalies, respectively, P = <0.05). Blais and colleagues[47] studied 13,280 pregnancies in women with asthma and found 1633 congenital anomalies, the most frequent being cardiac and musculoskeletal. High daily ICS use (>1000 μg/d beclomethasone equivalent) during the first trimester was associated with a significant risk of congenital anomalies (AOR = 1.63; 95% CI, 1.02–2.60), compared with women taking low- or medium-dose ICSs. These results must be interpreted with caution, however, because the number of women taking high-dose ICSs was small (n = 154, 1.1%), and the results were based on medication claims and not actual usage. Furthermore, the investigators could not out rule asthma severity, age, or socioeconomic group confounding the results. However, with respect to the first trimester, women who abstained from ICS use had a higher risk of congenital anomalies in their baby compared with women who used low- or moderate-dose ICS, supporting the belief that uncontrolled maternal asthma rather than ICS is associated with congenital anomalies. In addition, the ICS budesonide has been studied extensively in pregnancy with a large body of safety data showing no increased risk of congenital anomalies or stillbirths[34,48,49] and is considered first-line ICS if commencing therapy during pregnancy; however, if a patient is well controlled on an ICS before pregnancy this may be continued because changing formulations may threaten asthma control.

β-Agonists

SABAs provide symptom relief by rapidly reversing the effects of bronchoconstriction in asthma and are now recommended as an add-on therapy for patients taking ICSs.[9] LABAs are the second most widely used controller medication in asthma and compared with SABAs they provide more prolonged bronchodilation, with a greater reduction in symptoms, increased lung function, and reduced need for SABAs. SABAs are recommended as safe in pregnancy.[10] LABAs when used alone have previously been associated with increased asthma-related mortality in general,[50] and therefore they are only recommended as an add-on controller therapy in fixed-dose combination with ICSs to treat moderate to severe asthma.

A study examining more than 76,000 registrations of congenital abnormalities raised concerns finding an association between inhaled β-agonist exposure during the first trimester and congenital anomalies including cleft palate and gastroschisis.[17] However, a larger population-based cohort study of more than 519,242 infants, including 19,513 mothers with asthma medication exposure, found no significant association between inhaled β-agonists and cleft palate (AOR = 1.05; 95% CI: 0.44–2.51) or gastroschisis (AOR = 1.08; 95% CI, 0.37–3.15),[51] suggesting no association between β-agonists and congenital anomalies. A systematic review of 21 published studies that examined β-agonist use and congenital anomalies[52] found only 1 study that reported a significant risk of congenital anomalies with LABA, whereas 4 studies found a significantly higher risk of congenital anomalies with SABA and 1 reported a significantly lower risk of congenital anomalies with SABA. The investigators state, however, these results must be interpreted with caution because all studies except 2 used nonasthmatic women as the reference group, which could have confounded the underlying asthma disease and the effect of medication, and further studies are required.

Inhaled salbutamol is considered the first-line SABA therapy for pregnant women because it has been studied most extensively.[29] There is no preferred LABA therapy in pregnancy, and a previous study showed no difference in perinatal complications between salmeterol or formoterol exposure; however, congenital anomalies were not specifically examined.[53] Therefore, the goal of asthma management in pregnant women is to minimize the use of SABAs using ICSs, and if required, adding a LABA, to ensure adequate control and prevent severe exacerbations known to increase the risk of congenital anomalies. Ultra-LABAs (eg, indacaterol and vilanterol) are newer LABAs used in a once-daily fixed combination with ICSs. Although animal studies for ultra-LABAs suggest low risk of congenital anomalies, no human data are available. Thus, these agents are not our first choice in pregnancy unless a once-daily fixed combination regime is required to ensure adherence.

Combination Therapy

Asthma management for adolescents and adults is based on a stepwise approach. When asthma cannot be controlled with low-dose ICS alone, guidelines suggest adding LABA in a fixed-dose inhaler or increasing the ICS dose to the medium range.[9] As needed low-dose ICS-formoterol is now recommended as the first-line therapy for mild asthma instead of SABA[9] because it has been associated with reduced asthma exacerbations and improved peak flows and forced expiratory volume in the first second of expiration compared with as-needed SABA.[54] ICS-formoterol combination can also be used as a maintenance and reliever therapy and is effective at reducing exacerbation risk, and results in a simplified approach to asthma management.[55]

Pregnant women were excluded from clinical trials assessing the safety of ICS-formoterol combination therapy as needed and as a maintenance and reliever therapy, limiting our knowledge of safety in pregnancy. Physician's and patient's perception of medication risk of teratogenicity due to lack of clinical trial evidence for these agents may result in them changing treatment regimen during pregnancy. A Canadian retrospective cohort study of 1302 asthmatic pregnant women assessed the risk of congenital malformations in women using ICS-LABA combination versus high-dose ICS alone in the first trimester.[56] The use of ICS-LABA combination had a similar risk of congenital anomalies compared with high-dose ICS alone during the first trimester (AOR = 1.0; 95% CI, 0.6–1.7) in moderate to severe asthma. These results are reassuring and suggest that ICS-LABA combination therapy is safe in pregnancy with no increased congenital anomaly risk, and should provide reassurance to both women and physicians to continue their asthma combination medication during pregnancy.

Oral Corticosteroids

OCSs may be required for the treatment of acute exacerbations or used at low dose for management of persistent severe asthma. There are more data regarding the safety of prednisone for pregnant women because it has been studied more extensively.

There are conflicting data regarding the risk of congenital anomalies and OCS in pregnancy. Park-Wyllie and colleagues[57] performed a meta-analysis of 10 studies showing an increased risk of orofacial anomalies when OCS is used during the first trimester only (odds ratio [OR] = 3.35; 95% CI, 1.97–5.69). These results must be interpreted with caution because 7 studies included women with various underlying conditions requiring OCS use, whereas three studies did not describe the mother's indication for OCS. And this could have resulted in confounding, therefore further studies are required assessing the effect of OCS in asthma alone during pregnancy. Reassuringly data from the National Birth Defects Prevention Study of 1304 congenital anomaly births in women who reported any asthma medication use from 1997 to 2011 found no increased risk of cleft lip and prednisone use.[58,59] As a previous study found an association between first-trimester severe asthma exacerbation requiring hospitalization and congenital anomalies when compared with women with asthma who did not require a visit to the emergency department or hospitalization (OR = 1.64; 95% CI, 1.02–2.64),[60] the benefit of OCSs in the prevention of severe asthma exacerbations outweighs the potential risk of congenital anomalies associated with their use.

Antileukotrienes

Montelukast and zafirlukast are selective leukotriene receptor antagonists (LTRAs) indicated as maintenance controller therapies for asthma. Although data for the use of both agents are limited in pregnancy, montelukast is the first-line LTRA therapy during pregnancy because it has been studied most extensively. Zileuton is a leukotriene synthesis inhibitor that is not recommended in pregnancy due to fetal abnormalities in animal studies[61] with no evaluation of safety in human pregnancy.

Montelukast is indicated as an add-on therapy for asthma; however, a Danish cross-sectional observational study through a prescription-based database attempted to realize the risk of congenital abnormalities associated with montelukast in pregnant women when used as a single agent (n = 401) compared with its use simultaneously with other asthma medications (n = 426) during the first trimester of pregnancy.[62] Rates of major congenital anomalies were not different in the montelukast-only group (AOR = 1.4; 95% CI, 0.9–2.3) when compared with montelukast simultaneously with other asthma medications (AOR = 1.0; 95% CI, 0.6–1.8) or when compared with other asthma medications alone (AOR = 1.1; 95% CI, 1.0–1.2). This study did have several limitations because the number of congenital anomalies was low (16 in the montelukast alone group) reducing the statistical power. The study did not have sufficient power to look for associations with specific anomalies, the database did not include information regarding the pregnant women's indication for montelukast, and the extraction of information from a prescription database may be a poor proxy for actual use of medications. A separate prospective cohort study of 180 montelukast-exposed pregnancies reported the same findings that montelukast did not increase the risk of major congenital anomalies.[63] Although data about effects of montelukast on congenital abnormalities during pregnancy are limited, when combined these reports consistently suggest that montelukast is probably safe as an add-on controller medication to achieve good symptom control in pregnancy.

Anticholinergics

Anticholinergic agents include the short-acting muscarinic antagonist (SAMA) ipratropium and long-acting muscarinic antagonists (LAMAs) including tiotropium. Anticholinergics induce bronchodilation through the inhibition of muscarinic receptors in smooth muscle. LAMAs are recommended as add-on therapy for moderate to severe persistent asthma, due to their ability to reduce asthma exacerbations and improve asthma control.[64] Nebulized ipratropium with β-agonists has been recommended for the management of acute, severe asthma not responding to β-agonists alone.[65] No well-controlled clinical studies of tiotropium have been specifically performed in pregnant women.

Theophylline

Theophylline previously was a cornerstone of asthma medication because of its bronchodilator and anti-inflammatory activity; however, its use has decreased in recent decades due to the introduction of ICSs and concerns regarding its toxicity and side effect profile.[66] Thus, theophylline is no longer recommended as a first-line therapy for asthma and is only recommended as an alternative add-on controller therapy for moderate to severe asthma. Theophylline has previously been used in the treatment of asthma during pregnancy with no evidence of teratogenic effects; however, pregnant women were significantly more likely to discontinue theophylline than inhaled beclomethasone due to increased rate of side effects (6 of 194 discontinued in the beclomethasone group, 17 of 190 in the theophylline group; $P = 0.016$).[38] During theophylline treatment in all adults, however, blood levels should be monitored because the risk of toxic reactions increases when the serum theophylline level is higher than the therapeutic range of 10 to 20 µg/mL.[67]

Anti-IgE Therapy

Omalizumab is a recombinant monoclonal anti-IgE antibody that binds specifically to free human immunoglobulin E (IgE) in the blood and is approved as an add-on therapy for the treatment of moderate to severe allergic asthma despite adequate ICSs.[9] Animal studies using subcutaneous doses of omalizumab up to 10 times the maximum human dose found no evidence of fetal harm in cynomolgus monkeys.[68]

The Observational Study of the Use and Safety of Xolair (omalizumab) during Pregnancy Trial (EXPERT) examined the association between omalizumab and congenital anomalies in 230 pregnancies to compare exposed pregnancies with a disease-matched population of pregnant women with moderate to severe asthma.[69] The rates of major congenital anomalies were similar in both groups (8.1% in the omalizumab-exposed group vs 8.9% in the unexposed group) with the most common major congenital anomalies in the exposed group being torticollis (2.2%), hydronephrosis (1.3%), and hypospadias (0.9%), and the most common major congenital anomalies in the unexposed group being cardiac (2.8%), musculoskeletal (1.2%), and urinary system (1.1%) anomalies with no unique system anomaly found within the exposed group alone. Therefore, this study does provide reassurance regarding the lack of teratogenic risk of omalizumab and the safety of continued use of omalizumab in women with improved asthma control and reduced exacerbations before pregnancy. Therefore, for women established on omalizumab before pregnancy, if the benefits outweigh the risks, omalizumab therapy may be continued; however, it is not currently recommended to start omalizumab in pregnant women.

Anti-Interleukin-5, Anti-Interleukin-4/13, and Anti-Thymic Stromal Lymphopoietin Monoclonal Antibody Therapies

Interleukin (IL)-5 is a key cytokine involved in the recruitment, activation, and survival of eosinophils, and anti-IL-5 biological therapies reduce eosinophilic inflammation by inhibiting this pathway.[70] There are 3 monoclonal antibody (mAb) anti-IL-5 therapies that are approved for use in severe eosinophilic asthma uncontrolled despite maximal therapy (high-dose ICS or medium-dose ICS-LABA, and 2 or more exacerbations per year requiring OCS or chronic OCS use): mepolizumab and reslizumab, which bind to IL-5 preventing it from binding to its receptor on eosinophils, and benralizumab, which binds to the α subunit of the IL-5 receptor resulting in direct and rapid near depletion of eosinophils. Animal studies of mepolizumab (monkeys),[71] reslizumab (mice and rabbits),[72] and benralizumab (monkeys)[73] found no teratogenic effects. The safety and efficacy of all 3 anti-IL-5 agents in pregnant women is unknown because pregnancy was an exclusion criterion for all the clinical trials, and pregnancy registries are ongoing.

Dupilumab is an mAb that binds to the α subunit of the IL-4 receptor blocking signaling of both IL-4 and IL-13, which are key cytokines in type 2 airway inflammation. Dupilumab has been approved by the US Food and Drug Administration for the treatment of atopic dermatitis and severe oral steroid-dependent asthma. Animal studies of dupilumab up to 10 times the maximal human dose in cynomolgus monkeys found no fetal harm.[74] Three case reports of dupilumab used safely in the treatment of atopic dermatitis in pregnancy have been reported with no adverse fetal outcomes.[75–77] Pregnancy was an exclusion criterion for all the clinical trials of dupilumab, therefore the safety and efficacy in pregnant women is unknown. The European Medicines Agency completed a review in 2017 that reported 23 pregnancies in study patients treated with dupilumab resulting in 8 healthy births (1 twin birth), 2 induced abortions, 6 spontaneous abortions (with 2 of these 6 cases having at least 1 risk factor for abortion), 5 ongoing pregnancies, and 3 pregnancies lost to follow-up.[78] The risk of spontaneous abortion in pregnancy was similar to that of the general population (11%–24%).[79,80] The risk of medication-associated congenital anomalies could not be determined, however, due to the low numbers of pregnancies. The EMA report stated that dupilumab should only be used during pregnancy if the potential benefits outweigh the potential fetal risks.[81] A pregnancy registry for dupilumab in pregnancy is ongoing.

Thymic stromal lymphopoietin (TSLP) is a cytokine produced by the epithelium in response to external stimuli including viruses, bacteria, and allergens and drives allergic inflammation early in the inflammatory cascade and may be more suitable for a broader severe asthma population due to its earlier activity within the inflammatory cascade.[82] Tezepelumab is a human anti-TSLP immunoglobulin that binds to human TSLP and prevents interaction with its receptor[83] and has recently been granted approval by the US Food and Drug Administration for patients with severe asthma.[84] A randomized, double-blind, placebo-controlled study assessed the effect of tezepelumab on annualized rate of asthma exacerbations for patients with severe asthma with 2 or more asthma exacerbations in the year prior despite the use of medium- or high-dose ICSs and at least 1 additional controller medication, with or without OCSs.[85] The trial showed that annual asthma exacerbation rate was significantly reduced in the tezepelumab group compared with the placebo group (0.93; 95% CI, 0.8–1.07 with tezepelumab compared with 2.10; 95% CI, 1.84–2.39 with placebo; $P < 0.01$), with a significant reduction in exacerbations observed in the tezepelumab group irrespective of baseline blood eosinophil levels. These results were observed independent of baseline blood eosinophil count or other T2 inflammatory biomarkers. Pregnancy was an exclusion criterion for all studies to date; therefore no safety data are available. Animal studies of tezepelumab in cynomolgus monkeys up to 168 times the maximal human dose found no fetal harm.[84] A pregnancy registry for tezepelumab is yet to be created.

Given the lack of human data for anti-IL-5, anti-IL-4/13, and anti-TSLP biologics and the risk of teratogenic events, physicians prescribing these medications to women of reproductive age or pregnant should inform the woman regarding the potential effects of biologics on pregnancy and risks of congenital anomalies.

DISCUSSION

Managing asthma to control the underlying disease and optimizing fetal outcomes during pregnancy is a challenge, particularly in severe disease. Asthma may adversely affect both maternal quality of life and perinatal outcomes including congenital anomalies. Optimal management of asthma during pregnancy is imperative to reduce fetal risk of congenital anomalies associated with severe exacerbations. Owing to the increasing prevalence of asthma worldwide, it is imperative that physicians are aware of the potential teratogenic effect severe asthma with exacerbations can have on a developing fetus, as well as the potential teratogenic risk of antiasthma medications, to allow physicians determine the optimal therapy for their pregnant patient and ensure the pregnant women is educated regarding the importance of continuing therapy during pregnancy. Most human clinical drug trials exclude pregnant asthmatic women, thereby limiting our knowledge of the effect asthma medications can have on the developing fetus. This phenomenon is not unique to asthma, however, because more than 80% of pregnant women are prescribed at least 1 prescription or over-the-counter medication during pregnancy.[86] The lack of clinical trials in pregnant women with asthma can result in pregnant women and health care workers overestimating the teratogenic risk of asthma medications. A core part of improving the health of pregnant women is ensuring they are appropriately engaged and included in clinical research studies because this will allow future pregnant women to make evidence-based decisions regarding their disease and treatment.

Most small prospective studies showed no certain teratogenic effect of antiasthma medications. Several retrospective studies suggested associations with some specific malformations, but the scientific value of these studies is low. Some large studies demonstrated a relatively weak association between the use of antiasthma drugs and any congenital malformation and specifically ICS medications and cardiovascular anomalies and OCS and orofacial anomalies. There seems to be no specificity with regard to type of antiasthma drug, which makes it likely that a confounder such as maternal asthma or an asthma exacerbation causes anomalies most likely via hypoxia. A low priority should be placed on stepping down therapy in preparation for, or during pregnancy. Instead, pregnant women should be educated on the benefits and safety of usual controller medications particularly ICSs, and the increased risk of asthma exacerbations with poor adherence.

Women with severe asthma may require the use of biological therapies such as omalizumab, mepolizumab, reslizumab, benralizumab, dupilumab, and in the future tezepelumab to control their asthma, and the risk of continuing treatment during pregnancy or even commencing treatment in unwell pregnant women with severe asthma will need to be assessed. The randomized clinical trials that supported the approval of these medications for the treatment of severe asthma excluded pregnant women, therefore prospective data regarding their safety and efficacy are limited. Observational data for omalizumab shows no association between omalizumab treatment and increased risk of congenital anomalies; however, the interpretation of these data are limited due to small sample size and the presence of confounding factors such as asthma severity on perinatal outcomes. Pregnancy registries are ongoing for mepolizumab, reslizumab, benralizumab, and dupilumab; however, there are currently no published human data available, and therefore data are lacking regarding their teratogenic risks in pregnancy. Clinicians need to be aware of the risks of severe asthma in pregnant women, and the lack of available data regarding these agents to ensure they can appropriately consider the risks and benefits of these treatments during pregnancy, and relay this information to pregnant mothers and women of childbearing age. To adequately determine the safety of these medications in pregnancy, human data are critical, therefore clinicians are encouraged to enroll women who require or receive these treatments during pregnancy into the relevant pregnancy registries. High-quality randomized controlled trials of these agents in pregnancy are also required to strengthen the evidence base and inform future guidelines for asthma management in pregnancy.

SUMMARY

Although there are concerns regarding the use of any medications during pregnancy, particularly the first trimester, the benefits of actively treating asthma and reducing the risks of exacerbations markedly outweigh the risks of congenital anomalies. Given the evidence for adverse outcomes including congenital anomalies associated with un-controlled asthma during pregnancy, a low priority should be placed on stepping down therapy, and ICSs should not be stopped in preparation for or during pregnancy. High-quality randomized controlled trials are required to strengthen the evidence base and inform future guidelines for asthma management in pregnancy; specifically, safety studies regarding the use of biological therapies in severe asthma in pregnancy are needed urgently.

CLINICS CARE POINTS

- The available safety data for asthma medications in pregnancy and congenital anomaly risk are overall reassuring, particularly for ICSs and β-agonists
- The risk of congenital anomalies due to severe exacerbations and poorly controlled asthma can be reduced with good asthma control
- Pregnant women overestimate the risk of asthma medications resulting in congenital anomalies
- Physicians should discuss risk and benefit of asthma medications with women to ensure they understand the risks of discontinuing asthma medications during pregnancy and the risk of asthma exacerbations resulting in congenital anomalies
- Further studies for biological therapies in pregnant women with severe asthma are needed

---

DISCLOSURE

The authors have no relevant affiliations or financial involvement with any organization or entity with a financial interest in or financial conflict with the subject matter or materials discussed in the manuscript. This includes employment, consultancies, honoraria, stock ownership or options, expert testimony, grants or patents received or pending, or royalties.

REFERENCES

1. Cohen JM, Bateman BT, Huybrechts KF, et al. Poorly controlled asthma during pregnancy remains common in the United States. J Allergy Clin Immunol In Pract 2019;7(8):2672–80. e2610.
2. Sawicki E, Stewart K, Wong S, et al. Medication use for chronic health conditions by pregnant women attending an Australian maternity hospital. Aust N Z J Obstet Gynaecol 2011;51(4):333–8.
3. Rejnö G, Lundholm C, Gong T, et al. Asthma during pregnancy in a population-based study-pregnancy complications and adverse perinatal outcomes. PLoS One 2014;9(8).
4. Kwon HL, Belanger K, Bracken MB. Asthma prevalence among pregnant and childbearing-aged women in the United States: estimates from national health surveys. Ann Epidemiol 2003;13(5):317–24.
5. Hansen C, Joski P, Freiman H, et al. Medication exposure in pregnancy risk evaluation program: the prevalence of asthma medication use during pregnancy. Matern child Health J 2013;17(9):1611–21.
6. Wang G, Murphy VE, Namazy J, et al. The risk of maternal and placental complications in pregnant women with asthma: a systematic review and meta-analysis. J Maternal-Fetal Neonatal Med 2014;27(9):934–42.

7. Kim S, Kim J, Park SY, et al. Effect of pregnancy in asthma on health care use and perinatal outcomes. J Allergy Clin Immunol 2015;136(5):1215–23. e1216.

8. Murphy V, Namazy J, Powell H, et al. A meta-analysis of adverse perinatal outcomes in women with asthma. BJOG: An Int J Obstet Gynaecol 2011;118(11): 1314–23.

9. Global Strategy for Asthma Management and Prevention. Global Initiative for Asthma 2020.

10. Dombrowski M, Schatz M. ACOG practice bulletin: clinical management guidelines for obstetrician-gynecologists number 90, February 2008: asthma in pregnancy. Obstet Gynecol 2008;111(2 Pt 1):457–64.

11. Al Ghobain MO, AlNemer M. Assessment of knowledge and education relating to asthma during pregnancy among women of childbearing age. Asthma Res Pract 2018;4(1):1–5.

12. Powell H, McCaffery K, Murphy VE, et al. Psychosocial outcomes are related to asthma control and quality of life in pregnant women with asthma. J Asthma 2011;48(10):1032–40.

13. Chambers K. Asthma education and outcomes for women of childbearing age. Case manager 2003;14(6):58–61.

14. Lim AS, Stewart K, Abramson MJ, et al. Management of asthma in pregnant women by general practitioners: a cross sectional survey. BMC Fam Pract 2011;12(1):1–7.

15. Rocklin RE. Asthma, asthma medications and their effects on maternal/fetal outcomes during pregnancy. Reprod Toxicol 2011;32(2):189–97.

16. Yland JJ, Bateman B, Huybrechts KF, et al. Fetal Outcomes Among Women with Asthma during Pregnancy: Evidence from a Large Healthcare Database in the United States. J Allergy Clin Immunol 2019;143(2):AB422.

17. Garne E, Hansen AV, Morris J, et al. Use of asthma medication during pregnancy and risk of specific congenital anomalies: a European case-malformed control study. J Allergy Clin Immunol 2015;136(6):1496–502. e1497.

18. Blais L, Forget A. Asthma exacerbations during the first trimester of pregnancy and the risk of congenital malformations among asthmatic women. J Allergy Clin Immunol 2008;121(6):1379–84. e1371.

19. Crane JP, LeFevre ML, Winborn RC, et al. A randomized trial of prenatal ultrasonographic screening: impact on the detection, management, and outcome of anomalous fetuses. Am J Obstet Gynecol 1994;171(2):392–9.

20. Ramsay M. Genetic and epigenetic insights into fetal alcohol spectrum disorders. Genome Med 2010;2(4):1–8.

21. Torfs CP, Christianson RE, Iovannisci DM, et al. Selected gene polymorphisms and their interaction with maternal smoking, as risk factors for gastroschisis. Birth Defects Res A: Clin Mol Teratology 2006;76(10):723–30.

22. Mossey PA, Little J, Munger RG, et al. Cleft lip and palate. Lancet 2009; 374(9703):1773–85.

23. Hyoun SC, Običan SG, Scialli AR. Teratogen update: methotrexate. Birth Defects Res Part A: Clin Mol Teratology 2012;94(4):187–207.

24. Diav-Citrin O, Shechtman S, Tahover E, et al. Pregnancy outcome following in utero exposure to lithium: a prospective, comparative, observational study. Am J Psychiatry 2014;171(7):785–94.

25. Veroniki AA, Cogo E, Rios P, et al. Comparative safety of anti-epileptic drugs during pregnancy: a systematic review and network meta-analysis of congenital malformations and prenatal outcomes. BMC Med 2017;15(1):1–20.

26. Shanks N, Greek R, Greek J. Are animal models predictive for humans? Philos Ethics humanities Med 2009;4(1):1–20.
2.. Schardein JL. Drugs as teratogens. Cleveland: CRC press; 1976.
28. Robijn AL, Barker D, Gibson PG, et al. Factors Associated with Nonadherence to Inhaled Corticosteroids for Asthma During Pregnancy. The J Allergy Clin Immunol In Pract 2021;9(3):1242–52. e1241.
29. Schatz M, Dombrowski MP, Wise R, et al. The relationship of asthma medication use to perinatal outcomes. J Allergy Clin Immunol 2004;113(6):1040–5.
30. Murphy VE, Clifton VL, Gibson PG. Asthma exacerbations during pregnancy: incidence and association with adverse pregnancy outcomes. Thorax 2006; 61(2):169–76.
31. Abdullah K, Zhu J, Gershon A, et al. Effect of asthma exacerbation during pregnancy in women with asthma: a population-based cohort study. Eur Respir J 2020;55(2).
32. Breton M-C, Martel M-J, Vilain A, et al. Inhaled corticosteroids during pregnancy: a review of methodologic issues. Respir Med 2008;102(6):862–75.
33. Schatz M, Zeiger RS, Harden K, et al. The safety of asthma and allergy medications during pregnancy. J Allergy Clin Immunol 1997;100(3):301–6.
34. Silverman M, Sheffer A, Diaz PV, et al. Outcome of pregnancy in a randomized controlled study of patients with asthma exposed to budesonide. Ann Allergy Asthma Immunol 2005;95(6):566–70.
35. Bakhireva LN, Jones KL, Schatz M, et al. Asthma medication use in pregnancy and fetal growth. J Allergy Clin Immunol 2005;116(3):503–9.
36. Perlow JH, Montgomery D, Morgan MA, et al. Severity of asthma and perinatal outcome. Am J Obstet Gynecol 1992;167(4):963–7.
37. Alexander S, Dodds L, Armson BA. Perinatal outcomes in women with asthma during pregnancy. Obstet Gynecol 1998;92(3):435–40.
38. Dombrowski MP, Schatz M, Wise R, et al. Randomized trial of inhaled beclomethasone dipropionate versus theophylline for moderate asthma during pregnancy. Am J Obstet Gynecol 2004;190(3):737–44.
39. Dombrowski MP, Brown CL, Berry SM. Preliminary experience with triamcinolone acetonide during pregnancy. J Maternal-Fetal Med 1996;5(6):310–3.
40. Källén B, Rydhstroem H, Åberg A. Congenital malformations after the use of inhaled budesonide in early pregnancy. Obstet Gynecol 1999;93(3):392–5.
41. Källén B, Olausson PO. Use of anti-asthmatic drugs during pregnancy. 1. Maternal characteristics, pregnancy and delivery complications. Eur J Clin Pharmacol 2007;63(4):363–73.
42. Källén BA, Olausson PO. Maternal drug use in early pregnancy and infant cardiovascular defect. Reprod Toxicol 2003;17(3):255–61.
43. Namazy J, Schatz M, Long L, et al. Use of inhaled steroids by pregnant asthmatic women does not reduce intrauterine growth. J Allergy Clin Immunol 2004;113(3):427–32.
44. Blais L, Beauchesne M-F, Rey É, et al. Use of inhaled corticosteroids during the first trimester of pregnancy and the risk of congenital malformations among women with asthma. Thorax 2007;62(4):320–8.
45. Ericson A, Källén B. Use of drugs during pregnancy—unique Swedish registration method that can be improved. Inf Swedish Med Prod agency 1999;1:8–11.
46. Olesen C, Thrane N, Nielsen GL, et al. A population-based prescription study of asthma drugs during pregnancy: changing the intensity of asthma therapy and perinatal outcomes. Respiration 2001;68(3):256–61.

47. Blais L, Beauchesne M-F, Lemière C, et al. High doses of inhaled corticosteroids during the first trimester of pregnancy and congenital malformations. J Allergy Clin Immunol 2009;124(6):1229–34. e1224.
48. Norjavaara E, de Verdier MG. Normal pregnancy outcomes in a population-based study including 2968 pregnant women exposed to budesonide. J Allergy Clin Immunol 2003;111(4):736–42.
49. Gluck PA, Gluck JC. A review of pregnancy outcomes after exposure to orally inhaled or intranasal budesonide. Curr Med Res Opin 2005;21(7):1075–84.
50. Suissa S, Ernst P, Boivin J-F, et al. A cohort analysis of excess mortality in asthma and the use of inhaled beta-agonists. Am J Respir Crit Care Med 1994;149(3):604–10.
51. Garne E, Vinkel Hansen A, Morris J, et al. Risk of congenital anomalies after exposure to asthma medication in the first trimester of pregnancy–a cohort linkage study. BJOG: An Int J Obstet Gynaecol 2016;123(10):1609–18.
52. Eltonsy S, Kettani F-Z, Blais L. Beta2-agonists use during pregnancy and perinatal outcomes: a systematic review. Respir Med 2014;108(1):9–33.
53. Cossette B, Beauchesne M-F, Forget A, et al. Relative perinatal safety of salmeterol vs formoterol and fluticasone vs budesonide use during pregnancy. Ann Allergy Asthma Immunol 2014;112(5):459–64.
54. Satia I, Cusack R, O'Byrne P. Paradigm shift in the management of mild asthma: Focus toward a patient centered approach. Can J Respir Crit Care Sleep Med 2020;4(1):55–60.
55. Cusack RP, Satia I, O'Byrne PM. Asthma maintenance and reliever therapy: Should this be the standard of care? Ann Allergy Asthma Immunol 2020;125(2):150–5.
56. Eltonsy S, Forget A, Beauchesne M-F, et al. Risk of congenital malformations for asthmatic pregnant women using a long-acting β2-agonist and inhaled corticosteroid combination versus higher-dose inhaled corticosteroid monotherapy. J Allergy Clin Immunol 2015;135(1):123–30. e122.
57. Park-Wyllie L, Mazzotta P, Pastuszak A, et al. Birth defects after maternal exposure to corticosteroids: prospective cohort study and meta-analysis of epidemiological studies. Teratology 2000;62(6):385–92.
58. Skuladottir H, Wilcox AJ, Ma C, et al. Corticosteroid use and risk of orofacial clefts. Birth Defects Res Part A: Clin Mol Teratology 2014;100(6):499–506.
59. Howley MM, Papadopoulos EA, Van Bennekom CM, et al. Asthma Medication Use and Risk of Birth Defects: National Birth Defects Prevention Study, 1997–2011. J Allergy Clin Immunol In Pract 2020;8(10):3490–9.e9.
60. Blais L, Kettani F-Z, Forget A, et al. Asthma exacerbations during the first trimester of pregnancy and congenital malformations: revisiting the association in a large representative cohort. Thorax 2015;70(7):647–52.
61. Spector SL. Safety of antileukotriene agents in asthma management. Ann Allergy Asthma Immunol 2001;86(6):18–23.
62. Cavero-Carbonell C, Vinkel-Hansen A, Rabanque-Hernández MJ, et al. Fetal exposure to montelukast and congenital anomalies: a population based study in Denmark. Birth defects Res 2017;109(6):452–9.
63. Sarkar M, Koren G, Kalra S, et al. Montelukast use during pregnancy: a multicentre, prospective, comparative study of infant outcomes. Eur J Clin Pharmacol 2009;65(12):1259–64.
64. Kim LH, Saleh C, Whalen-Browne A, et al. Triple vs Dual Inhaler Therapy and Asthma Outcomes in Moderate to Severe Asthma: A Systematic Review and Meta-analysis. JAMA 2021;325(24):2466–79.

65. Busse WW. NAEPP expert panel report: managing asthma during pregnancy: recommendations for pharmacologic treatment—2004 update. J Allergy Clin Immunol 2005;115(1):34–46.

66. Weinberger M, Hendeles L. Theophylline in asthma. N Engl J Med 1996;334(21): 1380–8.

67. Barnes PJ. Theophylline. Am J Of Respir And Crit Care Med 2013;188(8):901–6.

68. Genentech. Xolair (omalizumab): full prescribing information. Available at: https://www.gene.com/download/pdf/xolair_prescribing.pdf. Accessed.

69. Namazy JA, Blais L, Andrews EB, et al. Pregnancy outcomes in the omalizumab pregnancy registry and a disease-matched comparator cohort. J Allergy Clin Immunol 2020;145(2):528–36, e521.

70. Yancey SW, Keene ON, Albers FC, et al. Biomarkers for severe eosinophilic asthma. J Allergy Clin Immunol 2017;140(6):1509–18.

71. Glaxosmithkline. Nucala (mepolizumab): summary of product characteristics. 2021.

72. Hom S, Pisano M. Reslizumab (Cinqair): an Interleukin-5 antagonist for severe asthma of the eosinophilic phenotype. P T 2017;42(9):564.

73. Astrazeneca. Fasenra (benralizumab): prescribing information. Available at: https://www.azpicentral.com/fasenra/fasenra.pdf#page=1. Accessed.

74. Regeneron. Dupixent (dupilumab): prescribing information. Available at: https://www.regeneron.com/sites/default/files/Dupixent_FPI.pdf. Accessed.

75. Kage P, Simon J, Treudler R. A case of atopic eczema treated safely with dupilumab during pregnancy and lactation. J Eur Acad Dermatol Venereol 2020;34(6): e256–7.

76. Mian M, Dunlap R, Simpson E. Dupilumab for the treatment of severe atopic dermatitis in a pregnant patient: A case report. JAAD Case Rep 2020;6(10):1051.

77. Lobo Y, Lee RC, Spelman L. Atopic Dermatitis Treated Safely with Dupilumab during Pregnancy: A Case Report and Review of the Literature. Case Rep Dermatol 2021;13(2):248–56.

78. European Medicines Agency (EMA): assessment report; dupilumab. 2017.

79. Knudsen UB, Hansen V, Juul S, et al. Prognosis of a new pregnancy following previous spontaneous abortions. Eur J Obstet Gynecol Reprod Biol 1991; 39(1):31–6.

80. Gray RH, Wu LY. Subfertility and risk of spontaneous abortion. Am J Public Health 2000;90(9):1452.

81. European Medicines Agency (EMA): Summary of product characteristics. 2020.

82. Cusack RP, Whetstone CE, Xie Y, et al. Regulation of Eosinophilia in Asthma—New Therapeutic Approaches for Asthma Treatment. Cells 2021;10(4):817.

83. Kabata H, Moro K, Fukunaga K, et al. Thymic stromal lymphopoietin induces corticosteroid resistance in natural helper cells during airway inflammation. Nat Commun 2013;4(1):1–10.

84. Astrazeneca. Tezspire™(tezepelumab) prescribing information: 2021.

85. Menzies-Gow A, Corren J, Bourdin A, et al. Tezepelumab in Adults and Adolescents with Severe, Uncontrolled Asthma. N Engl J Med 2021;384(19):1800–9.

86. Lupattelli A, Spigset O, Twigg MJ, et al. Medication use in pregnancy: a cross-sectional, multinational web-based study. BMJ open 2014;4(2):e004365.

Monoclonal Antibodies (Biologics) for Allergic Rhinitis, Asthma, and Atopic Dermatitis During Pregnancy and Lactation

Courtney L. Ramos, DO[a,b,*], Jennifer Namazy, MD[a,b]

KEYWORDS

- Asthma • Eczema • Allergic rhinitis • Biologics and safety • Pregnancy • Lactation
- Vaccines and medications during pregnancy surveillance studies • Mother to baby

KEY POINTS

- Poorly controlled allergies and eczema lead to significantly lower quality of life; poorly controlled asthma has increased the risk of adverse maternal and fetal outcomes.
- Asthma, eczema, chronic urticaria, and allergic rhinitis can worsen, improve, or stay the same with pregnancy.
- Obtaining safety data for biologics during pregnancy and lactation is challenging and reliant on cohort data obtained from Vaccines and Medications During Pregnancy Surveillance Studies.
- Omalizumab is the best studied with reassuring available safety data during pregnancy.
- There are insufficient safety data on mepolizumab, reslizumab, benralizumab, dupilumab, and tezepelumab use during pregnancy and lactation. More safety information is needed through registry data with matched controls.

INTRODUCTION

This article focuses on maternal health as affected by asthma, atopic dermatitis, and allergic rhinitis, and the use of biologics in women who are pregnant or lactating. The authors discuss indications of the medications, available safety information, as well as current knowledge gaps.

BACKGROUND AND SIGNIFICANCE

Maternal health in the United States is associated with higher morbidity and mortality when comparing it with other similar high-income countries.[1,2] Studies on the

[a] Division of Allergy, Asthma and Immunology, Scripps Clinic Medical Group, San Diego, CA, USA; [b] Scripps Clinic Mission Valley - 7565 Mission Valley Rd, Suite 200, San Diego, CA 92108, USA
* Corresponding author. 3811 Valley Drive, S99, San Diego, CA 92130.
E-mail address: DrCourtneyramos@gmail.com

Immunol Allergy Clin N Am 43 (2023) 187–197
https://doi.org/10.1016/j.iac.2022.07.001
0889-8561/23/© 2022 Elsevier Inc. All rights reserved.
immunology.theclinics.com

reasons for this have found it multifactorial, with the focus being complex socioeconomic factors coupled with cardiovascular diseases, such as hypertension, blood clots, diabetes, and obesity.[3] Asthma itself has an increased risk of adverse maternal and fetal outcomes, which include gestational hypertension, diabetes, preeclampsia, premature rupture of membranes, antepartum and postpartum hemorrhage as well as neonatal death, preterm birth, low birth weight, small for gestational size, and metabolic and cardiovascular disease.[4–6] Poorly controlled atopic dermatitis in pregnancy is associated with significant impacts on quality of life, but not adverse outcomes.[7,8] Allergic rhinitis on its own is not associated with worse outcomes, except as it goes hand in hand with asthma and can worsen its control, although it too is associated with lower quality of life when not well controlled.[9,10]

The allergist and immunologist have a role in assisting women with preconception concerns, pregnancy, and lactation as it pertains to management of allergic diseases: specifically, allergic rhinitis, asthma, atopic dermatitis, and chronic urticaria. A significant number of women who can become pregnant are affected by these conditions with frequency ranges between 18% and 30%; therefore, these conditions represent some of the most common coexisting conditions in pregnant women.[9]

Nasal symptoms in general are common in the pregnant population, affecting at least 30% of all pregnant women. Rhinitis during pregnancy can result from physiologic changes during pregnancy as well as allergic and nonallergic causes.[11] Allergic rhinitis is one of the most common allergic conditions, affecting around 20% of pregnant and lactating women.[12] Meanwhile, 8% to 17% of all adults under the age of 60 years carry the diagnosis of atopic dermatitis.[13] Pruritic disorders in pregnancy are common.[7] In one study of pruritic disorders, 49.7% were diagnosed as eczema, and 20% to 40% of those women had preexisting atopic dermatitis.[7,14] Finally, asthma represents the most common respiratory disease of pregnancy, with a prevalence of about 8.4% to 8.8%. In addition, about 4.1% had had an asthma exacerbation in the last year.[12] The implications of this are significant because based on the latest US birth information recording 3,605,201 live births for 2020, that translates to 721,040 (20%) pregnant women having allergies; 288,416 to 612,884 (8%–17%) have eczema, and around 288,416 (8%) women are affected by asthma. Notably, these numbers are likely larger because it only includes live births[15] and does not include the 10% of all known pregnancies that result in a miscarriage.[16]

During pregnancy, there is a relative shift toward type 2 inflammation, which could explain the deterioration in some but not all pregnant women with asthma, eczema, and allergic rhinitis.[8,17] Allergic rhinitis during pregnancy is known to improve, worsen, or remain the same.[9] Treatment includes both nonpharmacologic and pharmacologic treatment options.[10,11] For asthma, about 34% of pregnant women experience improvement in symptom control; 26% notice no difference, and a further 36% have worsening control of their asthma, while 4% is unknown.[18] Obese women and smokers are more likely to have poor asthma control.[19] It is known that better asthma control during pregnancy prevents adverse maternal and fetal outcomes.[20,21] Nonpharmacologic treatments as well as pharmacologic treatments have been reviewed separately.[6,22] In terms of eczema, for those with preexisting eczema who become pregnant, 25% have improvement, and 50% have worsening of control. Some women actually develop eczema during pregnancy either for the first time or after a period of prolonged remission.[7] Unfortunately, being pregnant can make it harder to achieve control owing to concern for teratogenic effects of steroid use.[8]

HOW THE SAFETY OF A MEDICATION DURING PREGNANCY IS DETERMINED

The use of medications is common in women of child-bearing years, defined as 15 to 44 years old. The Centers for Disease Control and Prevention (CDC) notes 1 in 4 women in this age range had used a medication in the last 30 days, and 9 out of 10 women used a medication during pregnancy.[23] Despite this frequency of use, pregnant women are generally excluded from drug development clinical trials.[23] Adherence to medications is another challenge: more than 30% of women on a prescribed inhaled corticosteroid for asthma stop taking it during pregnancy owing to concern of potential teratogenicity.[24]

When managing a pregnant woman with allergic rhinitis, asthma, and atopic dermatitis, assessing the safety and risks of a medication for both the pregnant mom and her developing fetus is necessary. Clear conversations about known and unknown evidence on specific medications should be provided so that the patient can make an informed decision.

What are the most common methods of studying medications in pregnant women? In the United States, there is no consensus on how medications should be studied.

During drug development, companies identify the medication dose that is therapeutic but not toxic. This dose can be determined via 2 different approaches based on animal data. Either dosing the drug to determine the minimum anticipated biological effect level (MABEL) and then confirmed in animals and converted to human dosing, or a more preferred method is to determine 2 levels on the toxicity curve beyond the therapeutic curve: no observed adverse effect level (NOAEL) and lowest observed adverse effect level (LOAEL) and scale down to efficacy level in humans that remains well below the toxicity level.[25] Drug companies will usually administer the medication to pregnant and lactating animals such as monkeys, but not to humans. In addition, when administered to animals, doses are given at much higher levels than seen in humans to look for potential teratogenic effects.

Without specific trials in pregnant women, human teratogens are identified through case reports. Nevertheless, further studies are needed to ensure reports of teratogens are more than coincident with background frequency of birth defects being more than 3% or 1 in 33 live births.[26] Congenital anomalies are structural or functional anomalies that occur during intrauterine life and therefore are present at birth. "Congenital anomalies" is used interchangeably with birth defects, congenital disorders, or congenital malformations.[27] These changes can affect appearance and/or function and range from mild to severe.

A common method used to classify congenital anomalies in studies is by using a birth defect categorization system based on Metropolitan Atlanta Congenital Defects Program (MACDP). This system does require some expertise, so in the Xolair Pregnancy Registry (EXPECT) study (see later discussion), they also used an independent, external teratology expert to apply MACDP.[28,29] For Vaccine Adverse Event Reporting System (VAERS), all US reports identified were reviewed by medical officers from the Food and Drug Administration (FDA) and CDC, who then characterized the adverse events, including classification of a birth defect.[30]

Observational studies have been used to help determine practice recommendations for pregnant and lactating women. There are 4 general observational studies, which include pregnancy registry, cohort, case-control, and database/claims data studies.[31] Pregnancy registries are important because they allow for prospectively collected exposure and outcome of a large cohort. One of the major registries used for biologics is MotherToBaby.[32] The FDA also keeps a list of open registries for various medications on their Web site.[33] An example of a successful use of the registries to confirm safety in pregnant women is VAERS, in which the registry collected data on women and their babies who received the influenza vaccine from 1990 to 2009.[30] This registry did not find any pattern to suggest increased risk of complications or fetal adverse outcomes with influenza vaccine administrations.

CURRENT BIOLOGICS APPROVED AND CURRENTLY AVAILABLE PREGNANCY AND LACTATION DATA

Biologics have a high target specificity, which lowers the risk for off target toxicity when compared with other drugs. Unfortunately, there is still potential for teratogenic effects, and so the study of these medications is imperative. Monoclonal antibodies are transported across the placenta during the third trimester of pregnancy; potential effects on a fetus are likely to be greater during the third trimester of pregnancy. In addition, immunoglobulin G (IgG) is found in breast milk. Whether this causes adverse effects short term or long term is discussed later.

Omalizumab (Xolair) was approved by the FDA in 2003.[34]

Mechanism of action: Blocks the binding of IgE to mast cells, basophils, and dendritic cells, thereby downregulating the IgE receptors, an unclear mechanism for chronic urticaria.
Effectiveness date: 12 to 16 weeks
Half-life: 26 days
Washout: 130 days = ~4.3 months
Approved conditions: Moderate to severe asthma, nasal polyps, chronic urticaria.
Human studies: The observational study EXPECT enrolled participants starting in 2006. Data were published in 2014 from 188 women who had been exposed to omalizumab during their first trimester. Of those, 169 had known outcomes with 160 live births, 11 had spontaneous abortions, 1 had elective termination, and there was 1 stillbirth. A total of 20 had congenital anomalies, and 7 had a single major defect. There was no pattern of anomalies observed.[28] A follow-up study was published in 2019, now including 250 women participants with 1153 disease-matched comparators (moderate to severe asthma pregnant participants).[35] There was no evidence of increased risk of major congenital anomalies for women exposed to omalizumab compared with unexposed disease-matched cohort.
Current registry information: Closed since it reached its target population.

Mepolizumab (Nucala) was approved in 2015.[36]

Mechanism of action: Interleukin-5 (IL-5) antagonist monoclonal antibody (IgG1 kappa)
Initial half-life: 2 days
Terminal half-life: 16 to 22 days (20 average)
Washout: 100 days or ~3.3 months
Approved conditions: Severe eosinophilic asthma, eosinophilic granulomatosis with polyangiitis, hypereosinophilic syndrome with nasal polyps.
Animal and human studies:
From the package insert animal data: In prenatal and postnatal development studies, pregnant cynomolgus monkeys received mepolizumab from gestation days 20 to 140 at doses that produced exposures up to 9 times the maximum recommended human dose (100 mg/kg once every 4 weeks). No adverse effects on fetal or neonatal growth (including immune function) were noted up to 9 months after birth. No teratogenic effects were observed. Mepolizumab crossed the

placenta in cynomolgus monkeys and persisted in the infants at 2.4 times higher levels than in the mother up to 178 days postpartum.[36]

Lactation: Levels of mepolizumab in milk were $\leq 0.5\%$ of maternal serum concentration.

CD-1 mice and wild-type mice were given a murine IL-5 antibody at intravenous (IV) dose 50 mg/kg weekly. There was no observed effect on fertility, on early embryonic development, and in an embryo-fetal development study.[36]

Two case reports have been published. In the first, the mother conceived while on mepolizumab, but upon learning she was pregnant stopped receiving mepolizumab injections at week 5 of pregnancy. Despite the pregnancy being complicated by poorly controlled asthma requiring high-dose steroids, she was able to deliver a healthy baby. In the second case report, the mother chose to terminate the fetus owing to unknown teratogenicity risk.[37]

Current registry information: www.mothertobaby.org/asthma.

Reslizumab (Cinqair) was approved in 2016.[38]

Mechanism of action: A humanized IL-5 antagonist monoclonal antibody
Half-life: 24 days
Washout: 120 days or ~ 4 months
Approved conditions: Severe eosinophilic asthma
Animal or human studies that have been done: Two separate embryo-fetal studies were done on pregnant mice and rabbits.

Mice (both CD-1 and wild type) received 6 times the maximum recommended human dose on days 16 and 18 (during period of organogenesis) and postnatal day 14. Rabbits (same days as mice) received 17 times the maximum recommended human dose. Reslizumab was not teratogenic in mice or rabbits. Reslizumab did not have any effects on fetal development up to approximately 4 months after birth. Reslizumab crossed the placenta of pregnant mice and was found to be 6% to 8% higher than in the parental female mice on postnatal day 14.[38]

Lactation: Reslizumab was present in the milk of lactating mice following dosing during pregnancy with levels approximately 5% to 7% of maternal serum concentrations.[38]

Current registry information: None

Benralizumab (Fasenra) was approved 2017.[39]

Mechanism of action: Binds to the IL-5 α receptor on eosinophils, signaling natural killer cells to induce eosinophilic apoptosis.
Half-life: 15 days
Washout: ~ 75 days or 2.5 months
Approved conditions: Eosinophilic asthma
Animal or human studies that have been done:
From the package insert of benralizumab: During the prenatal and postnatal development studies on pregnant cynomolgus monkeys, they were given IV benralizumab on gestational day 20 to 22, then day 35, and once every 14 days until 1-month postpartum. The levels were 310 times higher than the maximum recommended human dose. Benralizumab was not observed to be teratogenic or to elicit adverse effects on fetal or neonatal growth or immune function up to 6.5 months after birth. Benralizumab did cross the placenta, and its concentrations were about the same for mothers and infants on postpartum day 7 and then lower in infants at later time points. Eosinophil counts were suppressed in

infant monkeys with gradual recovery by 6 months postpartum; however, recovery of eosinophil counts was not observed for 1 infant monkey.[39]

A single case report describes an unexpected pregnancy while on benralizumab (week 128 of the drug trial) for hypereosinophilic syndrome with eosinophilic gastrointestinal disease. The baby was born late preterm (38 weeks) with normal APGAR scores by cesarean section. She was born with 0 eosinophils, which persisted until 7 months when she had 228 and 258 at 1 year (still below normal for age; normal, 700–1000).[40] She had no sick visits through her time followed at 1 year and was developing otherwise normally. She was not breastfed.[40]

Lactation

There is no information regarding the presence of benralizumab in human or animal milk, nor effects of benralizumab with milk production, and nor effects on the infant gastrointestinal track or systemic exposures.[39]

Current registry information: mothertobaby.org/Fasenra

Dupilumab (Dupixent) was approved in 2017 first for atopic dermatitis, in 2018 for asthma, and in 2019 for chronic rhinosinusitis with nasal polyps (CRSwNP).[41]

Mechanism of action: Fully human monoclonal antibody (IgG4) directed at the IL-4Rα subunit, so it inhibits IL-4 and IL-13 cytokine-induced responses, broadly suppressing type 2 inflammation, including the release of proinflammatory cytokines, chemokines, and IgE.

Human half-life: Variable, as it does not follow a linear curve. The antibody attacks the target quickly, resulting in a near instantaneous half-life, making calculating the terminal half-life not possible. If they saturate the receptors, it can be measured. In monkey models, it is reported as 26 days.[41]

Wash-out period, or time to nondetectable levels, depends on the maintenance dose. Once a steady state has been obtained while on 300 mg every 2 weeks, the washout is 10 to 12 weeks, but if on 200 mg every 2 weeks, the washout period is 9 weeks.

Approved conditions: Moderate to severe atopic dermatitis, moderate to severe asthma either eosinophilic, oral corticosteroid dependent, or chronic rhinosinusitis with nasal polyposis.

Animal or human studies that have been done:

Pregnant monkeys were given weekly injections through conception to birth as subcutaneous homologous antibody against IL-4Rα. The levels were 10 times the maximum recommended human dose. No embryo-fetal toxicity or malformations, including functional, or immunologic development, were observed in the infants from birth through 6 months of age.[41]

Lactation: There is no information regarding the presence of dupilumab in human or animal milk, nor effects of dupilumab with milk production, nor effects on the infant gastrointestinal track or systemic exposures.[41]

There are 5 published case reports or series,[42–46] and 1 report of data mining the World Health Organization's case reporting system on dupilumab.[47] In the case series, it included male or female parent on the medication.[42] All were prescribed the medication for atopic dermatitis, but when reported, most had asthma and allergic rhinitis as well. Some described continued use from conception to delivery. Others describe cessation upon learning they were pregnant; still others continued but stopped before the third trimester. Of those that reported it, none breastfed the infant while on the medication. Reassuringly, none reported teratogenic effects. All describe the infant as healthy. Of those that report the delivery, all babies were born term.[42–47]

Current registry information: www.mothertobaby.org/ongoing-study/dupixent/

Tezepelumab (Tezspire) was approved in 2021.[48]

Mechanism of action: A thymic stromal lymphopoietin blocker, human monoclonal antibody.
Elimination half-life: 26 days
Washout: 130 days, ~4.3 months
Approved conditions: Severe asthma
Animal or human studies that have been done:
Cynomolgus monkeys were administered tezepelumab at doses 168 times the exposure at the maximum recommended human dose (210 mg administered subcutaneously every 4 weeks). This was given during gestational days 20 to 22, which is the beginning of organogenesis, and then weekly until the end of gestation. No adverse effects on maternal health, pregnancy outcome, embryo-fetal development, or neonatal growth and development up to 6.5 months of age were reported. Tezepelumab crossed the placenta in cynomolgus monkeys and produced levels 0.5- to 6.7-fold higher in infants relative to maternal animals.[48]
Lactation
Tezepelumab concentrations in milk were 0.5% of the maternal serum concentrations after IV administration of tezepelumab at the above dosing. It does not appear the levels were assessed in the infant animals.[48]
Current registry information: There is no tezepelumab registry at this point.

KNOWLEDGE GAPS

There are several challenges with obtaining safety data for biologics during pregnancy and lactation. One key reason is the relative infrequency that these medications are prescribed because biologics are reserved for moderate to severe phenotypes of disease states. Therefore, it is difficult to make associations when the numbers are so low. Also, determining how to best study the safety of asthma medications is challenging. Although pharmacologic therapies are an uncommon cause for adverse pregnancy outcomes, they are preventable. Vaccines and Medications During Pregnancy Surveillance Studies are supported, but the American Academy of Allergy Asthma and Immunology goal is to monitor postmarketing surveillance of pharmacologic therapy in pregnancy.[49]

SUMMARY

Asthma, allergic rhinitis, and atopic dermatitis are common diseases that affect hundreds of thousands of pregnant women each year.[8,10,13,22] Asthma in particular has a documented increased risk of adverse outcomes for both mother and baby if not controlled.[6] Quality of life is significantly affected for patients, including pregnant mothers with poorly controlled allergic rhinitis and atopic dermatitis.[7,8] There are pregnant patients in which standard treatment options are either inadequate or contraindicated, so monoclonal antibodies (biologics) should be considered despite the unknown risk to the fetus. In terms of severe asthma, omalizumab is the best studied with reassuring available safety data. There are insufficient safety data on mepolizumab, reslizumab, benralizumab, dupilumab, and tezepelumab use during pregnancy and lactation. More safety information is needed through registry data with matched controls before routine use in this population.

CLINICS CARE POINTS

- In pregnant women with allergic rhinitis, asthma, and eczema, one-third will have worsening of their symptoms; one-third will show improvement, and one-third will have no change in their disease symptoms.
- When addressing severe asthma in a pregnant woman, omalizumab has the best-known safety data.
- During drug development, safety data are collected on animal models at significantly higher doses than administered to humans.
- There are ongoing cohort studies through Vaccines and Medications During Pregnancy Surveillance Studies and MotherToBaby for studies on the safety of biologics.

DISCLOSURE

C. Ramos has received consulting fees for Regeneron. J. Namazy has nothing to disclose.

REFERENCES

1. National Academies of Sciences, Engineering, and Medicine; Health and Medicine Division; Board on Population Health and Public Health Practice; McHugh K, Martinez RM, Alper J, editors. Advancing Maternal Health Equity and Reducing Maternal Morbidity and Mortality: Proceedings of a Workshop. Washington (DC): National Academies Press (US); 2021 Oct 28. Available from: https://www.ncbi.nlm.nih.gov/books/NBK575264/ doi: 10.17226/26307.
2. Chinn JJ, Eisenberg E, Artis Dickerson S, et al. Maternal mortality in the United States: research gaps, opportunities, and priorities. Am J Obstet Gynecol 2020;223(4):486–492 e6.
3. What are examples and causes of maternal morbidity and mortality?. 2020. Available at: https://www.nichd.nih.gov/health/topics/maternal-morbidity-mortality/conditioninfo/causes#f1. Accessed date May 14 2020.
4. Breton MC, Beauchesne MF, Lemiere C, et al. Risk of perinatal mortality associated with asthma during pregnancy. Thorax 2009;64(2):101–6.
5. Murphy VE, Wang G, Namazy JA, et al. The risk of congenital malformations, perinatal mortality and neonatal hospitalisation among pregnant women with asthma: a systematic review and meta-analysis. BJOG 2013;120(7):812–22.
6. Namazy JA, Schatz M. Contemporary management and treatment strategies for asthma during pregnancy. Expert Rev Respir Med 2021;15(9):1149–57.
7. Ambros-Rudolph CM. Dermatoses of pregnancy - clues to diagnosis, fetal risk and therapy. Ann Dermatol 2011;23(3):265–75.
8. Mawhirt SL, Fonacier L. Atopic Dermatitis and allergic Contact Dermatitis in pregnancy. Asthma, allergic and immunologic diseases during pregnancy 2018.
9. Pali-Scholl I, Namazy J, Jensen-Jarolim E. Allergic diseases and asthma in pregnancy, a secondary publication. World Allergy Organ J 2017;10(1):10.
10. Carroll MP, Bulkhi AA, Lockey RF. Rhinitis and Sinusitis. In: Namazy J, Schatz M, editors. Asthma, Allergic and Immunologic Diseases During Pregnancy. Springer, Cham. 2019. https://doi.org/10.1007/978-3-030-03395-8_5.
11. Brauer DL, Woessner KM. Non-pharmacologic aspects of management: asthma and allergic and immunologic diseases during pregnancy a guide to management asthma. Allergic and Immunologic Diseases During Pregnancy 2018.

12. Kwon HL, Triche EW, Belanger K, et al. The epidemiology of asthma during pregnancy: prevalence, diagnosis, and symptoms. Immunol Allergy Clin North Am 2006;26(1):29–62.
13. Weatherhead S, Robson SC, Reynolds NJ. Eczema in pregnancy. BMJ 2007; 335(7611):152–4.
14. Ambros-Rudolph CM, Mullegger RR, Vaughan-Jones SA, et al. The specific dermatoses of pregnancy revisited and reclassified: results of a retrospective two-center study on 505 pregnant patients. J Am Acad Dermatol 2006;54(3):395–404.
15. Martin JA, Hamilton BE, Osterman M. Births in the United States, 2020. NCHS Data Brief 2021;(418):1–8.
16. Early Pregnancy Loss. 2022 January 2022; November 2021:Available at: https://www.acog.org/womens-health/faqs/early-pregnancy-loss. Accessed January 1, 2022.
17. Wang W, Sung N, Gilman-Sachs A, et al. T Helper (Th) Cell Profiles in Pregnancy and Recurrent Pregnancy Losses: Th1/Th2/Th9/Th17/Th22/Tfh Cells. Front Immunol 2020;11:2025.
18. Kircher S, Schatz M, Long L. Variables affecting asthma course during pregnancy. Ann Allergy Asthma Immunol 2002;89(5):463–6.
19. Ali Z, Nilas L, Ulrik CS. Postpartum airway responsiveness and exacerbation of asthma during pregnancy - a pilot study. J Asthma Allergy 2017;10:261–7.
20. Bain E, Pierides KL, Clifton VL, et al. Interventions for managing asthma in pregnancy. Cochrane Database Syst Rev 2014;(10):CD010660.
21. Yoo EJ, Most JF, Lee NL, et al. Improving Asthma Symptoms Among Inner-City Women During Pregnancy: A Prospective Cohort Intervention. J Allergy Clin Immunol Pract 2021;9(10):3672–8.
22. Namazy JA. Asthma: management. Asthma, allergic and immunologic diseases during pregnancy 2018.
23. Division of Pediatric and Maternal Health - Clinical Trials in Pregnant Women. Available at: https://www.fda.gov/drugs/development-resources/division-pediatric-and-maternal-health-clinical-trials-pregnant-women. Accessed date January 10 2022.
24. Wangberg H, Namazy J. Predicting Who Will Stop Medications During Pregnancy: A Complex Issue. J Allergy Clin Immunol Pract 2021;9(3):1253–4.
25. Suh HY, Peck CC, Yu KS, et al. Determination of the starting dose in the first-in-human clinical trials with monoclonal antibodies: a systematic review of papers published between 1990 and 2013. Drug Des Devel Ther 2016;10:4005–16.
26. Birth Defects are Common, Costly, and Critical. 2019. Available at: https://www.cdc.gov/ncbddd/birthdefects/infographic.html. Accessed date December 5 2019.
27. World Health Organization. Congenital anomalies. 2022. Available at: https://www.who.int/health-topics/congenital-anomalies#tab=tab_1. Accessed January 1, 2022.
28. Namazy J, Cabana MD, Scheuerle AE, et al. The Xolair Pregnancy Registry (EXPECT): the safety of omalizumab use during pregnancy. J Allergy Clin Immunol 2015;135(2):407–12.
29. Scheuerle A, Tilson H. Birth defect classification by organ system: a novel approach to heighten teratogenic signalling in a pregnancy registry. Pharmacoepidemiol Drug Saf 2002;11(6):465–75.
30. Moro P, Baumblatt J, Lewis P, et al. Surveillance of Adverse Events After Seasonal Influenza Vaccination in Pregnant Women and Their Infants in the Vaccine Adverse Event Reporting System. Drug Saf 2017;40(2):145–52.

31. Chambers C. *Safety of Asthma and Allergy medications during pregnancy.* Asthma. Allergic and Immunologic Diseases During Pregnancy; 2018.
32. MotherToBaby [internet]; Available at: https://mothertobaby.org/ongoing-study/asthma/. Accessed January 1, 2022.
33. List of Pregnancy Exposure Registries. Available from: https://www.fda.gov/science-research/womens-health-research/list-pregnancy-exposure-registries. Accessed date January 9 2022.
34. Genentech, Novartis. Omalizumab (Xolair) [package insert]. *U.S. Food and Drug Administration website.* Available at: https://www.accessdata.fda.gov/drugsatfda_docs/label/2016/103976s5225lbl.pdf. Accessed January 1, 2022.
35. Namazy JA, Blais L, Andrews EB, et al. Pregnancy outcomes in the omalizumab pregnancy registry and a disease-matched comparator cohort. J Allergy Clin Immunol 2020;145(2):528–536 e1.
36. GSK. Mepolizumab (Nucala) [package insert]. U.S. Food and Drug Administration website. Available at: https://gskpro.com/content/dam/global/hcpportal/en_US/Prescribing_Information/Nucala/pdf/NUCALA-PI-PIL-IFU-COMBINED.PDF. Accessed January 1, 2022.
37. Ozden G, Pinar Deniz P. May mepolizumab used in asthma correct subfertility? Ann Med 2021;53(1):456–8.
38. TEVA. Reslizumab (Cinqair) [package insert]. U.S. Food and Drug Administration website. Available at: https://www.accessdata.fda.gov/drugsatfda_docs/label/2016/761033lbl.pdf. Accessed January 1, 2022.
39. AstraZeneca. Benralizumab (Fasenra) [package insert]. U.S. Food and Drug Administration website. Available at: https://www.accessdata.fda.gov/drugsatfda_docs/label/2017/761070s000lbl.pdf. Accessed January 1, 2022.
40. Manetz S, Maric I, Brown T, et al. Successful pregnancy in the setting of eosinophil depletion by benralizumab. J Allergy Clin Immunol Pract 2021;9(3):1405–1407 e3.
41. Sanofi and Regeneron Pharmaceuticals. Dupilumab (Dupixent) [package insert]. U.S. Food and Drug Administration website. Available at: https://www.accessdata.fda.gov/drugsatfda_docs/label/2017/761055lbl.pdf. Accessed date January 13, 2022.
42. Bosma AL, Gerbens LAA, Middelkamp-Hup MA, et al. Paternal and maternal use of dupilumab in patients with atopic dermatitis: a case series. Clin Exp Dermatol 2021;46(6):1089–92.
43. Mian M, Dunlap R, Simpson E. Dupilumab for the treatment of severe atopic dermatitis in a pregnant patient: A case report. JAAD Case Rep 2020;6(10):1051–2.
44. Gracia-Darder I, Pons De Ves J, Reyero Cortina M, et al. Patient with atopic dermatitis, hyper IgE syndrome and ulcerative colitis, treated successfully with dupilumab during pregnancy. Dermatol Ther 2021;e15237.
45. Costley M, Murphy B. Successful treatment of a pregnant mother with dupilumab therapy for severe atopic dermatitis throughout pregnancy. Clin Exp Dermatol 2021.
46. Lobo Y, Lee RC, Spelman L. Atopic Dermatitis Treated Safely with Dupilumab during Pregnancy: A Case Report and Review of the Literature. Case Rep Dermatol 2021;13(2):248–56.
47. Khamisy-Farah R, Damiani G, Kong JD, et al. Safety profile of Dupilumab during pregnancy: a data mining and disproportionality analysis of over 37,000 reports from the WHO individual case safety reporting database (VigiBase). Eur Rev Med Pharmacol Sci 2021;25(17):5448–51.

48. AstraZeneca. Tezepelumab (Tezspire) [package insert]. U.S. Food Drug Administration website. Available at: https://www.accessdata.fda.gov/drugsatfda_docs/label/2021/761224s000lbl.pdf. Accessed January 1, 2022.
49. Vaccines and Medications in Pregnancy Surveillance System (VAMPSS). 2022. Available at: https://www.aaaai.org/about/strategic-relationships/vampss. Accessed date February 23 2022.

Improving Asthma Outcomes During Pregnancy in Underserved Communities

Alan Gandler, MD[a], Edward S. Schulman, MD[b],
Erika J. Yoo, MD, FCCP[c],*

KEYWORDS

- Pregnancy • Asthma • Underserved

KEY POINTS

- There is a paucity of data examining strategies to improve asthma control specifically among pregnant women from vulnerable populations.
- Barriers to adequate asthma care in this underserved group of women may necessarily be extrapolated from data from other vulnerable populations with asthma.
- Interventions may be addressed on both individual and population levels through targeted interventions, multidisciplinary health care outreach, and policy advocacy.

BACKGROUND

The prevalence of asthma in pregnancy has increased over the decades, with data between 1997 and 2001 estimating that up to 8.4% to 8.8% of pregnant women in the United States are affected by asthma.[1,2] More recent data show a sustained increase in asthma prevalence in pregnancy, which may be even higher at 12%.[3] Asthma in general is more common in underserved communities and is characterized by poorer control, more often requiring emergency visits or culminating in asthma-related deaths.[4] These outcomes are particularly problematic among pregnant women in whom there are tremendous implications for both mother and baby.

[a] Department of Medicine, Division of Pulmonary, Allergy, and Critical Care, Perelman School of Medicine, University of Pennsylvania, 800 Walnut Street, 9th floor, Philadelphia, PA, 19107, USA; [b] Department of Medicine, Division of Pulmonary, Allergy and Critical Care, Allergy and Sleep Medicine, Drexel University College of Medicine, Philadelphia, PA, USA; [c] Division of Pulmonary, Allergy and Critical Care Medicine, Jane and Leonard Korman Respiratory Institute, TJU and NJH, Sidney Kimmel Medical College, Thomas Jefferson University, 834 Walnut Street, Suite 650, Philadelphia, PA 19107, USA
* Corresponding author.
E-mail address: Erika.yoo@jefferson.edu

Immunol Allergy Clin N Am 43 (2023) 199–208
https://doi.org/10.1016/j.iac.2022.07.002   immunology.theclinics.com

Nature of the Problem

It is known that poor asthma control is common in pregnancy overall. Conventional wisdom has been that asthma follows the "rule of thirds" in this population, with one-third of women experiencing symptomatic improvement, one-third experiencing a deterioration, and one-third having no change in symptoms.[5] A more recent study of gestational asthma demonstrated worse control in 40% of women, similar control in 60%, and none with improvement, challenging the rule of thirds.[6] Up to 45% of pregnant asthmatics have been shown to have moderate to severe exacerbation requiring medical intervention during pregnancy.[7]

Poor control of asthma in pregnancy has been linked to multiple obstetric complications, including preeclampsia and pregnancy-induced hypertension.[8,9] In addition, women with asthma exacerbations during pregnancy have higher odds of preterm labor and a higher prevalence of low birthweight offspring. An increased prevalence of congenital malformations has been seen in children born of women with severe asthma in the first trimester, and a higher frequency of bronchiolitis has been reported in children born of mothers suffering more frequent asthma exacerbations during pregnancy.[10,11] Therefore, irrespective of demographics or socioeconomic status, asthma control in pregnancy is paramount. In fact, the Global Initiative for Asthma in its most recent update highlights that the benefits of active asthma management during pregnancy outweigh any potential risks. The statement focuses on maintenance of therapy until after delivery and regular monitoring of symptom control throughout pregnancy.[12]

The impact of asthma in pregnancy specifically in underserved communities, however, is less clearly defined, although the aforementioned risks for poor outcomes among both mothers and their babies are more than likely to be relevant. In a cohort study of asthma-related morbidity in pregnancy using data from Tennessee's Medicaid Program, Carroll and colleagues[13] reported that black women were more likely to receive corticosteroids, have an emergency department visit (16.7% versus 8.7%), or experience asthma-related hospitalizations (9% versus 5.2%) compared with white women. In the same data set, it was noted that maternal race did not change the relationship between maternal asthma and adverse pregnancy and perinatal outcomes. However, maternal asthma exacerbations were significantly more frequent in black women compared with white women despite lower rates of smoking in black women and similar rates of inhaled corticosteroid use.[14] This higher rate of asthma exacerbation among minority women during pregnancy undoubtedly leads to more maternal and perinatal complications and is therefore critical to address.

The relationship between asthma and race is complex, with structural inequities and social determinants being important drivers of disparities. Blacks have 1.25 times the asthma prevalence and twice the asthma-related mortality compared with the general population.[4] Asthma prevalence is noted to be higher among those with higher poverty levels; national data estimates show an asthma prevalence of 11.8% below the poverty threshold and a prevalence of 5.9% in groups at least 4.5 times the poverty threshold. Asthma-related hospitalizations in Philadelphia were increased in poverty area residence, with those of black race having increased hospitalizations across all poverty levels.[15] Lower socioeconomic status has been linked to worse asthma control, greater emergency health service use, and worse asthma self-efficacy.[16] In the general population, non-Hispanic blacks are 2 to 3 times more likely to die of asthma compared with other race groups.[17] In Pennsylvania, asthma prevalence, hospitalizations, and mortality have been shown to be higher among black non-Hispanics than white, and among women compared with men.[18] Data specific to Philadelphia have shown that higher rates of mortality are associated with black race, female residents, and poverty.[15,17,19]

DISCUSSION
Current Evidence for Management of Asthma During Pregnancy

In light of the far-reaching consequences of poor asthma control during pregnancy in general, efforts have been made to design interventions specific to this population. In a cohort intervention, Murphy and colleagues[20] identified that 40% of pregnant asthmatics were nonadherent with inhaled corticosteroids, less than 50% had optimal inhaler technique, and 42% had inadequate medication knowledge. By targeting these deficiencies through structured educational sessions, investigators were able to achieve measurable improvements in asthma self-management skills.[20] Similarly, a pharmacist-led multidisciplinary intervention conducted in Australia that included education, monitoring, feedback, and follow-up resulted in better asthma control among pregnant women as noted by significantly improved Asthma Control Questionnaire (ACQ) scores at 6 months.[21] Active asthma management in pregnancy guided by measurement of the fraction of nitric oxide in expired air (FeNO) has resulted in improvements in exacerbation rates, maternal quality of life, and neonatal hospitalizations compared with controls.[22] Such interventions have shown that collaborative efforts to improve the care of women with asthma during pregnancy have measurable benefits.[22]

Asthma Care During Pregnancy in Underserved Populations

Unfortunately, there is a remarkable dearth of interventional studies targeting asthma outcomes specifically among underserved women during pregnancy. Yoo and colleagues[23] conducted a prospective cohort study of 85 pregnant asthmatics in Philadelphia, more than 80% of whom were black and more than 60% of whom resided in ZIP codes of the city where at least 30% of the local community were below the poverty line. Women were enrolled in a physician-driven, antenatal asthma management program integrated into routine obstetric care. In this intervention, pulmonologists provided education, regular monitoring, and focused follow-up. The investigators discovered a high proportion of women with poor baseline asthma control, with 34% to 43% requiring systemic corticosteroids in the year preceding and an associated high proportion of those needing step-up therapy (85%) at their initial visit. Only 15% to 21% of women were taking controller medicines, and the majority reported short-acting beta-agonist use alone. Only 62% attended at least 1 follow-up visit, and of those, 32% required further step-up therapy. There was a significant improvement in Asthma Control Test scores between initial visits and first follow-up visits, and for those with follow-up Mini Asthma Quality of Life Questionnaire data, there was also a significant improvement.[23]

BARRIERS TO ASTHMA CARE IN UNDERSERVED COMMUNITIES
Medication Hesitance and Health Illiteracy

Although the study by Yoo and colleagues[23] did not specifically query reasons for medication nonadherence in their underserved population, fear of medications has been frequently reported among pregnant women in general (**Table 1**). A study in Saudi Arabia reported nearly half of pregnant asthmatic patients had stopped their medications and believed asthma medication would harm them and their babies more than asthma. However, the vast majority reported willingness to use asthma medications if their safety was physician confirmed.[24] Similarly, in a prospective study of 80 pregnant women with asthma conducted in the United States, the reasons for uncontrolled asthma during pregnancy were most often lack of knowledge of asthma medications (30%) and fear of side effects of inhaled corticosteroids (19%). In

Table 1
Potential barriers to optimal asthma care and proposed solutions

Barrier	Solution
Medication hesitancy Health illiteracy	Targeted education on medication safety and adherence (in-person or remotely by computer or phone)[20–23,32,33] Multidisciplinary (eg, utilizing pharmacists, nurses, and/or physicians) structured programs[20–23]
Lack of in-person care continuity	Care coordinators[40] Home visits[41] Using technology to reach patient[32,33]
Underinsured or uninsured status	Revised health care incentive models[36]
Cultural incompetence	Culturally competent interventions[38] Utilization of primary language[34,37] Peer-led groups[39]
Community disengagement	Recruitment of community health care workers[30,31,40,41]
Poor control of environmental triggers	Home-based evaluations with interventions[41,43] Policies to reduce asthma triggers[46]

addition, investigators found 64% of women had incorrect inhaler technique, whereas only 38% knew the difference between controller and rescue medications.[25]

Specifically addressing medication knowledge, adherence, and inhaler technique can lead to improved asthma care in pregnancy.[20,21] The impact of these interventions may be especially robust among women from underserved communities. Review of public and private insurance claims among pregnant women shows that despite a higher proportion of poorly controlled asthma, a lower percentage of women with public insurance are dispensed controller medications.[26] Therefore, targeting appropriateness of prescribed medications and educating on the importance of medication adherence may be a particularly effective means of improving asthma outcomes among vulnerable women during pregnancy.

Lack of In-Person Care Continuity

The high no-show rate for follow-up visits also among the cohort of Yoo and colleagues[23] suggests that there may be social and/or structural barriers to care continuity unique to vulnerable populations that impede optimal asthma management. For example, parking costs, childcare, and time off work have been suggested as indirect costs of health care that may lead to unmet medical care continuity even when such care is available and covered.[27] This is supported by high rates of financial hardship among pregnant women regardless of insurance coverage status.[27] Transportation to medical visits has been similarly identified as a barrier to optimal pediatric asthma care in underserved communities.[28] Poor attendance at office visits may be further exacerbated by poor symptom self-perception, as nearly 10% of pregnant women with uncontrolled asthma misclassify their asthma as mild.[25] In other underserved, albeit nonpregnant populations, subjective symptoms have been shown to poorly correlate with objective measurements of asthma control, which may further support difficulty in self-perception of asthma severity as a contributing barrier to optimal asthma management.[29,30]

Thus, patient outreach outside the office setting may have promise in improving asthma care in underserved communities.[31] In a randomized trial of inner-city children with asthma, researchers compared the impact of using a computer-based educational program (Health Buddy) with usual care with an asthma diary on measures of functional status. They found that self-reported limitations in activity, which were then validated against a nurse's knowledge of the patient, were significantly lower in the children randomized to the Health Buddy.[32] Similarly, among young-adult African American patients with persistent asthma, a text message–based intervention for medication reminders was found to decrease asthma symptoms.[33] Although neither study was specifically conducted in pregnant women, interventions that are independent of office visits may help overcome the patient, family, or structural barriers to care continuity characteristic of women during pregnancy as well.

Uninsured or Underinsured Health Status

Health insurance status has been shown to impact asthma self-care and may be yet another area of focus for improving asthma control in underserved communities that include pregnant women. Ejebe and colleagues[34] uncovered lower self-efficacy in non-white and low-income individuals with asthma and found health insurance status to be 1 mediator to explain this difference. Patients without insurance were least likely to have high self-efficacy, and those with public insurance fared worse than those with private insurance in an analysis of health interview surveys in California. US families with lower cost-sharing requirements on their insurance plans have been shown to be less likely to delay care for physician visits compared with those with higher cost sharing.[35] Insurances with higher cost sharing may be chosen by lower-income individuals because of lower premiums. Disparities in health care access are a contributor to poorer health outcomes; however, they do not fully explain different outcomes in lower socioeconomic groups. Large-scale interventions have been suggested, such as moving away from fee-for-service care and promoting care coordination through incentive models and using multilevel preventative programs to help underserved communities.[36]

Cultural Incompetence

To improve care for underserved women with asthma during pregnancy, cultural competency is likely also essential. Multiple studies have shown that communicating in the patient's language of choice is needed for optimal health care. Patients without proficiency in English have worse asthma self-management skills.[34] In a prestudy and poststudy looking at low socioeconomic adult asthmatics in Bronx, New York, an asthma education program that included a bilingual respiratory therapist as well as written educational material in the participant's preferred language resulted in reductions in emergency room visits and hospital admissions.[37] A randomized trial by La Roche and colleagues[38] worked to overcome barriers to equal care in underserved communities by using culturally competent asthma management interventions, including multilingual resources. Investigators hypothesized that certain underserved communities may see themselves through a more allocentric or interpersonal lens than typical American individualistic culture, which prompted them to target education guided by perceived educational preferences. They used multifamily asthma group treatment strategies in lieu of stand-alone psychoeducational asthma interventions, which yielded a decrease in emergency room visits and an increase in parental asthma knowledge. Other programs have worked with peer-led community health workshops for refugees in order to help overcome cultural barriers to the US health care system.[39] Understanding the specific cultural/language needs of underserved communities is essential to improve asthma care for pregnant women.

Inadequate Community Outreach

Community-based interventions have been shown to improve asthma control in underserved communities in general and are likely applicable to women during pregnancy. Community programs can range from awareness campaigns, neighborhood support groups, care coordinators, and government or local organizational involvement. Studies to date in this area have largely been conducted in children. Improving care coordination by linking families to health services, facilitating patient clinician-communication, or deploying community health workers to provide asthma education in underserved pediatric asthma patients can reduce symptoms and emergency department visits.[40] This coordination and education have been performed by professionals from variegated training backgrounds, including nurses, health educators, and community health workers.[40]

A recent meta-analysis of publications between 2000 and 2019 focused on community-based asthma interventions in children from ethnic minorities demonstrated that comprehensive asthma programs with multicomponent interventions were associated with less asthma-related emergency room visits, hospitalizations, and asthma symptoms.[31] In low-income adults with uncontrolled asthma, a randomized parallel group study showed in-home asthma self-management support by community health workers improved asthma quality of life. Moreover, such an intervention could be easily replicated at low cost.[31,41] Community health care workers play a valuable role in improving the reach of health care to marginalized groups and may help to navigate specific challenges faced by underserved communities better than the health care system at large. A systematic review found community health workers to be effective in improving equitable care, disease prevention, and medical services. Program promotion is necessary to ensure efficacy, and recruitment of poor communities, closeness to facilities, and free services are associated with equitable outcomes.[42]

Insufficient Environmental Protections

Indoor air pollution and allergen exposures characteristic of housing conditions in vulnerable health populations are known triggers of asthma and may be a targetable area for improving respiratory health in underserved women during pregnancy. Residential environmental assessment among lower-income older adults with asthma and chronic obstructive pulmonary disease followed by intervention plans targeting pest management, mattress encasements for dust mites, cleaning supplies, and improved ventilation or plumbing were effective in improving quality of life and asthma control scores.[41,43] Although these types of interventions can be effective, they are also often labor-intensive, expensive, and difficult to conduct on a larger scale.

Government, policy, and culture can shape intermediate social determinants, such as housing, to impact underserved populations more broadly. For instance, increased housing code violation density has been linked to population-level asthma morbidity independent of poverty.[44] Targeting these communities with interventions that address environmental asthma triggers may be a means by which asthma control can be improved. Another simple intervention that has positively impacted asthma outcomes is the implementation of a smoke-free policy for public multifamily housing.[45] In addition, population-based efforts, such as the one led by the Centers for Disease Control and Prevention aimed at addressing air pollution, have the potential to achieve measurable improvements in asthma control.[46] Such an initiative could have broad reach in underserved communities, as increased air pollution has been distinctly linked to areas of lower socioeconomic residence.[47] Pregnant women are equally as likely to benefit from advocacy that promotes pollutant reduction or safe housing development as other asthmatics from underserved communities.

SUMMARY

There is a striking paucity of direct evidence addressing how to improve asthma care for underserved women during pregnancy. Many of the aforementioned suggestions are extrapolated from other studies conducted in underserved children with asthma or in other vulnerable asthma populations. In light of the far-reaching consequences of poor asthma control among pregnant women, and the higher incidence of inadequate asthma control in underserved populations overall, further quality improvement initiatives targeting barriers to care specific to vulnerable women with asthma during pregnancy are necessary. Successful interventions need not be led solely by medical professionals. Efforts that also engage community activists, policy leaders, and government agencies and seek to address education, access, affordability, and sociocultural and environmental disparities are likely to have the greatest impact in changing the trajectory of poor asthma control in women during pregnancy.

CLINICS CARE POINTS

- It is essential to consider structural inequities and social determinants that drive disparities in the care of pregnant women with asthma from underserved communities.
- Specifically addressing medication knowledge, adherence, and inhaler technique can lead to improved asthma control in this vulnerable population.
- Attention to the provision of culturally competent, accessible health care can likely optimize asthma outcomes among pregnant women who experience unique barriers to care continuity.

CONFLICTS OF INTEREST

The authors have no relevant conflicts of interest to disclose.

REFERENCES

1. Kwon HL, Belanger K, Bracken MB. Asthma prevalence among pregnant and childbearing-aged women in the United States: estimates from national health surveys. Ann Epidemiol 2003;13(5):317–24.
2. Kwon HL, Triche EW, Belanger K, et al. The epidemiology of asthma during pregnancy: prevalence, diagnosis, and symptoms. Immunol Allergy Clin N Am 2006; 26(1):29–62.
3. Flores KF, Bandoli G, Chambers CD, et al. Asthma prevalence among women aged 18 to 44 in the United States: national health and nutrition examination survey 2001–2016. J Asthma 2020;57(7):693–702.
4. Most recent national asthma data | CDC. 2021. Available at: https://www.cdc.gov/asthma/most_recent_national_asthma_data.htm. Accessed Dec 13, 2021.
5. Schatz M, Harden K, Forsythe A, et al. The course of asthma during pregnancy, post partum, and with successive pregnancies: a prospective analysis. J Allergy Clin Immunol 1988;81(3):509–17.
6. Stevens DR, Perkins N, Chen Z, et al. Determining the clinical course of asthma in pregnancy. J Allergy Clin Immunol Pract 2021.
7. Murphy VE. Managing asthma in pregnancy. Breathe (Sheff) 2015;258–67.
8. Bonham CA, Patterson KC, Strek ME. Asthma outcomes and management during pregnancy. Chest 2018;153(2):515.

9. Abdullah K, Zhu J, Gershon A, et al. Effect of asthma exacerbation during pregnancy in women with asthma: a population-based cohort study. Eur Respir J 2020;55(2).

10. Blais L, Kettani FZ, Forget A, et al. Asthma exacerbations during the first trimester of pregnancy and congenital malformations: revisiting the association in a large representative cohort. Thorax 2015;70(7).

11. Carroll KN, Gebretsadik T, Griffin MR, et al. Maternal asthma and maternal smoking are associated with increased risk of bronchiolitis during infancy. Pediatrics 2007;119(6):1104–12.

12. 2021 GINA main report. Global initiative for asthma - GINA Web site. Available at: https://ginasthma.org/gina-reports/. Accessed Nov 21, 2021.

13. Carroll KN, Griffin MR, Gebretsadik T, et al. Racial differences in asthma morbidity during pregnancy. Obstet Gynecol 2005;106(1):66–72.

14. Enriquez Rachel, Griffin, et al. Effect of maternal asthma and asthma control on pregnancy and perinatal outcomes. J Allergy Clin Immunol 2007;120(3):625–30.

15. Lang DM, Polansky M, Sherman MS. Hospitalizations for asthma in an urban population: 1995-1999. Ann Allergy Asthma Immunol 2009;103(2):128–33.

16. Bacon SL, Bouchard A, Loucks EB, et al. Individual-level socioeconomic status is associated with worse asthma morbidity in patients with asthma. Respir Res 2009;10:125.

17. Asthma as the underlying cause of death | CDC. Available at: https://www.cdc.gov/asthma/asthma_stats/asthma_underlying_death.html. Accessed Nov 18, 2021.

18. Pennsylvania department of health programs, services and health information. Department of Health Web site. Available at: https://www.health.pa.gov:443/Pages/default.aspx. Accessed Dec 15, 2021.

19. Lang DM, Polansky M. Patterns of asthma mortality in Philadelphia from 1969 to 1991. N Engl J Med 1994;331(23):1542–6.

20. Murphy VE, Gibson PG, Talbot PI, et al. Asthma self-management skills and the use of asthma education during pregnancy. Eur Respir J 2005;26(3):435–41.

21. Lim AS, Stewart K, Abramson MJ, et al. Multidisciplinary approach to management of maternal asthma (MAMMA): A randomized controlled trial. Chest 2014; 145(5):1046–54.

22. Powell H, Murphy VE, Taylor DR, et al. Management of asthma in pregnancy guided by measurement of fraction of exhaled nitric oxide: a double-blind, randomized controlled trial. Lancet 2011;378(9795):983–90.

23. Yoo EJ, Most JF, Lee NL, et al. Improving asthma symptoms among inner-city women during pregnancy: A prospective cohort intervention. J Allergy Clin Immunol Pract 2021.

24. Al Ghobain MO, AlNemer M, Khan M. Assessment of knowledge and education relating to asthma during pregnancy among women of childbearing age. Asthma Res Pract 2018;4:2.

25. Ibrahim WH, Rasul F, Ahmad M, et al. Asthma knowledge, care, and outcome during pregnancy: the QAKCOP study. Chron Respir Dis 2019;16. 1479972318767719.

26. Cohen JM, Bateman BT, Huybrechts KF, et al. Poorly controlled asthma during pregnancy remains common in the United States. J Allergy Clin Immunol Pract 2019;7(8):2672–80.e10.

27. Taylor K, Compton S, Kolenic GE, et al. Financial hardship among pregnant and postpartum women in the United States, 2013 to 2018. JAMA Netw Open 2021; 4(10):e2132103.

28. Mansour ME, Lanphear BP, DeWitt TG. Barriers to asthma care in urban children: Parent perspectives. Pediatrics 2000;106(3):512–9.
29. Chan M, Sitaraman S, Dosanjh A. Asthma control test and peak expiratory flow rate: Independent pediatric asthma management tools. J Asthma 2009;46(10): 1042–4.
30. Khalili B, Boggs PB, Shi R, et al. Discrepancy between clinical asthma control assessment tools and fractional exhaled nitric oxide. Ann Allergy Asthma Immunol 2008;101(2):124–9.
31. Mei Chan, et al. Community-based interventions for childhood asthma using comprehensive approaches: a systematic review and meta-analysis. Allergy Asthma Clin Immunol 2021.
32. Guendelman S, Meade K, Benson M, et al. Improving asthma outcomes and self-management behaviors of inner-city children: a randomized trial of the Health Buddy interactive device and an asthma diary. Arch Pediatr Adolesc Med 2002;156(2):114–20.
33. Kolmodin MacDonell K, Naar S, Gibson-Scipio W, et al. The Detroit young adult asthma project: Pilot of a technology-based medication adherence intervention for African American emerging adults. J Adolesc Health 2016;59(4):465–71.
34. Ejebe IH, Jacobs EA, Wisk LE. Persistent differences in asthma self-efficacy by race, ethnicity, and income in adults with asthma. J Asthma 2015;52(1):105–13.
35. Fung V, Graetz I, Galbraith A, et al. inancial barriers to care among low-income children with asthma: Health care reform implications. JAMA Pediatr 2014; 168(7):649–56.
36. Sullivan K, Thakur N. Structural and social determinants of health in asthma in developed economies: a scoping review of literature published between 2014 and 2019. Curr Allergy Asthma Rep 2020;20(2):5.
37. Mishra R, Kashif M, Venkatram S, et al. Role of adult asthma education in improving asthma control and reducing emergency room utilization and hospital admissions in an inner city hospital. Can Respir J 2017;2017:e5681962.
38. La Roche MJ, Koinis-Mitchell D, Gualdron L. A culturally competent asthma management intervention: a randomized controlled pilot study. Ann Allergy Asthma Immunol 2006;96(1):80–5.
39. Im H, Rosenberg R. Building social capital through a peer-led community health workshop: a pilot with the Bhutanese refugee community. J Community Health 2016;41(3):509–17.
40. Janevic MR, Stoll S, Wilkin M, et al. Pediatric asthma care coordination in underserved communities: a quasiexperimental study. Am J Public Health 2016; 106(11):2012–8.
41. Krieger J, Song L, Philby M. Community health worker home visits for adults with uncontrolled asthma: the HomeBASE Trial randomized clinical trial. JAMA Intern Med 2015;175(1):109–17.
42. McCollum R, Gomez W, Theobald S, et al. How equitable are community health worker programmes and which programme features influence equity of community health worker services? A systematic review. BMC Public Health 2016; 16:419.
43. Turcotte DA, Woskie S, Gore R, et al. Asthma, COPD, and home environments: Interventions with older adults. Ann Allergy Asthma Immunol 2019;122(5):486–91.
44. Beck AF, Huang B, Chundur R, et al. Housing code violation density associated with emergency department and hospital use by children with asthma. Health Aff (Millwood) 2014;33(11):1993–2002.

45. Department of housing and urban development 2017, implementing HUD's smoke-free policy in public housing. Available at: Https://www.hud.gov/sites/documents/SMOKEFREE_GUIDEBK.PDF.
46. National asthma control program | CDC. 2020. Available at: https://www.cdc.gov/asthma/nacp.htm. Accessed Nov 21, 2021.
47. O'Neill MS, Jerrett M, Kawachi I, et al. Workshop on Air Pollution and Socioeconomic Conditions. Health, wealth, and air pollution: advancing theory and methods. Environ Health Perspect 2003;111(16):1861–70.

Moving?

Make sure your subscription moves with you!

To notify us of your new address, find your **Clinics Account Number** (located on your mailing label above your name), and contact customer service at:

Email: journalscustomerservice-usa@elsevier.com

800-654-2452 (subscribers in the U.S. & Canada)
314-447-8871 (subscribers outside of the U.S. & Canada)

Fax number: 314-447-8029

Elsevier Health Sciences Division
Subscription Customer Service
3251 Riverport Lane
Maryland Heights, MO 63043

*To ensure uninterrupted delivery of your subscription, please notify us at least 4 weeks in advance of move.

Printed and bound by CPI Group (UK) Ltd, Croydon, CR0 4YY

16/10/2024

01775080-0001